Robotics in Knee and Hip Arthroplasty

Jess H. Lonner

Editor

Robotics in Knee and Hip Arthroplasty

Current Concepts, Techniques and Emerging Uses

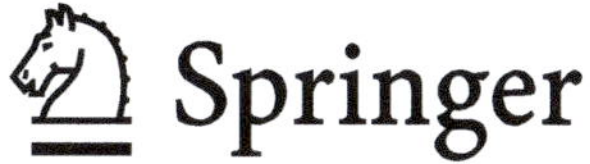

Editor
Jess H. Lonner
Department of Orthopaedic Surgery
Rothman Orthopaedic Institute,
Sidney Kimmel Medical College,
Thomas Jefferson University
Philadelphia, PA
USA

ISBN 978-3-030-16595-6   ISBN 978-3-030-16593-2   (eBook)
https://doi.org/10.1007/978-3-030-16593-2

This Springer imprint is published by the registered company Springer Nature Switzerland AG
The registered company address is: Gewerbestrasse 11, 6330 Cham, Switzerland

*To the surgeons, engineers, industry leaders, and executives
who have contributed tremendous time and energy to the
advancement of robotic science and technology in surgery and
who recognize that this is just the beginning of a field that will
continue to evolve and expand throughout all aspects of
healthcare.*

*To my mentors, role models, and former partners – Drs. Paul
Lotke and the late Richard Rothman – who encouraged my
intellectual curiosity in the robotic space.*

*To our fellows and residents whom I hope will further explore
and develop the field of robotics into the future, in ways that we
are not yet considering.*

*Most importantly, to my wife, Ami, and our children, Carson
and Jared – my greatest joys in life.*

Foreword

In the past few decades, there have been great changes in the science related to knee and hip replacement surgery. *Robotics in Knee and Hip Arthroplasty* is a testament to the newest advances in this ever-emerging process.

When total hips and total knees were first introduced four decades ago, the acetabular reaming was guided with a drill hole in the bottom of the acetabulum, in the knee the proximal tibial osteotomy was guided with the wide osteotome placed along the long axis of the tibia, and the femoral osteotomy was guided with an angular rod slide under the quadriceps muscles. It did not take long to appreciate that consistent techniques for perfect position and alignment were essential for the long-term success of a prosthesis.

We can now appreciate the evolutionary changes that have occurred during the past few decades. These changes in techniques started with instruments that allowed reproducible acetabular reaming and position, well-placed femoral neck osteotomies in the hip, as well as accurate tibial and femoral cuts for a total knee arthroplasty. Over the years, instrument sets have evolved, creating reasonably reproducible results. Smaller instrumentation for smaller incisions evolved; there has been a gradual introduction into computer-assisted surgery; and we now have robotic-assisted surgery. This latest advancement will allow joint replacement surgeries to achieve a level of consistency and efficiency never even considered a decade ago, let alone when joint arthroplasties were first introduced.

This text gives the reader a comprehensive synthesis of the state of the art in robotic hip and knee surgery. It is superbly written and edited. It first outlines the history and evolution of robotics in healthcare and hip and knee arthroplasty. There is a review of the advantages and disadvantages of robotics. The entire second and third sections are devoted to techniques and are a "how-to" for a variety of different hip and knee robotic applications.

This excellent, up-to-date text will serve as a testament to the emerging science of robotic surgery: it will be a classic in this field and a guide for the next generation of arthroplasty surgery.

Paul A. Lotke
Emeritus Professor of Orthopaedic Surgery
University of Pennsylvania School of Medicine
Philadelphia, PA, USA

Preface

While manufacturing and warehousing have enjoyed longer-term use of robotic technology to enhance their industries, healthcare – and particularly orthopaedic surgery – has been slower to embrace robotic technologies, until recently. The field of robotics is now hitting an inflection point in healthcare in general, as well as arthroplasty and other sectors of orthopaedics in particular, with tremendous recent growth. When considering the dynamic trends and attitudes toward robotics in joint arthroplasty, early scepticism was the norm for nearly a decade when it came to robotics, and other than a relative handful of us who were innovating in and advocating for robotics, few others were using robotic methods. When I first began presenting on robotics at national meetings in 2008, there were many who doubted the need for this sort of advanced technology. After all, there were decades of reasonable outcomes after joint arthroplasties performed with conventional tools. Happily, the past few years have experienced a paradigm shift. A recent informal poll of the members in attendance at the 2018 annual meeting of the American Association of Hip and Knee Surgeons found that 30% use robotic assistance for unicompartmental knee arthroplasty. Additionally, in some regions in the United States, 30% of hospitals now offer robotic technology for knee or hip arthroplasty, and some hospitals have several orthopaedic robots in their operating rooms. Robotic technologies have expanded into their third generation, and each major company has a robot either in use or in development. As technologies evolve, efficiencies improve, and costs are better contained, it is likely that robotic assistance will continue to grow as a surgical tool and beyond the operating table to improve perioperative processes within our hospitals.

This text is designed to give a broad descriptive overview of available robotic technologies, primarily for knee and hip arthroplasty procedures, as well as spinal surgery. While some are available worldwide, others are emerging and at various stages of approval by regulatory bodies. By virtue of the fact that the same technologies may be used for various kinds of procedures, there may be some redundancy among chapters with regard to system descriptions, but it is intended that each chapter can stand alone. Additionally, a section on the emerging field of robotics for hospital process improvement is included as a window into advances that may become more commonplace in the next 5–10 years.

While using this text, please recognize that each surgeon contributor is describing their personal perspective on a particular use of a particular robotic technology or the field of robotics in general. These perspectives may not be completely shared by the broader robotics community as a whole; subtle differences may exist between surgeons' preferences, protocols, and techniques based on personal or institutional experiences and philosophies. This text is geared toward providing the reader with a foundation upon which build their knowledge base for the current and emerging robotic platforms. Given the rapid evolution of robotic technologies, I suspect the next edition of this book will need to be written in the near term.

Philadelphia, PA, USA   Jess H. Lonner

Acknowledgement

I am grateful to my colleagues who shared their valuable insight into, and experiences with, the growing field of robotics for this book and indebted to each of you for the time you took from your families, orthopaedic practices, and other endeavours to participate in this project.

I would like to thank the professionals at Springer, but particularly Kristopher Spring, the visionary editor who saw value in a text on robotics in orthopaedics, and Margaret Burns, the developmental editor, who kept us on task and put in countless hours to see this book through to completion.

Contents

Contributors

Mark W. Allen, DO Department of Adult Reconstruction, The CORE Institute, Phoenix, AZ, USA

William L. Bargar, MMAE, MD Department of Orthopaedic Surgery, University of California at Davis School of Medicine, Sutter General Hospital, Sacramento, CA, USA

Cécile Batailler, MD Department of Orthopedic Surgery, Hôpital de la Croix Rousse, Lyon, France

Christopher P. Bechtel, MD Department of Orthopedics, University Hospitals Westlake Health Center, Westlake, OH, USA

Joseph A. Bosco, MD Department of Orthopaedic Surgery, NYU Langone Medical Center, Hospital for Joint Diseases, New York, NY, USA

Anthony E. Bozzio, MD Texas Back Institute, Plano, TX, USA

Kevin K. Chen, MA Department of Orthopaedic Surgery, NYU Langone Medical Center, Hospital for Joint Diseases, New York, NY, USA

Pak Lin Chin, MD The Orthopaedic Centre, Mount Elizabeth Medical Centre, Singapore, Singapore

Marius Dettmer, PhD Memorial Bone and Joint Research Foundation, Houston, TX, USA

Ameer M. Elbuluk, MD Department of Orthopaedic Surgery, NYU Langone Medical Center, Hospital for Joint Diseases, New York, NY, USA

Michael J. Feldstein, MD Department of Orthopaedic Surgery, Kaiser Permanente, San Francisco, CA, USA

James F. Fraser, MD, MPH Department of Orthopedic Surgery, Novant Health, Charlotte, NC, USA

Kenneth Gustke, MD Florida Orthopaedic Institute, Tampa, FL, USA

Department of Orthopaedic Surgery, University of South Florida College of Medicine, Tampa, FL, USA

Brian Hamlin, MD Department of Orthopaedics, Magee Womens Hospital of UPMC, Pittsburgh, PA, USA

Aaron Hofmann, MD Department of Orthopaedic Surgery, Center for Precision Joint Replacement, Salt Lake Regional Medical Center/Hofmann Arthritis Institute, Salt Lake City, UT, USA

Xiaobang Hu, PhD Scoliosis and Spine Tumor Center, Texas Back Institute, Texas Health Presbyterian Hospital, Plano, TX, USA

Richard Iorio, MD Department of Orthopaedic Surgery, Brigham and Women's Hospital, Boston, MA, USA

David J. Jacofsky, MD Department of Orthopedics, The CORE Institute, Phoenix, AZ, USA

Dugal James, MBBS FRACS (Orth) Bendigo Orthopaedic & Sports Medicine Practice, Bendigo, VIC, Australia

Seth A. Jerabek, MD Department of Orthopaedic Surgery, Hospital for Special Surgery, New York, NY, USA

Alexander H. Jinnah, MD Department of Orthopaedic Surgery, Wake Forest School of Medicine, Winston Salem, NC, USA

Riyaz H. Jinnah, MD, FRCS Department of Orthopaedic Surgery, Wake Forest School of Medicine, Winston Salem, NC, USA

Department of Orthopaedic Surgery, Southeastern Regional Medical Center, Lumberton, NC, USA

Kelvin Y. Kim, BA Department of Orthopaedic Surgery, NYU Langone Medical Center, Hospital for Joint Diseases, New York, NY, USA

Laura J. Kleeblad, MD Department of Orthopedic Surgery, Noordwest Hospital Group, Alkmaar, The Netherlands

Gregg R. Klein, MD Hartzband Center for Hip and Knee Replacement, Paramus, NJ, USA

Department of Orthopedic Surgery, Hackensack University Medical Center, Hackensack, NJ, USA

Department of Orthopaedic Surgery, Hackensack Meridian School of Medicine at Seton Hall, Hackensack, NJ, USA

Jan A. Koenig, MD Department of Orthopaedic Surgery, NYU-Winthrop Hospital, Mineola, NY, USA

Stefan W. Kreuzer, MD, MSc INOV8 Orthopedics/Memorial Bone and Joint Research Foundation, Houston, TX, USA

Jesua Law, DO Department of Orthopedics, Valley Orthopedic Surgery, Modesto, CA, USA

Isador H. Lieberman, MD, MBA, FRCSC Scoliosis and Spine Tumor Center, Texas Back Institute, Texas Health Presbyterian Hospital, Plano, TX, USA

Ming Han Lincoln Liow, MBBS, FRCSEd Department of Orthopaedic Surgery, Singapore General Hospital, Singapore, Singapore

Jess H. Lonner, MD Department of Orthopaedic Surgery, Rothman Orthopaedic Institute, Sidney Kimmel Medical College, Thomas Jefferson University, Philadelphia, PA, USA

T. David Luo, MD Department of Orthopaedic Surgery, Wake Forest School of Medicine, Winston Salem, NC, USA

Sébastien Lustig, MD, PhD Department of Orthopedic Surgery, Hôpital de la Croix Rousse, Lyon, France

Stefany J. K. Malanka, MD Memorial Bone and Joint Research Foundation, Houston, TX, USA

David J. Mayman, MD Department of Orthopaedic Surgery, Hospital for Special Surgery, New York, NY, USA

Patrick A. Meere, MD Department of Orthopaedic Surgery, NYU Langone Medical Center, Hospital for Joint Diseases, New York, NY, USA

Alexandria Myers, BS Hofmann Arthritis Institute, Salt Lake City, UT, USA

Nathan A. Netravali, PhD Think Surgical, Inc., Fremont, CA, USA

P. Neyret, MD Albert Trillat Center, Orthopedic Surgery, Lyon North University Hospital, Lyon, France

Michael J. O'Malley, MD Department of Orthopaedic Surgery, University of Pittsburgh Medical Center, Pittsburgh, PA, USA

Douglas E. Padgett, MD Department of Orthopaedic Surgery, Hospital for Special Surgery, New York, NY, USA

Andrew D. Pearle, MD Department of Orthopedic Surgery, Sports Medicine, and Shoulder Service, Hospital for Special Surgery, New York, NY, USA

Christopher Plaskos, PhD Technology and Clinical Research, Omni/Corin-Group, Raynham, MA, USA

Johannes F. Plate, MD, PhD Department of Orthopaedic Surgery, Wake Forest School of Medicine, Winston Salem, NC, USA

Martin Roche, MD Department of Orthopedic Surgery, Holy Cross Orthopedic Institute, Fort Lauderdale, FL, USA

Sundeep Saini, DO Department of Orthopaedic Surgery, Rowan University School of Osteopathic Medicine, Stratford, NJ, USA

E. Servien, MD Albert Trillat Center, Orthopedic Surgery, Lyon North University Hospital, Lyon, France

Richard Southgate, MD Department of Orthopaedic Surgery, Division of Adult Reconstruction, University of California, San Francisco, CA, USA

Bradley Stevens, BS, MPAS Hofmann Arthritis Institute, Salt Lake City, UT, USA

Jonathan M. Vigdorchik, MD Department of Orthopaedic Surgery, NYU Langone Medical Center, Hospital for Joint Diseases, New York, NY, USA

Derek Ward, MD Department of Orthopaedic Surgery, University of California, San Francisco, CA, USA

Nathan White, B Physio, MBBS, FRACS Park Clinic Orthopaedics, Melbourne, VIC, Australia

Seng Jin Yeo, MBBS, FRCSEd Department of Orthopaedic Surgery, Singapore General Hospital, Singapore, Singapore

Julian Zangrilli, DO Department of Orthopaedic Surgery, Rowan University School of Osteopathic Medicine, Stratford, NJ, USA

Jason P. Zlotnicki, MD Department of Orthopaedic Surgery, University of Pittsburgh, Pittsburgh, PA, USA

Part I

Basic Principles

A Brief History of Robotics in Surgery

Jess H. Lonner and James F. Fraser

The word "robot," derived from the Czech word *robata*, which means "forced labor," was first introduced to popular culture in 1917 by Joseph Capek in the science fiction story Opilec [1]. In the contemporary Oxford Dictionary, a robot is defined as a "machine capable of carrying out a complex series of actions automatically, especially one programmable by a computer" [2]. The modern concept of robotics was advanced in the science fiction writings of Isaac Asimov in the 1940s, who coined, among other things, The First Law of Robotics, which admonished that "A robot may not injure a human being or, through inaction, allow a human being to come to harm" [3]. These concerns are particularly germane in the healthcare realm, where the focus on robotic interventions has not only been on their potential efficacy in performing "complex series of actions" but also the safety of those tools vis-a-vis both the patients and surgical teams working in collaboration with the robots.

Visionaries in computer science and automation have stated that the emergence of robotics in various industries [and perhaps even more so in healthcare] has lagged behind where the personal computer was three decades ago [4]. Nonetheless, having gained an early foothold in the industrial arena [5], robots are now proving useful in many sectors, ranging from transportation to manufacturing to warehousing and beyond. Indeed, we are in the midst of the "Second Machine Age" – a time marked by exponential and impactful growth of digitalization, artificial intelligence, robotics, and other highly advanced smart technologies, which are creating unparalleled growth and impacting so many areas, including healthcare [6]. As Brynjolfsson and McAfee point out, just as the introduction of the steam engine in 1775 was a dramatic "inflection point" in the Industrial Revolution, recent advances in computer technologies and robotics in a variety of industries are having a comparable dramatic, even extraordinary, impact on vast sectors of society [6]. Ninety-nine percent of farm workers have been replaced by automation, and it is anticipated that by the end of this century, 70% of today's occupations – manufacturing, assembly, transport, warehousing, military, inventory, and healthcare – will likewise be replaced, or more likely augmented, by automated technologies [7, 8]. Since the use of robotic technologies has expanded across a broad swath of industries and increasingly used alongside humans – collaborating with, and augmenting our capabilities,

J. H. Lonner (✉)
Department of Orthopaedic Surgery, Rothman Orthopaedic Institute, Sidney Kimmel Medical College, Thomas Jefferson University, Philadelphia, PA, USA
e-mail: jess.lonner@rothmanortho.com

J. F. Fraser
Department of Orthopedic Surgery, Novant Health, Charlotte, NC, USA

© Springer Nature Switzerland AG 2019
J. H. Lonner (ed.), *Robotics in Knee and Hip Arthroplasty*,
https://doi.org/10.1007/978-3-030-16593-2_1

rather than replacing them – there is no doubt why numerous surgical procedures are now identified as optimally suited for robotic assistance. After years of slow, measured, almost undetectable advances in robotics in healthcare, the last 5–10 years have seen more dramatic growth and progress in surgery. In fact, taking joint arthroplasty surgery as an example, recent patent activity in robotics is greater than most other areas of surgical technology development at this time, highlighting the tremendous interest in, and resource allocation toward, the field of robotics [9].

In addition to the drive to improve outcomes and surgical efficiencies, economic pressures and regional competition have been major drivers of robotic technology acquisition [10]. The main benefit of robots to augment human capabilities in surgery is their ability to perform repetitive, predictable, and often "complex" tasks with unmatched accuracy and consistency while also improving the ergonomics of the surgery for the surgeon user [11]. The story of the evolution of robotics in arthroplasty and other surgical specialties is a study in the characteristic patterns that define technological progress and innovation, in general, whereby initial skepticism questions the role of the intervention, after which exponential developments occur along with data on the class of interventions, followed by declining capital and maintenance costs, smaller space requirements, broadening access, and increased utilization [6, 12, 13]. Although additive costs of robotic surgery with the current predominant systems are currently high, increased competition from manufacturers and wider dissemination of alternative technologies should drive costs down, as we have observed with orthopedic robotic systems [6, 12–14].

Despite the "promise" of robot assistance, there will naturally be surgeon adopters on the one hand and nonusers on the other [15, 16]. Simplifying the unified theory of acceptance and use of technology, it can be argued that one's perceptions regarding the usefulness and ease of use of the technology, as well as extrinsic factors such as regional competition, patient requests, technology costs, and learning curves, may at once serve as either motivators or deterrents to using robotics in surgery [10, 11, 15, 17, 18]. Indeed, in healthcare, the decision to acquire and implement a new technology is largely based on the perceived "value" of that technology, which is traditionally determined by considering the applicable costs and benefits [17]. However, while these factors are often concrete and well defined, the unclear net costs and uncertainty regarding the long-term benefits of robotically assisted surgery challenge this assessment.

Notwithstanding those competing interests and biases for or against surgical robots, the emergence of robotics in the medical space, while initially quite slow, is now growing parabolically. Over the past decade, robots have augmented nearly two million surgical operations worldwide [19]. In addition to the intrinsic and extrinsic motivators described above, the global market for medical robotic systems is driven by other factors such as technological advancement in the automation of the healthcare industry, increase in elderly population, increased volumes of all sorts of surgeries, and pursuit of precision in the setting of less invasive surgical techniques. Certainly, the prevalence of knee and hip arthroplasty is experiencing tremendous growth, with no end in sight [20]. The global surgical robotics market is expected to increase substantially, growing from $4.9 billion in 2016 to $12.8 billion in 2021 and $16.74 billion by 2023, a cumulative annual growth rate of over 20% [21, 22]. Intuitive Surgical – the dominant surgical robot company – estimates that in 2017 alone, surgeons throughout the world completed approximately 877,000 surgical procedures using its technology, compared to roughly 80,000 in 2007. Similarly, albeit slower to the robotics space, the knee and hip arthroplasty robotics market has grown from $84 million in 2015 to $375 million in 2017, and the global orthopedic medical robots market is anticipated to reach between $2 billion and $4.6 billion over the next 5–6 years as a new generation of robotic devices, systems, and instruments is introduced to manage a rising number of musculoskeletal conditions in a growing orthopedic population [23, 24].

History of Robotic Surgery

Early surgical robot development can be traced to the mid-1980s when innovative surgeons and engineers worked to advance the field in neurosurgery and orthopedics, taking advantage of the rigidity of fixed bony landmarks to serve as landmarks from which to guide early robotic tools [11]. The first surgical robot, Puma 560 (Unimate, New Jersey, US), was introduced in 1985 and was designed to be used in conjunction with computed tomography (CT) guidance for obtaining neurosurgical biopsies [25]. The next-generation neurosurgical robot, Minerva, was introduced in the early 1990s. It was a stereotactical neurosurgical robot and utilized an intraoperative CT scanner and a head frame attached to the robot that allowed for increased rigidity and precision [26, 27]. Each of these systems combined information from three-dimensional scans with fiducial markers affixed to rigid points of the cranium to determine exactly where in space the tip of a biopsy device was located [11]. In addition to their ongoing use in obtaining brain biopsies, modern robots have assisted with other neurosurgical operations ranging from glioma resections to pedicle screw insertion [28, 29]. In 1988, ROBODOC (Integrated Surgical Systems, Delaware, US) was introduced to allow precision planning and milling for the femoral component in total hip arthroplasty. Also in 1988, the earliest robotic procedure in urology was performed at Imperial College (London, UK) with the use of the PROBOT in a clinical trial. In 1993, a robotic arm to assist in laparoscopic camera holding and positioning called AESOP (Automated Endoscopic System for Optimal Positioning) was released by Computer Motion, Inc. (Santa Barbara, CA). While the earliest robotic interventions were in orthopedics, neurosurgery, and cardiac surgery, it was in urologic applications where the broadest and most widespread adoption occurred throughout the world before expanding to other specialties like general surgery, gynecology, and head and neck surgery and ultimately seeing greater recent use in orthopedics and neurosurgery [30].

The year 1998 was a seminal period in the field of surgical robotics, with the introduction to the market of both the ZEUS Robotic Surgical System (Computer Motion, Inc.) and the da Vinci Surgical System (Intuitive Surgical, Inc., Sunnyvale [CA], US), both with remote surgical consoles manipulating their articulated robotic arms. The initial da Vinci robotic surgical procedure was a robot-assisted heart bypass, performed in Germany in 1998 [31]. In 2000 the first reported robot-assisted radical prostatectomy was performed in Paris, France [32]. The US Food and Drug Administration (FDA) approved the da Vinci robot for general laparoscopic surgery (cholecystectomy and gastroesophageal reflux surgery) in July 2000, for prostate surgery in 2001, for mitral valve repair surgery in November 2002, and for gynecological surgeries in 2005 [1]. Intuitive Surgical, Inc., is now the primary player worldwide in the non-orthopedic robotic surgical market, although newer entrants into the space are emerging, with the prospects of lower costs, improved efficiencies, and portability.

Early on it was observed that robots were well-suited to assist with laparoscopic surgeries, where complex tasks were being performed in confined spaces with precision, but which were plagued by long learning curves, ergonomic and dexterity challenges, compromised sensory feedback, and visualization challenges compared to open techniques [33]. The ability of the surgeon to control laparoscopic tools with haptic sensors while seated at a control console that magnified the field in three dimensions enhanced the ability to manipulate tissues with extreme precision and dexterity through minimally invasive approaches in a way that enhanced the ease and ergonomics for the surgeon users, thereby improving on the limitations of conventional laparoscopic techniques [34].

Across a number of disciplines, compared to open surgery, robotic assistance has been shown to decrease length of stay and reduce complications such as bleeding and in-hospital mortality [35–37]. However, in its current iteration, robot-assisted laparoscopic surgery is costlier, and often more time consuming, than laparoscopic surgery and open surgery, adding as much as 13% ($3200) to the total average procedural costs across 20 surgical procedures when using robotic assistance [17]. Despite the additional costs, robot assistance has been utilized in over 1.5 million operations in the fields of general surgery, gynecology, head and neck surgery, cardiothoracic surgery, and urology and over 130,000 cases in orthopedic surgery.

Urology

The vast majority of radical prostatectomies in the United States – roughly 80% – are now performed with a robot [38]. This has resulted in measurable reductions in surgical blood loss, hospital length of stay, and complication rates compared to open prostatectomies [36]. Despite these potential benefits, a number of studies have found equivalent cancer cure rates and no significant differences between open and robotic techniques in potency or urinary continence [39]. While the vast majority of robot-assisted urological cases relate to prostate disease, in some centers, robotics has expanded into the treatment of bladder and kidney disease as well, resulting in quicker discharge, less bleeding, and equivalent cure rates compared to open treatments [40–43].

Colorectal, General, and Gynecological Surgery

Robotics has been shown to be effective and safe for a myriad of other conditions and surgical procedures such as bariatric surgery, fundoplication, cholecystectomy, and hysterectomy, with comparable blood loss, clinical outcomes, conversion rate to open surgery, length of hospitalization, and overall morbidity compared to conventional laparoscopic techniques. The longer surgical times and higher costs of robotic surgery have tempered broader enthusiasm for the use of robots for these surgeries [44–49]. Admittedly, there is a relative paucity of high-quality studies evaluating the health outcomes of robotic technology in non-orthopedic- and non-prostate-related conditions, which make

definitive conclusions about the role of robotics across the spectrum of surgeries difficult [50]. Natural orifice robotic techniques may further refine robotic applications in general surgery and other applications in the future [51].

Cardiothoracic Surgery

One of the earliest robotic-assisted procedures was a coronary artery bypass grafting (CABG) performed endoscopically in the United States in 1999 [52]. Robotics has since been used not only for CABG but also to repair and replace the mitral valve, close atrial septal defects, implant left ventricular pacing leads, and resect myocardial tumors. Robotics has also been used to treat thoracic conditions, including resection of primary lung cancers, esophageal tumors, thymic diseases, and mediastinal tumors. While some metrics appear to be improved with robotic assistance, including reduced morbidity and mortality, shorter hospital and intensive care unit length of stay, and less blood loss, the lengthy and risky learning curves and additional surgical time are likely reasons that robotics is mostly limited to select centers for treating cardiothoracic diseases [53–56].

Head and Neck Surgery

Otolaryngology, which also benefits from the relative rigidity of the cranium and its surrounding structures, has proven to be another fertile ground for the introduction of robotic surgical techniques. In the 1990s, a robotically controlled device for drilling the footplate of the stapes was developed [11]. Robots have also been shown to be safe and effective at removing benign and malignant thyroid lesions [57] and are now venturing into the realm of retinal surgery, inner and middle ear surgery, and head and neck surgeries where exacting precision is paramount to optimal success [58–60]. More recent robotic systems have been utilized to perform minimally invasive transoral thyroidectomies, with mixed results [61, 62].

Robots in Orthopedics

Despite being first to the field, widespread use of robotic technology for joint arthroplasty and particularly spine surgery is a relatively recent phenomenon. Similar to cranial surgery, robots in orthopedics benefit from the structural rigidity of the human skeleton [11]. This rigidity allows robots to integrate information from preoperative imaging studies or intraoperative surface mapping methods with fiducial markers and fixed anatomic landmarks during surgery [11, 63]. Some orthopedic robotic systems are imageless, having been designed to function without the need for additional advanced imaging studies, whereas others require preoperative computer tomography scanning for planning [11, 63, 64].

The main advantage of robots over conventional techniques in knee and hip arthroplasty procedures is the accurate and precise cutting and reaming of bone in preparation for implant placement, resulting in fewer errors and outliers. The ability to quantitatively balance the soft tissues through a range of motion in knee arthroplasty using several currently available semiautonomous robotic technologies may further optimize kinematics and functional recovery and prove to be equally, or more, important than component alignment for achieving maximal durability. While we rely on component alignment and position as surrogate determinants of the benefit of robotic technology, data are limited as to whether there is a measurable influence on clinical outcomes and durability in knee or hip arthroplasty with robotics [65–69]. Current data suggest that robotics that include algorithms for both bone and implant alignment and soft tissue balance may indeed have an impact on function and early durability in UKA, whereas midterm and longer-term studies analyzing robotic systems devoid of a soft tissue balancing algorithm for TKA have not shown a measurable impact on either function or durability. Newer robotic systems that emphasize both precision of implant position and soft tissue balance may prove to be more beneficial in TKA, but further study is necessary before we can fully determine the importance of robotics in

TKA and THA, other than satisfying the desire to get closer to some chosen "target."

In fact, there may be a need to change our mindset on how we judge the role of robotic technologies. No studies in knee and hip arthroplasty have found that assistance from semiautonomous robots is detrimental to outcomes. Even if we do not eventually convincingly show that robotics has an impact on durability or functional outcomes with "optimized" alignment and balance in some procedures, the technology may still prove beneficial if we can show equivalence of outcomes, particularly if by using a robotic tool we can reduce inventory, eliminate instruments and surgical trays, improve workflow and surgical efficiency, and show net cost neutrality or even cut costs. We are beginning to approach the latter goal with newer enabling robotic technologies. In the end, it may turn out that robotics may be more beneficial for some procedures than others (like UKA over TKA) or have a greater role for novice or lower volume surgeons, who may have difficulty achieving adequate precision and balance with conventional instrumentation [69–71]. It may also be possible that although robotic systems are effective for both achieving alignment and soft tissue balance, the relative importance of those capabilities may differ between procedures. For instance, in UKA, the need for both precision of implant alignment and soft tissue balance is established; in TKA, on the other hand, recent data suggests that variability in component alignment is well tolerated as long as the soft tissues are balanced. The issue of how we think about robots in TKA, THA, and UKA conjures a story about Abraham Wald, an Eastern European mathematician who worked for the American government during World War II. Concerned about the state of fighter planes which were returning from overseas combat missions with their fuselage and tails riddled with bullet holes, the military leadership sought a solution to reinforce and protect the planes' tails and fuselage without weighing the planes down and impairing their ability to fly. Wald's response based on clever statistical analyses and his abundance of common sense was that their perception of the problem was misguided. As he explained, the planes struck with bullets in the tails or fuselage were making it back safely; the concern should have been for the planes struck in their noses and engines, as those were the ones which weren't returning, and thus it was the engines and noses of the planes which needed reinforcement [72, 73]. With this unconventional wisdom in mind, unlike UKA, it may be that we should acknowledge that our efforts to optimize component alignment within in 1–2 degrees of a target in TKA is an attainable, but misguided, goal. Perhaps, our objective for the robot in TKA should be to better quantify soft tissue balance and enhance surgical efficiency, ergonomics, and economies of scale.

Regardless of the ideal use of robots for knee and hip arthroplasty, what is clear is that during the past decade, the use of robotic technology has grown exponentially in the field of joint arthroplasty, as data has emerged, pricing improved, additional robotic options entered the space, and utilization expanded beyond UKA into total knee arthroplasty (TKA) and total hip arthroplasty (THA) [74, 75]. Analysts suggest that once robotic penetration in the joint arthroplasty market achieves a 35% level, orthopedic surgeons and hospitals will demand access for the procedures [74]. Given a recent informal poll of the members in attendance at the 2018 annual meeting of the American Association of Hip and Knee Surgeons, which found that 30% use robotic assistance for unicompartmental knee arthroplasty, we may soon reach that threshold. Between 2008 and 2015, utilization of robotics in knee arthroplasty alone increased from 15.3% to 27.4% of hospitals and 6.8–17.7% of surgeons in the New York state alone [76]. It is anticipated that the role of robotics will further expand over the next decade, particularly as our focus shifts beyond component and limb alignment in TKA and more toward the role of robotics in soft tissue balancing, reduction in instrumentation and inventory and its attendant cost savings, and surgical efficiencies. One semiautonomous robotic technology first used in 2006 (MAKO, Stryker, Mahwah, NJ, USA) reported a 130% increase in robotic volume from 2011 to 2012; another, first used in 2013, reported growth of 480% between

2013 and 2014, due to its improved cost structure, ease of use, smaller footprint, image-free platform, and applicability in ambulatory surgery centers (Navio, Smith and Nephew, Memphis, TN), demonstrating the growing popularity of robotic technology [77, 78]. Further, a recent analysis of potential market penetration over the next decade projected that nearly 37% of UKA's and 23% of TKA's will be performed with robotics in 10 years [79]. As of January 2019, these robots, as well as newer emerging systems, are expanding usage worldwide, while others are in various stages of development.

Spine Surgery

Robots for spine surgery have expanded beyond Puma and Minerva [11, 25–29], and more recently there has been tremendous growth in the robotics market for spine surgery worldwide [80]. Current ramp-up with FDA-approved spinal surgery robots – Mazor SpineAssist, Mazor X, and Renaissance (Mazor Robotics, Orlando, FL) approved in 2004 with subsequent approval of updates in 2011 and 2017; Rosa Robotics (Zimmer Biomet, Warsaw, IN) approved in 2016; and Excelsius (Globus Medical, Audubon, PA) approved in 2017 – is occurring [81]. Mazor robotic systems, for instance, have been used in 36,000 surgical cases [82], with the other systems growing in market share. According to one analysis, by the year 2022, the worldwide market for spinal surgical robots is anticipated to increase from $26 million to $2.77 billon [83]. Indeed, in the coming years, the accessibility and the number of spine surgeries performed with robotic technology is expected to increase substantially.

Summary

The relative proliferation of robotic systems in surgery and orthopedics in the last decade or two is the natural progression of a robotic evolution that began in the industrial realm in the middle of the twentieth century. The 1960s and 1970s witnessed rapid advances and widespread adoption of robotic technologies in various manufacturing settings. Robots have become more impactful after the development of collaborative robots that perform side-by-side *with* workers, rather than *instead* of them. The collaborative nature of robots is perfectly suited for use in the operating room. Despite the recent expansion of robotics into modern surgery, the additional cost and surgical times accrued as a result of the technologies must be reconciled with both the proven and heretofore unrealized benefits of the various available and emerging robotic systems across a variety of specialties. The critical stakeholders – physician/surgeons, hospital administrators, patients, regulators, and payers – may argue the role for robotics in healthcare; however, advocates and critics alike cannot help but to recognize that robotic technology is becoming more pervasive in many surgical specialties.

References

1. Faust RA. Robotics in surgery: history, current and future applications. New York: Nova Publishers; 2007.
2. Oxford Dictionary. Definition of robot in English. Oxford Dictionaries|English. https://en.oxforddictionaries.com/definition/robot. Accessed 11 Mar 2017.
3. Asimov I. Runaround. I, Robot (The Isaac Asimov Collection ed.). New York City: Doubleday; 1950. p. 40.
4. Bill Gates. A robot in every home: the leader of the PC revolution predicts that the next hot field will be robotics. Sci Am. 2007;2961.
5. Pearce J. George Devol, Developer of Robot Arm, Dies at 99. The New York Times. http://www.nytimes.com/2011/08/16/business/george-devol-developer-of-robot-arm-dies-at-99.html. Published 15 Aug 2011. Accessed 11 Mar 2017.
6. Brynjolfsson E, McAfee A. The second machine age: work, progress, and prosperity in a time of brilliant technologies. New York: W.W. Norton & Company; 2014.
7. Kelly K. Better than human. Wired Magazine. pp 70–83, Jan 2013.
8. Daugherty PR, Wilson HJ. Human + machine: reimagining work in the age of AI. Boston: Harvard Business Review Press; 2018.
9. Dalton DM, Burke TP, Kelly EG, Curtin PD. Quantitative analysis of technological innovation in knee arthroplasty: using patent and publication metrics to identify developments and trends. J Arthroplast. 2016;31:1366e72.
10. Barbash GI, Friedman B, Glied SA, Steiner CA. Factors associated with adoption of robotic surgical technology in US hospitals and relationship to radical prostatectomy procedure. Ann Surg. 2014;259:1–6.
11. Lonner JH. Robotically-assisted unicompartmental knee arthroplasty with a hand-held image-free sculpting tool. Oper Tech Orthop. 2015;25:104–13.
12. Buckingham RA, Buckingham RO. Robots in operating theatres. BMJ. 1995;311(7018):1479–82.
13. Lonner JH, Moretti VM. The evolution of image-free robotic assistance in unicompartmental knee arthroplasty. Am J Orthop. 2016;45:249–54.
14. Ahmed K, Ibrahim A, Wang TT, et al. Assessing the cost effectiveness of robotics in urological surgery: a systematic review. BJU Int. 2012;110:1544–56.
15. BenMessaoud C, Kharrazi H, MacDorman KF. Facilitators and barriers to adopting robotic-assisted surgery: contextualizing the unified theory of acceptance and use of technology. PLoS One. 2011;6(1):e16395. https://doi.org/10.1371/journal.pone.0016395.
16. Yarbrough AK, Smith TB. Technology acceptance among physicians: a new take on TAM. Med Care Res Rev. 2007;64:650–72.
17. Barbash GI, Glied SA. New technology and health care costs – the case of robotic-assisted surgery. N Engl J Med. 2010;363:701–4.
18. Blute ML, Prestipino AL. Factors associated with adoption of robotic surgical technology in US hospitals and relationship to radical prostatectomy procedure volume. Ann Surg. 2014;259:7–9.
19. Cole AP, Trinh QD, Sood A, Menon M. The rise of robotic surgery in the new millennium. J Urol. 2017;197(2S):S213–5. https://doi.org/10.1016/j.juro.2016.11.030.
20. Kurtz SM, Ong KL, Lau E, Bozic KJ. Impact of the economic downturn on total joint replacement demand in the United States: updated projections to 2021. J Bone Joint Surg Am. 2014;96(8):624–30. https://doi.org/10.2106/JBJS.M.00285.
21. https://www.marketresearchengine.com/medical-robots-market. Accessed 3 Sept 2018.
22. https://www.researchandmarkets.com/research/8p4b2q/global_medical?w=5. Accessed 3 Sept 2018.
23. https://www.reportlinker.com/p05653781/Orthopedic-Medical-Robots-Market-to-Global-Analysis-and-Forecasts.html. Accessed 25 Dec 2018.
24. https://www.researchmoz.us/hip-and-knee-orthopedic-surgical-robots-market-shares-strategy-and-forecasts-worldwide-2016-to-2022-report.html. Accessed 12 Sept 2018.
25. Davies B. A review of robotics in surgery. Proc Inst Mech Eng H. 2000;214(1):129–40. https://doi.org/10.1243/0954411001535309.
26. Glauser D, Fankhauser H, Epitaux M, Hefti JL, Jaccottet A. Neurosurgical robot Minerva: first results and current developments. J Image Guid Surg. 1995;1(5):266–72.

27. Fankhauser H, Glauser D, Flury P, et al. Robot for CT-guided stereotactic neurosurgery. Stereotact Funct Neurosurg. 1994;63(1–4):93–8.
28. Schatlo B, Molliqaj G, Cuvinciuc V, Kotowski M, Schaller K, Tessitore E. Safety and accuracy of robot-assisted versus fluoroscopy-guided pedicle screw insertion for degenerative diseases of the lumbar spine: a matched cohort comparison. J Neurosurg Spine. 2014;20(6):636–43. https://doi.org/10.3171/2 014.3.SPINE13714.
29. Maddahi Y, Zareinia K, Gan LS, Sutherland C, Lama S, Sutherland GR. Treatment of Glioma using neuroArm surgical system. Biomed Res Int. 2016;2016:9734512. https://doi.org/10.1155/2016/9734512.
30. Menon M, Tewari A, Baize B, Guillonneau B, Vallancien G. Prospective comparison of radical retropubic prostatectomy and robot-assisted anatomic prostatectomy: the Vattikuti urology institute experience. Urology. 2002;60:864–8.
31. Pugin F, Bucher P, Morel P. History of robotic surgery: from AESOP® and ZEUS® to da Vinci®. J Visc Surg. 2011;148(5 Suppl):e3–8.
32. Abbou CC, Hoznek A, Salomon L, et al. Remote laparoscopic radical prostatectomy carried out with a robot. Report of a case [in French]. Prog Urol. 2000;10:520–3.
33. Oleynikov D. Robotic surgery. Surg Clin North Am. 2008;88:1121–30. https://doi.org/10.1016/j. suc.2008.05.012.
34. Peters BS, Armijo PR, Krause C, Choudhury SA, Oleynikov D. Review of emerging surgical robotic technology. Surg Endosc. 2018;32:1636–55. https://doi.org/10.1007/s00464-018-6079-2.
35. Yu HY, Hevelone ND, Lipsitz SR, Kowalczyk KJ, Hu JC. Use, costs and comparative effectiveness of robotic assisted, laparoscopic and open urological surgery. J Urol. 2012;187:1392–8.
36. Trinh QD, Sammon J, Sun M, et al. Perioperative outcomes of robot-assisted radical prostatectomy compared with open radical prostatectomy: results from the nationwide inpatient sample. Eur Urol. 2012;61:679–85.
37. Smith JA Jr, Herrell SD. Robotic-assisted laparoscopic prostatectomy: do minimally invasive approaches offer significant advantages? J Clin Oncol. 2005;23:8170–5.
38. Skarecky DW. Robotic-assisted radical prostatectomy after the first decade: surgical evolution or new paradigm. ISRN Urol. 2013;2013:157379.
39. Jackson MA, Bellas N, Siegrist T, Haddock P, Staff I, Laudone V, Wagner JR. Experienced open vs early robotic-assisted laparoscopic radical prostatectomy: a 10-year prospective and retrospective comparison. Urology. 2016;91:111–8. https://doi.org/10.1016/j. urology.2015.12.072.
40. Benway BM, Bhayani SB, Rogers CG, et al. Robot-assisted partial nephrectomy versus laparoscopic partial nephrectomy for renal tumors: a multi-institutional analysis of perioperative outcomes. J Urol. 2009;182:866–72.
41. Luciani LG, Chiodini S, Mattevi D, Cai T, Puglisi M, Mantovani W, Malossini G. Robotic-assisted partial nephrectomy provides better operative outcomes as compared to the laparoscopic and open approaches: results from a prospective cohort study. J Robot Surg. 2017;11(3):333–9. https://doi.org/10.1007/s11701-016-0660-2. Epub 2016 Dec 20
42. Kader AK, Richards KA, Krane LS, Pettus JA, Smith JJ, Hemal AK. Robot-assisted laparoscopic vs open radical cystectomy: comparison of complications and perioperative oncological outcomes in 200 patients. BJU Int. 2013;112:E290–4.
43. Sathianathen NJ, Kalapara A, Frydenberg M, Lawrentschuk N, Weight CJ, Parekh D, Konety BR. Robotic-assisted radical cystectomy vs open radical cystectomy: systematic review and meta-analysis. J Urol. 2018. pii: S0022-5347(18)43984-5. https://doi.org/10.1016/j.juro.2018.10.006. [Epub ahead of print].
44. Delaney CP, Lynch AC, Senagore AJ, Fazio VW. Comparison of robotically performed and traditional laparoscopic colorectal surgery. Dis Colon Rectum. 2003;46:1633–9.
45. Pinar I, Fransgaard T, Thygesen LC, Gögenur I. Long-Term Outcomes of Robot-Assisted Surgery in Patients with Colorectal cancer. Ann Surg Oncol. 2018;25(13):3906–12. https://doi.org/10.1245/s10434-018-6862-2. Epub 2018 Oct 11
46. deSouza AL, Prasad LM, Park JJ, Marecik SJ, Blumetti J, Abcarian H. Robotic assistance in right hemicolectomy: is there a role? Dis Colon Rectum. 2010;53:1000–6.
47. Wright JD, Ananth CV, Lewin SN, et al. Robotically assisted vs laparoscopic hysterectomy among women with benign gynecologic disease. JAMA. 2013;309:689–98.
48. Liu H, Lu D, Wang L, Shi G, Song H, Clarke J. Robotic surgery for benign gynecological disease. Cochrane Database Syst Rev. 2012;(2):CD008978.
49. Swenson CW, Kamdar NS, Harris JA, Uppal S, Campbell DA Jr, Morgan DM. Comparison of robotic and other minimally invasive routes of hysterectomy for benign indications. Am J Obstet Gynecol. 2016;215(5):650.e1–8. https://doi.org/10.1016/j. ajog.2016.06.027. Epub 2016 Jun 22
50. Tan A, Ashrafian H, Scott AJ, Mason SE, Harling L, Athanasiou T, Darzi A. Robotic surgery: disruptive innovation or unfulfilled promise? A systematic review and meta-analysis of the first 30 years. Surg Endosc. 2016;30(10):4330–52.
51. Minjares-Granillo RO, Dimas BA, LeFave JJ, Haas EM. Robotic left-sided colorectal resection with natural orifice IntraCorporeal anastomosis with extraction of specimen: the NICE procedure. A pilot study of consecutive cases. Am J Surg. 2018. pii: S0002-9610(18)31234-0. https://doi.org/10.1016/j. amjsurg.2018.11.048.
52. Loulmet D, Carpentier A, d'Attellis N, et al. Endoscopic coronary artery bypass grafting with the aid of robotic assisted instruments. J Thorac Cardiovasc Surg. 1999;118:4–10.

53. O'Sullivan KE, Kreaden US, Hebert AE, Eaton D, Redmond KC. A systematic review and meta-analysis of robotic versus open and video-assisted thoracoscopic surgery approaches for lobectomy. Interact Cardiovasc Thorac Surg. 2018. https://doi.org/10.1093/icvts/ivy315.

54. Wang A, Brennan JM, Zhang S, Jung SH, Yerokun B, Cox ML, Jacobs JP, Badhwar V, Suri RM, Thourani V, Halkos ME, Gammie JS, Gillinov AM, Smith PK, Glower D. Robotic mitral valve repair in older individuals: an analysis of the Society of Thoracic Surgeons database. Ann Thorac Surg. 2018;106(5):1388–93. https://doi.org/10.1016/j.athoracsur.2018.05.074. Epub 2018 Jun 30

55. Cerfolio RJ, Bryant AS, Skylizard L, Minnich DJ. Initial consecutive experience of completely portal robotic pulmonary resection with 4 arms. J Thorac Cardiovasc Surg. 2011;142:740–6.

56. Doulamis IP, Spartalis E, Machairas N, Schizas D, Patsouras D, Spartalis M, Tsilimigras DI, Moris D, Iliopoulos DC, Tzani A, Dimitroulis D, Nikiteas NI. The role of robotics in cardiac surgery: a systematic review. J Robot Surg. 2018. https://doi.org/10.1007/s11701-018-0875-5.

57. Roizenblatt M, Grupenmacher AT, Belfort Junior R, Maia M, Gehlbach PL. Robot-assisted tremor control for performance enhancement of retinal microsurgeons. Br J Ophthalmol. 2018. pii: bjophthalmol-2018-313318. https://doi.org/10.1136/bjophthalmol-2018-313318.

58. Caversaccio M, Gavaghan K, Wimmer W, Williamson T, Ansò J, Mantokoudis G, Gerber N, Rathgeb C, Feldmann A, Wagner F, Scheidegger O, Kompis M, Weisstanner C, Zoka-Assadi M, Roesler K, Anschuetz L, Huth M, Weber S. Robotic cochlear implantation: surgical procedure and first clinical experience. Acta Otolaryngol. 2017;137(4):447–54. https://doi.org/10.1080/00016489.2017.1278573. Epub 2017 Feb 1

59. Ahn D, Sohn JH, Lee GJ, Hwang KH. Feasibility of using the retroauricular approach without endoscopic or robotic assistance for excision of benign neck masses. Head Neck. 2017;39(4):748–53. https://doi.org/10.1002/hed.24678. Epub 2017 Jan 9.

60. Chai YJ, Lee KE, Youn Y-K. Can robotic thyroidectomy be performed safely in thyroid carcinoma patients? Endocrinol Metab (Seoul). 2014;29(3):226–32. https://doi.org/10.3803/EnM.2014.29.3.226.

61. Russell JO, Noureldine SI, Al Khadem MG, et al. Transoral robotic thyroidectomy: a preclinical feasibility study using the da Vinci Xi platform. J Robot Surg. 2017. https://doi.org/10.1007/s11701-016-0661-1.

62. Lang BH-H, Wong CKH, Tsang JS, Wong KP, Wan KY. A systematic review and meta-analysis evaluating completeness and outcomes of robotic thyroidectomy. Laryngoscope. 2015;125(2):509–18. https://doi.org/10.1002/lary.24946.

63. Jacofsky DJ, Allen M. Robotics in arthroplasty: a comprehensive review. J Arthroplasty. 2016. https://doi.org/10.1016/j.arth.2016.05.026.

64. Bargar WL. Robots in orthopaedic surgery: past, present, and future. Clin Orthop Relat Res. 2007;463:31–6.

65. Yang HY, Seon JK, Shin YJ, Lim HA, Song EK. Robotic total knee arthroplasty with a Cruciate-Retaining implant: a 10-year follow-up study. Clin Orthop Surg. 2017;9(2):169.

66. Gilmour A, MacLean AD, Rowe PJ, Banger MS, Donnelly I, Jones BG, Blyth MJG. Robotic-arm-assisted vs conventional unicompartmental knee arthroplasty. The 2-year clinical outcomes of a randomized controlled trial. J Arthroplast. 2018;33(7S):S109–15. https://doi.org/10.1016/j.arth.2018.02.050. Epub 2018 Feb 21

67. Liow MHL, Goh GS, Wong MK, Chin PL, Tay DK, Yeo SJ. Robotic-assisted total knee arthroplasty may lead to improvement in quality-of-life measures: a 2-year follow-up of a prospective randomized trial. Knee Surg Sports Traumatol Arthrosc. 2017;25(9):2942.

68. Bargar WL, Parise CA, Hankins A, Marlen NA, Campanelli V, Netravali NA. Fourteen year follow-up of randomized clinical trials of active robotic-assisted total hip arthroplasty. J Arthroplast. 2018;33(3):810–4. https://doi.org/10.1016/j.arth.2017.09.066. Epub 2017 Oct 6

69. Lonner JH, Fillingham YA. Pros and cons: a balanced view of robotics in knee arthroplasty. J Arthroplast. 2018;33:2007–13.

70. Ritter MA, Davis KE, Meding JB, Pierson JL, Berend ME, Malinzak RA. The effect of alignment and BMI on failure of total knee replacement. J Bone Joint Surg Am. 2011;93(17):1588.

71. Parratte S, Pagnano MW, Trousdale RT, Berry DJ. Effect of postoperative mechanical axis alignment on the fifteen-year survival of modern, cemented total knee replacements. J Bone Joint Surg Am. 2010;92(12):2143.

72. https://blogs.dnvgl.com/software/2017/11/thinking-outside-of-the-box/

73. Mangel M, Samaniego FJ. Abraham Wald's work on aircraft survivability. J Am Stat Assoc. 1984;79:259–67.

74. https://www.cnbc.com/2016/05/23/globe-newswire-orthopedic-surgical-and-surgical-assist-robots-market%2D%2Dhip-and-knee-orthopedic-surgical-robot-device-markets-will-reach-5.html

75. Conditt MA, Bargar WL, Cobb JP, Dorr LD, Lonner JH. Current concepts in robotics for the treatment of joint disease. London, UK: Hindawi Publishing Corporation. 2013.

76. Boylan M, Suchman K, Vigdorchik J, Slover J, Bosco J. Technology-assisted hip and knee arthroplasties: an analysis of utilization trends. J Arthroplast. 2017;33:1019e23.

77. MAKO Surgical Corp Fact Sheet. http://www.makosurgical.com/assets/files/Company/newsroom/Corporate_Fact_Sheet_208578r00.pdf; 2013. Accessed 7 Mar 2016.

78. Navio data courtesy of Smith and Nephew, Memphis, TN.

79. Medical Device and Diagnostic Industry, 5 Mar 2015. http://www.mddionline.com
80. Fiani B, Quadri SA, Farooqui M, Cathel A, Berman B, Noel J, Siddiqi J. Impact of robot-assisted spine surgery on health care quality and neurosurgical economics: a systemic review. Neurosurg Rev. https://doi.org/10.1007/s10143-018-0971-z.
81. Joseph JR, Smith BW, Liu X, Park P. Current applications of robotics in spine surgery: a systematic review of the literature. Neurosurg Focus. 2017;42:E2.
82. https://mazorrobotics.com/en-us/resources/for-surgeons/faq-for-surgeons. Accessed 3 Jan 2019.
83. OpenPR. Global Surgical Robots for the Spine Industry Trend, Growth, Shares, Strategy and Forecasts 2016 to 2022; 2017. https://www.openpr.com/news/442943/Global-Surgical-Robots-for-the-Spine-Industry-Trend-Growth-Shares-Strategy-and-Forecasts-2016-to-2022.html

Evolution of Robotics in Arthroplasty

2

Mark W. Allen and David J. Jacofsky

Robotic-assisted orthopedic surgery has improved total joint arthroplasty by enhancing the surgeon's ability to reproduce alignment; this technology has been available for over 20 years. As more surgical procedures are being performed with robotic assistance, and surgical indications and techniques are expanding, a growing body of supporting literature is emerging [1, 2]. The evolution of arthroplasty from past to present is reviewed in this chapter.

Over the long term, robotic technologies introduced in various industries have shown an increase in production capacity, improved accuracy and precision, and lower overall costs. As in all development efforts, robotics in other industries generally undergoes a period of development and refinement prior to rapid adoption, which occurs after the benefits of the technology become clear. Robotic surgery has become an increasingly popular tool for orthopedic surgeons in the operative suite. During unicompartmental knee arthroplasty (UKA), total knee arthroplasty (TKA), and total hip arthroplasty (THA), these robotic platforms have been shown to increase accuracy and precision of component placement. Improved alignment has been shown to increase implant

survival and decrease revision surgery [3]. The future of robotics in orthopedics appears bright.

History of Robotics

Several definitions of "robot" exist. According to the Robot Institute of America, a robot is defined as a reprogrammable, multifunctional manipulator designed to move material, parts, tools, or specialized devices through various programmed motions for the performance of a variety of tasks [4]. *Webster's Dictionary* describes a robot as an automatic device that performs functions normally ascribed to humans or a machine in the form of a human [5].

Devol, from Louisville, KY, created the first robots in the early 1950s by inventing and patenting a reprogrammable manipulator called "Unimate" [6]. In the late 1960s, the "Father of Robotics," Joseph Engelberger, acquired Devol's robot patent, modified it into an industrial robot, and formed a company called Unimation [6]. This robot was the standard hydraulic robot in the industry until electrically driven robots were developed.

The work completed in the 1950s and 1960s led to robotic advancements in the surgical field. In 1985, Puma 560 was the first robotic surgical system created which allowed neurosurgical biopsies to be done with greater precision using CT guidance [7]. In 1988, the same system was used for a transurethral resection of a prostate. This eventually led to the development of the PROBOT system,

M. W. Allen
Department of Adult Reconstruction, The CORE Institute, Phoenix, AZ, USA

D. J. Jacofsky (✉)
Department of Orthopedics, The CORE Institute, Phoenix, AZ, USA
e-mail: David.Jacofsky@thecoreinstitute.com

© Springer Nature Switzerland AG 2019
J. H. Lonner (ed.), *Robotics in Knee and Hip Arthroplasty*,
https://doi.org/10.1007/978-3-030-16593-2_2

designed to specifically aid in the resection of prostatic tissue, proving that predictable soft tissue surgery was feasible with robotics [8]. Since then, the field of medical robotics has grown tremendously.

Much of the initial field of robotics has focused on advancing laparoscopic surgical techniques. In 2000, the FDA approved the first robotic surgical system – the da Vinci surgical system. This is considered a sophisticated robotic platform designed to expand a surgeon's capabilities and offer a state-of-the art minimally invasive option for major surgery. Physicians have used the da Vinci system successfully worldwide in approximately 1.5 million various surgical procedures to date in multiple surgical fields including cardiac, colorectal, general, head and neck, and thoracic surgery, gynecology, and urology [9]. The da Vinci system is a passive, remote, tele-manipulator system that allows the surgeon to sit at the da Vinci console and view a magnified, high-resolution 3D image of the patient's anatomy. The surgeon is actively controlling the robotic arms without a preoperative plan in place, thus allowing for intraoperative variability.

The field of orthopedics has focused on hard tissue models in the advancing robotic field. Knee and hip arthroplasty surgeries require a very high degree of precision when preparing and placing implants [10]. Bony landmarks are static structures, thus allowing preoperative imaging and intraoperative mapping for reliable and precise anatomic positioning of bone resection. In contrast to the da Vinci system, the orthopedic systems are able to be modified by the surgeon to develop the final planned outcome before an incision is even made and then can accurately produce that outcome.

Historical Systems

CASPAR

CASPAR (Ortho-Maquet/URS Ortho Rastatt, Germany) was an early autonomous system. The CASPAR system was an image-guided active robot used for THA and TKA similar to ROBODOC [11]. Initial results focused on improving and decreasing the variability in the mechanical axis of the leg during TKA. Many studies have demonstrated the importance of the mechanical axis in TKA function, outcomes, and longevity [12, 13]. A study performed by Siebert et al. using CASPAR for TKA noted improved tibiofemoral alignment [14]. However, despite improving tibiofemoral alignment, the CASPAR system was somewhat restrictive. Femoral and tibial bone screws had to be placed preoperatively (during an initial first surgery) as fiducial markers for registration of the preoperative CT scan allow for intraoperative robotic function. No major adverse events related to the CASPAR system were found.

CASPAR for THA has been shown to increase the accuracy of femoral preparation and position of the cementless prosthesis in the femoral cavity [15]. Conversely, CASPAR has been shown to have a low accuracy of postoperative anteversion angles of the femoral stem compared to the preoperative plan [16]. A prospective trial compared the clinical outcome of both conventional (35 hips) and robotic milling (36 hips) procedures using the CASPAR system and demonstrated that the CASPAR system surgeries lasted about 50 minutes longer and patients showed increased blood loss, had significantly lower hip abductor function, had an increased incidence of Trendelenburg's sign, and had a higher complication rate [17]. The authors recommended critical consideration of possible complications prior to initiating robotic-assisted THA [17]. These early attempts at robotics, with less advanced systems, clearly showed that robotics can have the potential to portend risks greater than their benefits. The CASPAR robotic system is no longer available for clinical use, and the company is no longer in business.

Acrobot

Acrobot, an acronym for active constraint robot, was developed largely at the Imperial College of London. The Acrobot utilized CT-based software to accurately plan TKAs preoperatively. Intraoperatively, the surgeon guided a small, special-purpose robot called Acrobot, which was mounted on a gross positioning device. The Acrobot used active constraint control, limiting motion to a pre-defined region and allowed the surgeon to safely resect the bone to accept a TKA prosthesis with high precision. A noninvasive anatomical registration method was used, and this was a predicate to more modern haptic systems. The company was acquired by Stanmore Implants Worldwide in 2010 and subsequently withdrew from robotics. MAKO Surgical acquired the assets as part of a confidential patent infringement settlement in 2013.

Contemporary Systems

The steps performed during a robotically assisted surgery typically involve (1) creating a patient-specific model preoperatively (in image-based systems); (2) intraoperatively registering the patient to create a final model and developing a plan based on the patient's anatomy; and (3) using robotic assistance to make bone cuts and carry out the procedure. Many robotic systems have been developed and prototyped, but only a handful have been successfully used in a clinical setting. More recent and commonly utilized systems for arthroplasty surgery (Table 2.1) include the Navio PFS (Smith and Nephew, London and Hull, UK), the iBlock robotic cutting guide (OMNIlife Science, East Taunton, MA), the MAKO Robotic Arm Interactive Orthopedic System (RIO; MAKO Surgical Corporation, Fort Lauderdale, FL, USA), and ROSA Knee Robot (Zimmer Biomet, Warsaw, IN).

ROBODOC/TSolution One™ Surgical System

In the early 1990s, Howard A. Paul, DVM, and William L. Bargar, MD, teamed up to develop a system to prepare the femoral side of a THA to facilitate the use of cementless stems and improve bony ingrowth [18]. In 1992, the ROBODOC system (initially by Curexo Technology, Fremont, CA) designed by Drs. Paul and Bargar made history by being the first robot used clinically in orthopedic surgery (Fig. 2.1). ROBODOC was an image-based, active, autonomous, milling

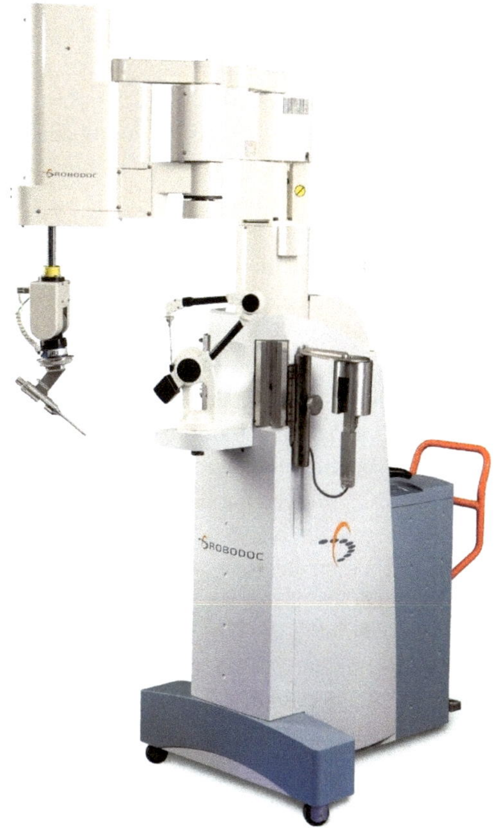

Fig. 2.1 THINK surgical robot. (Courtesy of Curexo Technology, Fremont, CA)

Table 2.1 Current robotic platforms

System	Corporation	Arthroplasty	Preoperative planning	Control	Platform	Bone resection
TSolution One (Robodoc)	Think Surgical, Fremont, CA, USA	TKA, THA (femur)	CT scan	Autonomous	Open	Mill
iBlock	OMNIlife Science, East Taunton, MA, USA	TKA	None	Autonomous	Closed	Saw
MAKO	Stryker Corporation, Mahwah, NJ, USA	UKA, PFA, TKA, THA	CT scan	Semiautonomous, haptic	Closed	Burr, Saw
Navio PFS	Smith and Nephew, Memphis, TN, USA	UKA, PFA,TKA	None	Semiautonomous	Open	Burr, Saw
ROSA Knee	Zimmer Biomet, Warsaw, IN, USA	TKA	None	Semiautonomous	Closed	Saw

TKA total knee arthroplasty, *UKA* unicompartmental knee arthroplasty, *THA* total hip arthroplasty

robotic system. The system operates with an open implant platform. Once the system was positioned and fixed to the patient, markers in the surgical field (fiducials) were then used as a reference for image guidance. After anchoring in the bone, the robot would automatically mill a cavity in the femur for the stem. Initial pilot studies were performed in dogs, and human trials began in 1992 [18]. The European Union approved ROBODOC for sale in 1994, and the first system was installed in Germany [19]. Worldwide, the system has been used for more than 24,000 joint arthroplasties. More recently, the system has been improved and expanded the focus beyond THA, to also include TKA using a similar technical approach.

Initial clinical trials began in 1994 and were approved for THA by the FDA in 2008 [19–21]. The FDA has not yet approved it for TKA or partial knee arthroplasty. As in the early ROBODOC system design, it remains CT based, but it is now a computer-aided, robotic milling device that allows cavity preparation for hip arthroplasty and surface preparation for TKA. The "ORTHODOC" workstation transfers data, completes the segmentation, and plans the implant positioning before engaging and operating the robot intraoperatively. A series of clinical trials have proven clinical success and utility [21, 22]. Overall implant positioning and alignment are consistently within 1° of error in all planes and radiographic improvements in accuracy with robotic-assisted arthroplasty compared to conventional techniques [2, 13, 23]. The company was formerly known as Curexo Technology Corporation and changed its name to Think Surgical, Inc. in September 2014.

In cementless primary hip arthroplasty, a randomized multicenter study conducted from 1994–1998 showed statistically improved fit, fill, and alignment with ROBODOC as compared to manual THA [18], and ROBODOC milling has shown a decrease in intraoperative embolic events compared to standard femoral broach preparation [24].

The first 100 ROBODOC TKA procedures were performed by Professor Martin Börner at the Berufsgenossenschaftliche Unfallklinik (BGU) in Frankfurt, Germany [25]. The ROBODOC system made cuts that were good enough to allow cementless implantation for both the tibia and femur in 76% of the patients. In 97% of the cases, the alignment of the knee was restored to the planned ideal mechanical axis (0° error). In two different prospective studies comparing ROBODOC-assisted to manual TKA, the robot had more accuracy and less variation in the mechanical axis and had no difference in patient-reported outcome measures [23, 26]. In both studies, the ROBODOC-assisted TKA procedures averaged 25 minutes longer than the manual procedures, but they demonstrated less postoperative bleeding.

The ROBODOC system requires increased time for planning, registration, and milling. The increase in operative time is a known potential risk factor for prosthetic joint infection [27]. If the robot monitoring system detects an error (such as movement of the bone), the robot will stop, and the recovery process is a series of steps that must be completed to allow the procedure to safely continue. The current hip application is limited to femoral preparation only; however, it can assist in acetabular positioning by providing the calculated femoral anteversion to provide an appropriate estimate of combined anteversion and decrease component impingement. Neither live kinematic joint assessment nor final implant position information is currently available with the ROBODOC platform.

Navio PFS

Navio PFS (Smith and Nephew, Memphis, TN), initially FDA approved in 2012 for UKA and later for TKA, is a handheld and imageless device that uses an open platform and provides freehand sculpting for unicondylar, patellofemoral, and total knee arthroplasty (Fig. 2.2). The interactive, surgeon-controlled, handheld cutting tool has an end-cutting burr that extends and retracts so that only the planned bone is removed. As a semi-autonomous system, it monitors the surgeon's movements of the burring tool, with safeguards in place to optimize both accuracy and safety via the retraction of the burr tip when the edge of the desired bone removal volume is approached. Navio utilizes optical-based navigation with an

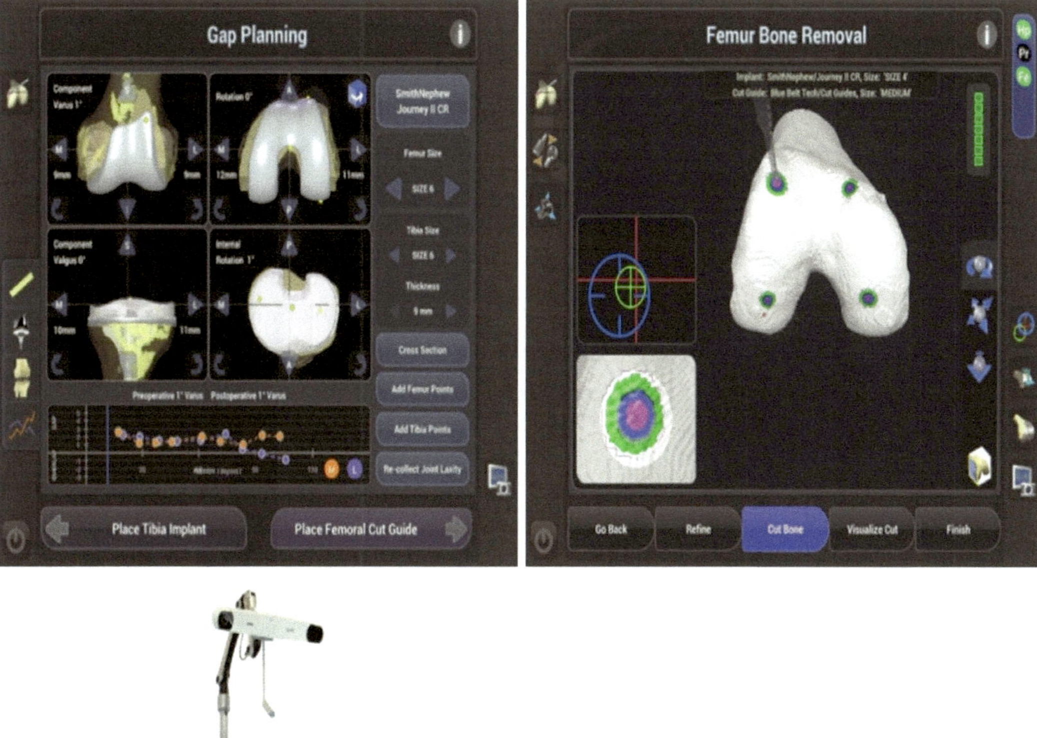

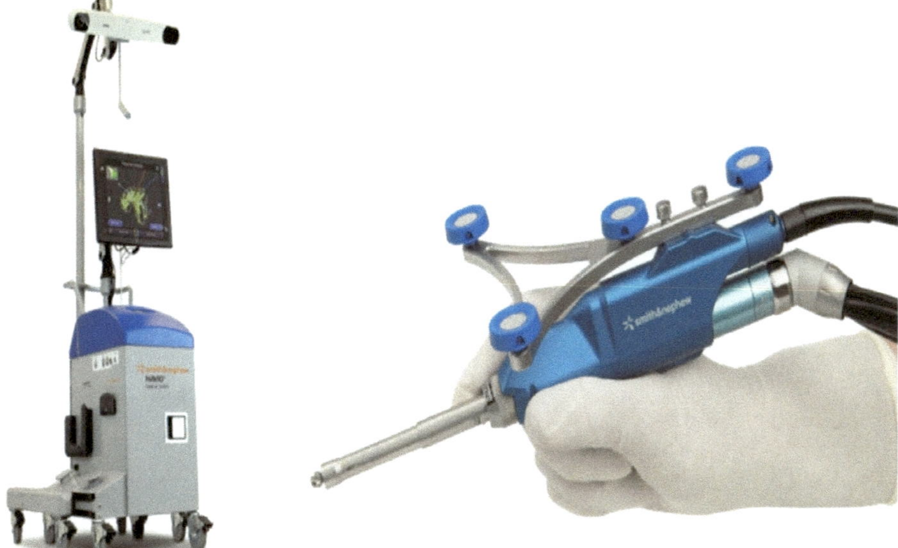

Fig. 2.2 Navio TKA planning and instrumentation. (Courtesy of Smith & Nephew, Andover, MA, USA)

imageless system to provide 3D morphed images and views of the procedure, thus creating a virtual model of the osseous knee. The system continuously tracks the position of the patients' lower limb and the handheld burr, so that the limb position and degree of knee flexion can be changed constantly during the surgical procedure to gain exposure to different parts of the knee during registration and bone preparation.

As the Navio system is imageless, it eliminates the risk of radiation exposure and the associated cost with preoperative imaging. However, Navio does not rely on haptic feedback. Rather, it provides protective control against inadvertent bone removal by modulating the exposure and speed of the motorized burr. The safety of the burr retraction is limited to its sensitivity and retraction speed.

A cadaveric study of the medial UKA Navio system investigated implant accuracy and was able to demonstrate implant position within the expected target with low rotational, angular, and translational errors [28]. Navio improved post-surgical mechanical axis alignment, decreased cutting phase time, and improved Oxford Knee Scores from preoperative to 6 weeks postoperative, and the mean mechanical axis deformity was reduced in the Navio group [29].

There is a fairly rapid learning curve with this technology [30, 31]. There is limited published complication and outcome data available; however, a number of clinical trials and studies are currently in press or at various stages of completion.

iBlock

The iBlock robotic cutting guide (OMNIlife Science, East Taunton, MA), previously known as Praxiteles, was FDA approved in 2010 [32] for femoral resections in TKA (Fig. 2.3). It is an imageless, motorized, bone-mounted cutting guide that positions itself for femoral resections according to the surgeon's plan, allowing the surgeon to then use a standard oscillating saw. iBlock is paired with the NanoBlock, a separate, adjustable, resection block used for tibial resection. The OmniBiotics computer station utilizes bone morphing technology to generate a unique 3D digital model of the patient's knee intraoperatively, allowing for planning of implant positioning and sizing intraoperatively and visualizing planned bone cuts before they are made.

Compared to conventional navigated instrumentation, iBlock's mean femoral preparation time was shorter, the average deviation in the final bone resections was more accurate, and the adjustable cutting block was found to provide equal or better component alignment while decreasing postoperative mechanical alignment

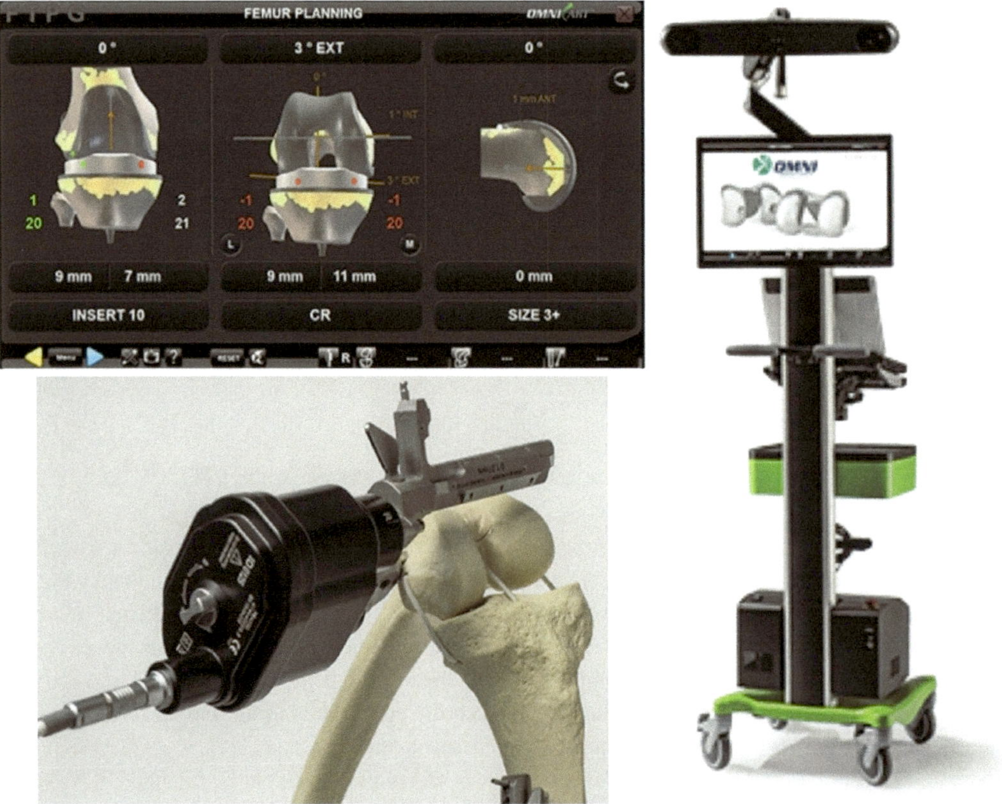

Fig. 2.3 OmniBiotics total knee system with iBlock. (Courtesy of OMNIlife science, Inc., Raynham, MA, USA)

and tourniquet time [33, 34]. The femoral resections were also compared using a robotic cutting guide vs. conventional techniques, and the robotic guide allowed for significantly more accurate and repeatable bone resections [35].

There is limited clinical data on iBlock available. A retrospective review of the first 100 cases used with iBlock at a single institution was performed, allowing one surgeon to make bone resections within 3° of neutral in 98% of cases [34]. The iBlock system is limited by having no haptic feedback, available only for TKA applications on a closed platform, and having limited kinematic assessment after implantation of trials and/or implants. Many believe that this is best characterized as a motorized, computer-navigated, adjustable jig rather than a "robot."

MAKO

The Robotic Arm Interactive Orthopedic System (RIO; MAKO Stryker, Fort Lauderdale, Florida) is a haptic system available in clinical practice for UKA, THA, and TKA (Fig. 2.4). As an image-based system, a preoperative CT is used in surgical planning to help determine component sizing, positioning, and bone resection which is then confirmed and adjusted preoperatively and/or intraoperatively based on the patient's specific kinematics prior to any surgical resection. The robotic system provides haptic feedback during the procedure to prevent bone resection outside of the desired plan [36].

MAKO robotic arm-assisted procedures have been shown to overcome technical challenges associated with manual partial and/or multi-compartmental knee procedures. A series of studies demonstrated that, as compared to manual techniques, the robotic system has increased accuracy in placing the tibial component [10, 37–40] and significantly decreases the learning curve during the adoption of UKAs with traditional instrumentation [41–44]. Data supports improved outcomes with bicompartmental arthroplasty using robotic assistance and preservation of the cruciate ligaments as well [45]. One study reviewed patellofemoral resurfacing in combination with medial or lateral compartment resurfacing in 29 patients (30 knees) who were, on average, 63.6 years old and demonstrated 83% good to excellent results [46].

MAKO robotic-arm assisted UKA resulted in shorter hospital stays, significantly lower postoperative pain, greater functionality, and decreased office visits to general practitioners and hospital-

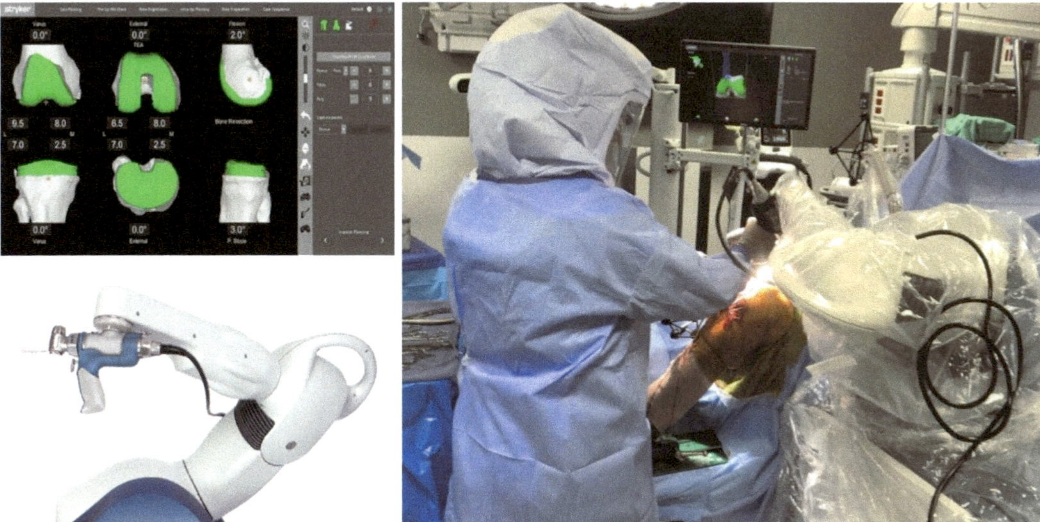

Fig. 2.4 MAKO planning, instrumentation, and intraoperative use for distal femur resection. (Operative photo courtesy of Steven Myerthall, MD, The CORE Institute; MAKO photo courtesy of Stryker, Kalamazoo, MI, USA)

izations within 3 months following surgery [47]. MAKO-assisted UKA procedures had a cumulative revision rate of 1.2%, a substantially lower rate than historically reported rates for manual UKR of 4.5% and 4.8% at a 2-year follow-up (Swedish and Australian national registries, respectively) [48]. Recently, Pearl reported a survivorship of 98.8% at 2.5 years for 909 robotically assisted unicompartmental arthroplasty procedures with 92% of patients either very satisfied or satisfied with their knee function [49]. A single-center study of 65 medial UKA and 8 lateral UKA performed with MAKO robotic assistance showed 91 and 88% satisfactory postoperative results with 1 case of overcorrection of HKA angle in a lateral UKA [50].

The use of manual THA with traditional instruments is associated with complications including dislocation, impingement, and wear, leading to patient discomfort and walking complications. In a recent study evaluating patients undergoing posterior-approach THA, individuals receiving manual THA experienced more dislocations at 6 months as compared to those undergoing MAKO robotic-assisted THA [51]. In a study comparing manual THA to THA using robotic-assisted alignment, 50 MAKO-assisted THAs were matched to historical manual THAs conducted between 2008 and 2012 [52]. 100% of the MAKO-assisted THAs were placed within the Lewinnek safe zone for anteversion and inclination (vs. only 80% of manual), and 92% of the MAKO-assisted THAs were within the Callanan safe zone (vs. only 62% of manual) [52]. In a multicenter study of MAKO-assisted THA cases, planned cup placement was compared with cup orientation after impaction and immediately postoperatively, and in 95% of cases, cup placements were recorded to be within 5° of the surgical plan. This demonstrates that MAKO robotic assistance provides surgeons with optimal measures to facilitate patient-specific planning [53]. In a cadaveric investigation, 12 acetabular components were implanted into 6 cadaveric pelvises: MAKO-assisted THA on one side and manual THA on the other side. Hips implanted with the MAKO assistance had four to six times greater accuracy in version and inclination vs. manual THA [54]. The use of MAKO-assisted THA has been shown to improve accuracy in achieving desired leg length and offset compared with manual THA based on a cadaveric investigation of 21 hips [55]. In a matched-pair controlled study, the size of the acetabular cup relative to that of the femoral head was used as a surrogate measure of acetabular bone resection. In this study, MAKO-guided THA allowed for the use of smaller acetabular cups in relation to the patient's femoral head size compared to conventional THA, indicating greater preservation of acetabular bone stock [56].

Improved component positioning leads to better range of motion, decreased impingement, and more stability, potentially improving function and outcome in primary THAs. MAKO-assisted THA improved accuracy for both acetabular abduction angles and acetabular anteversion leading to lower dislocation rates with 0% dislocations in the robotic THA group within the first 2 years postoperatively [51]. At 1-year follow-up, patients who had received MAKO-guided THA demonstrated significantly higher modified Harris Hip scores and UCLA activity level compared with manual THA [57].

MAKO has received 510(k) market clearances of the MAKO total knee application and is in clinical use (Fig. 2.4). Early studies have shown improved safety as it relates to soft tissue and ligamentous damage from the saw when comparing MAKO assisted to manual TKA [58]. The total knee application expands the MAKO offering by providing a comprehensive solution in the robotic reconstructive service line (i.e., UKA, TKA, and THA). The total knee application utilizes the MAKO Integrated Cutting System (MICS). The MICS powers a saw blade specifically designed for the MAKO platform. Given the 3D planning capabilities of the system and the ability of the system to predictably reproduce an intended surgical plan, it is expected that the safety and precision of this application will prove to be similar to the published results of other applications on the MAKO platform.

ROSA Knee Robot®

ROSA robot has been used for cranial surgery, but recent adaptation of the system for TKA

(ROSA Knee Robot, Zimmer Biomet, Warsaw, IN) has led to its use initially in Australia in 2018 and now in the United States, having received 510 K approval by the US Food and Drug Administration in early 2019. The ROSA Knee Robot system (Fig. 2.5) does not require advanced preoperative imaging, such as CT scanning; planning can be done exclusively intraoperative by registering bony and cartilage landmarks for three-dimensional modeling, intraoperative decisionmaking, and resection plans. It is a semi-autonomous surgical system that haptically positions a resection guide, but not the cutting saw, to augment the precision of bone resections, and assesses the balance of the soft tissue envelope in TKA surgery. Early data demonstrates precision of bone resections and implant positioning, with reductions in outliers compared to conventional methods.

Other Systems

In addition to TSolution One (ROBODOC), Navio, iBlock, ROSA, and MAKO, there has been development of miniature bone-mounted robots [10]. For example, PiGalileo (Plus Orthopedics AG, Smith & Nephew, Switzerland)

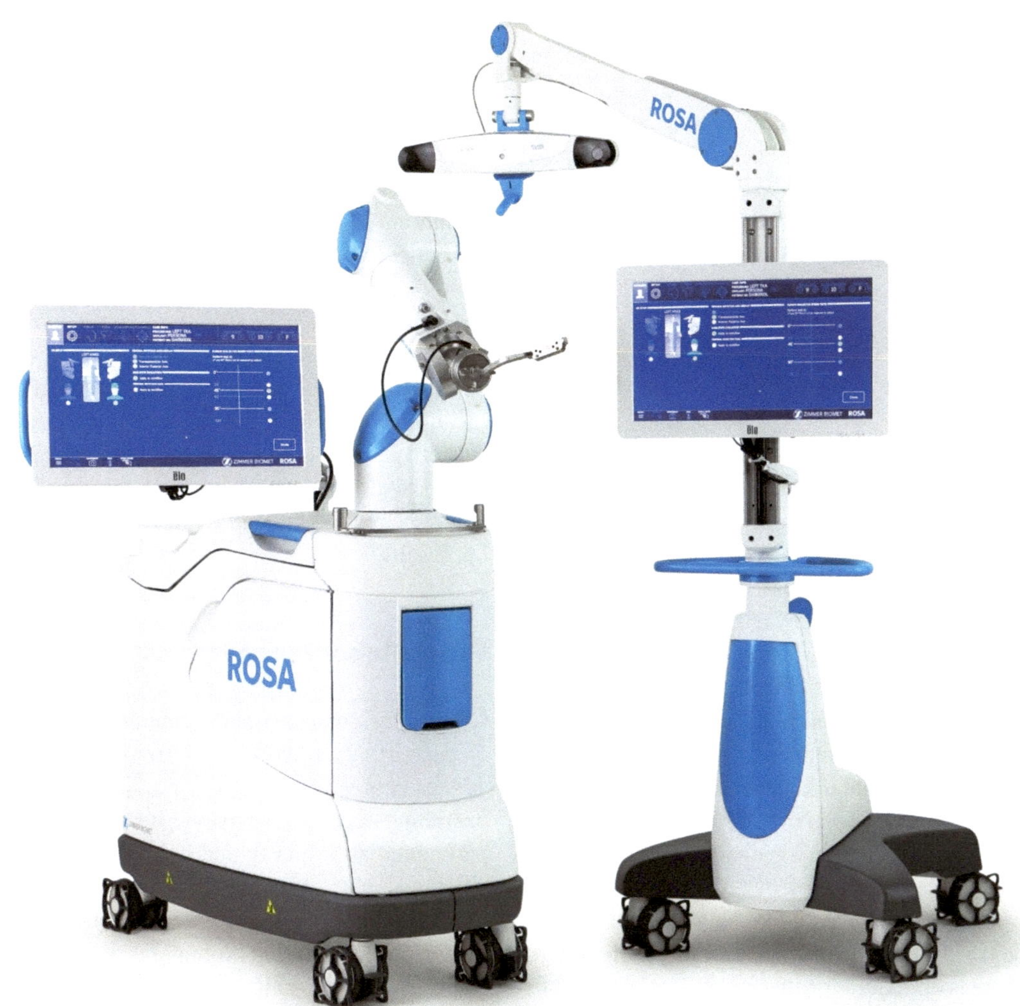

Fig. 2.5 ROSA Knee Robot. (Courtesy of Zimmer Biomet, Warsaw, IN)

is a passive system that uses a hybrid navigated robotic device that clamps onto the mediolateral aspects of the distal femoral shaft [10]. The MBARS (Mini Bone-Attached Robotic System) was an active system developed for patellofemoral joint arthroplasty procedures [59]. Plaskos et al. presented Praxiteles in 2005 as a miniature bone-mounted robotic cutting guide for TKA [60], the predecessor to the modern iBlock. Song et al. have developed an active system consisting of a hybrid bone-attached robot for joint arthroplasty (HyBAR) that uses hinged prismatic joints to provide a structurally rigid robot for minimally invasive joint arthroplasty [61]. It is important to begin to carefully define the definitions of "robot" and "robotic tools," as compared to "navigated jigs" and/or "smart instruments" as the industry advances and the space begins to fill with various products all claiming to be "robotic." Further, several robotic systems are currently in early use or development for spinal applications, such as Mazor X (Mazor Robotic Ltd., Caesarea, Israel), ROSA Spine robotic system (Zimmer Biomet, Warsaw, IN), and Excelsus system (Globus Medical, Audubon, PA).

Discussion

Robotic surgery is changing the landscape of orthopedics. Robots were initially introduced into orthopedic operating rooms to improve precision, accuracy, and patient's overall outcome and satisfaction rates. Robotic-assisted surgery is already achieving these goals by enhancing the surgeon's ability to generate reproducible techniques through an individualized surgical approach. Anatomic restoration with optimized soft tissue balancing, reproducible alignment, and restoration of normal joint kinematics has already demonstrated advantages of robotically assisted total knee surgery, partial knee surgery [62–65], and total hip arthroplasty [57, 66]. Although experts may argue about the ideal target in arthroplasty (e.g., ideal posterior slope and ideal alignment), there is little question that robotics allows the surgeon to more accurately hit whatever target they may set.

Limitations of Robotics

In addition to the cost associated with robotics in the operating room, there is also a significant amount of education required for surgeons and staff to optimize the safety, efficiency, and usefulness of robotics. Operative time with the use of robotic systems may be longer, especially during the learning curve, and the preferred robotic system of a surgeon may not be compatible with their preferred implant system. The systems are currently unable to directly perform soft tissue balancing, despite the ability of certain systems to provide gap balancing feedback to the surgeon in very accurate ways (e.g., similar to navigation). Additionally, these systems will make cuts in the planned location regardless of what they may be cutting. Despite improved soft tissue safety with haptic systems when tissue retraction is performed properly, the surgeon must still retract the soft tissues, or the tissues in the planned path can be damaged. Future designs will likely include an evolution of failsafe mechanisms and navigated retractors to prevent such inadvertent injury to soft tissues. Finally, the robot will cut based on a plan designed around the registration data provided to it. Although image-based systems provide additional safety by more easily recognizing errors in registration, both image-based and imageless systems are only as good as the data provided to them. Therefore, grossly incorrect registration can lead to potentially devastating results.

Future Robotic Innovations

Current design in the field of robotics has focused on decreasing outliers and improving accuracy in TJA radiographic outcomes. Early data is demonstrating decreased revision rates with unicompartmental arthroplasty and improved functional outcomes with THA. Future innovations will likely continue to improve the planning, setup, and workflow during robotic-assisted arthroplasty. These innovations will be implemented in a way that simplifies the process and minimizes the learning curve. Critical areas for improvement include preoperative analysis, intraoperative sensors, and robotically controlled instrumentation. Currently, image-based systems rely on preoperative CT scans to evaluate the patient's anatomy, but the next step would be to go beyond imaging to appreciate the kinematics of the operative joint before it has been altered by the pathology of arthritis. The preoperative plan will be used to recreate the desired anatomic and kinematic framework. Whereas prior implant design was limited by the preparation possible with traditional jigs, traditional visualization requirements, and traditional instruments, the future of implant development may look very different.

Conclusion

To date, robotics has improved consistency and decreased variability at the cost of initial increased operative time. There is growing evidence proving better alignment and a better margin of safety with robotic arthroplasty and emerging evidence supporting improved clinical outcomes and patient satisfaction. Although additional research will be required to fully define the costs and benefits of robotics, one thing is clear: robotics is here to stay.

References

1. Banerjee S, Cherian JJ, Elmallah RK, Pierce TP, Jauregui JJ, Mont MA. Robot-assisted total hip arthroplasty. Expert Rev Med Devices. 2016;13:47–56.
2. Banerjee S, Cherian JJ, Elmallah RK, Jauregui JJ, Pierce TP, Mont MA. Robotic-assisted knee arthroplasty. Expert Rev Med Devices. 2015;12: 727–35.
3. de Steiger RN, Liu Y-L, Graves SE. Computer navigation for Total knee arthroplasty reduces revision rate for patients less than sixty-five years of age. J Bone Joint Surg Am. 2015;97:635–42.
4. NBS/RIA Robotics Research Workshop: Proceedings of the NBS/RIA Workshop on Robotic Research.
5. Merriam-Webster. Merriam-Webster's collegiate dictionary. Merriam-Webster, 2004.
6. Robotics History. http://cs.stanford.edu/people/eroberts/courses/soco/projects/1998-99/robotics/history.html. Accessed 9 Apr 2017.
7. Davies B. A review of robotics in surgery. Proc Inst Mech Eng H J Eng Med. 2006;214:129–40.
8. Murphy D, Challacombe B, Khan MS, Dasgupta P. Robotic technology in urology. Postgrad Med J. 2006;82:743–7.
9. Gourin G, Terris J. History of robotic surgery. In: Faust RA, editor. Robotics in surgery history. New York: Current and Future Applications; 2007. p. 3–12.
10. Netravali NA, Shen F, Park Y, Bargar WL. A perspective on robotic assistance for knee arthroplasty. Adv Orthop. 2013;2013:970703–9.
11. Kazanzides P. Robotics for Orthopaedic Joint Reconstruction. Robotics in surgery: history, current and future applications; 2007.
12. Tew M, Waugh W. Tibiofemoral alignment and the results of knee replacement. J Bone Joint Surg Br. 1985;67:551–6.
13. Bellemans J, Vandenneucker H, Vanlauwe J. Robot-assisted total knee arthroplasty. Clin Orthop Relat Res. 2007;464:111–6.
14. Siebert W, Mai S, Kober R, Heeckt PF. Technique and first clinical results of robot-assisted total knee replacement. Knee. 2002;9:173–80.
15. Wu L-D, Hahne HJ, Hassenpflug J. The dimensional accuracy of preparation of femoral cavity in cementless total hip arthroplasty. J Zheijang Univ Sci A. 2004;5:1270–8.
16. Mazoochian F, Pellengahr C, Huber A, Kircher J, Refior HJ, Jansson V. Low accuracy of stem implantation in THR using the CASPAR-system: anteversion measurements in 10 hips. Acta Orthop Scand. 2009;75:261–4.
17. Siebel T, Käfer W. Clinical outcome following robotic assisted versus conventional total hip arthroplasty: a controlled and prospective study of seventy-one patients. Z Orthop Ihre Grenzgeb. 2005;143: 391–8.
18. Bargar WL, Bauer A, Borner M. Primary and revision total hip replacement using the Robodoc system. Clin Orthop Relat Res. 1998;354:82–91.
19. Bargar WL. Robots in orthopaedic surgery. Clin Orthop Relat Res. 2007;463:31–6. https://doi.org/10.1097/BLO.0b013e318146874f.
20. Chun YS, Kim KI, Cho YJ, Kim YH, Yoo MC, Rhyu KH. Causes and patterns of aborting a robot-assisted arthroplasty. J Arthroplast. 2011;26:621–5.
21. Jakopec M, Harris SJ, Rodriguez y Baena F, Gomes P, Cobb J, Davies BL. The first clinical application of a "hands-on" robotic knee surgery system. Comput Aided Surg. 2010;6:329–39.
22. Park SE, Lee CT. Comparison of robotic-assisted and conventional manual implantation of a primary total knee arthroplasty. J Arthroplast. 2007;22:1054–9.
23. Song E-K, Seon J-K, Park S-J, Jung WB, Park H-W, Lee GW. Simultaneous bilateral total knee arthroplasty with robotic and conventional techniques: a prospective, randomized study. Knee Surg Sports Traumatol Arthrosc. 2011;19:1069–76.
24. Hagio K, Sugano N, Takashina M, Nishii T, Yoshikawa H, Ochi T. Effectiveness of the ROBODOC system in preventing intraoperative pulmonary embolism. Acta Orthop Scand. 2003;74:264–9.

25. Börner M, Wiesel U, Ditzen W. Clinical experiences with ROBODOC and the Duracon total knee. In: Navigation and robotics in Total joint and spine surgery. Berlin, Heidelberg: Springer; 2004. p. 362–6.

26. Song E-K, Seon J-K, Yim J-H, Netravali NA, Bargar WL. Robotic-assisted TKA reduces postoperative alignment outliers and improves gap balance compared to conventional TKA. Clin Orthop Relat Res. 2012;471:118–26.

27. Pugely AJ, Martin CT, Gao Y, Schweizer ML, Callaghan JJ. The incidence of and risk factors for 30-day surgical site infections following primary and revision total joint arthroplasty. J Arthroplast. 2015;30:47–50.

28. Lonner JH, Smith JR, Picard F, Hamlin B, Rowe PJ, Riches PE. High degree of accuracy of a novel image-free handheld robot for unicondylar knee arthroplasty in a cadaveric study. Clin Orthop Relat Res. 2014;473:206–12.

29. Gregori A, Picard F, Bellemans J, Smithi J, Simone A. Handheld precision sculpting tool for unicondylar knee arthroplasty: a clinical review: th EFFORT Congress; 2014.

30. Wallace D, Gregori A, Picard F, Bellemans J, Lonner JH, Marquez R. The learning curve of a novel handheld robotic system for unicondylar knee arthroplasty. International Society of Computer Assisted Orthopedic Surgery; 2014.

31. Simons M, Riches P. The learning curve of robotically-assisted unicondylar knee arthroplasty. Bone Joint J. 2014;96-B:152.

32. Plaskos C, Cinquin P, Lavallée S, Hodgson AJ. Praxiteles: a miniature bone-mounted robot for minimal access total knee arthroplasty. Int J Med Rob Comput Assisted Surg. 2005;1:67–79.

33. Koulalis D, O'Loughlin PF, Plaskos C, Kendoff D, Cross MB, Pearle AD. Sequential versus automated cutting guides in computer-assisted total knee arthroplasty. Knee. 2011;18:436–42.

34. Suero EM, Plaskos C, Dixon PL, Pearle AD. Adjustable cutting blocks improve alignment and surgical time in computer-assisted total knee replacement. Knee Surg Sports Traumatol Arthrosc. 2012;20:1736–41.

35. Ponder CE, Plaskos C, Cheal EJ. Press-fit total knee arthroplasty with a robotic-cutting guide: proof of concept and initial clinical experience. Bone Joint J. 2013;95-B:61.

36. Lang JE, Mannava S, Floyd AJ, Goddard MS, Smith BP, Mofidi A, Seyler TM, Jinnah RH. Robotic systems in orthopaedic surgery. J Bone Joint Surg Br. 2011;93-B:1296–9.

37. Lonner JH, John TK, Conditt MA. Robotic arm-assisted UKA improves tibial component alignment: a pilot study. Clin Orthop Relat Res. 2010;468: 141–6.

38. RK SINHA. Outcomes of robotic arm-assisted unicompartmental knee arthroplasty. Am J Orthop. 2009;38:20–2.

39. Pearle AD, O'Loughlin PF, Kendoff DO. Robot-assisted unicompartmental knee arthroplasty. J Arthroplast. 2010;25:230–7.

40. Citak M, Suero EM, Citak M, Dunbar NJ, Branch SH, Conditt MA, Banks SA, Pearle AD. Unicompartmental knee arthroplasty: is robotic technology more accurate than conventional technique? Knee. 2013;20:268–71.

41. Hamilton WG, Ammeen D, Engh CA, Engh GA. Learning curve with minimally invasive unicompartmental knee arthroplasty. J Arthroplast. 2010;25:735–40.

42. Lonner JH. Indications for unicompartmental knee arthroplasty and rationale for robotic arm-assisted technology. Am J Orthop. 2009;38:3–6.

43. Coon TM. Integrating robotic technology into the operating room. Am J Orthop. 2009;38:7–9.

44. Jinnah RH, Horowitz S, Lippincott C, Conditt M. The learning curve of robotically assisted UKA. Annual Congress of ISTA; 2009.

45. Conditt M, Coon T, Hernandez A, Branch S. Short term survivorship and outcomes of robotically assisted bicompartmental arthroplasty. Bone Joint J. 2016;98-B:49.

46. Tamam C, Plate JF, Augart M, Poehling GG, Jinnah RH. Retrospective clinical and radiological outcomes after robotic assisted Bicompartmental knee arthroplasty. Adv Orthop. 2015;2015:1–7.

47. Jones B, Blyth MJ, MacLean A, Anthony I, Rowe P. Accuracy of UKA implant positioning and early clinical outcomes in a RCT comparing robotic assisted and manual surgery. th Annual CAOS Meeting; 2013.

48. Coon T. MAKOplasty medial UKA demonstrates low two-year revision rate in multicenter study. From short to mid term survivorship of robotically assisted UKA: a multicenter study. ISTA th Annual Congress; 2014.

49. Pearle AD, van der List JP, Lee L, COON TM, Borus TA, Roche MW. Survivorship and patient satisfaction of robotic-assisted medial unicompartmental knee arthroplasty at a minimum two-year follow-up. Knee. 2017;24:419–28.

50. Marcovigi A, Zambianchi F, Sandoni D, Rivi E, Catani F. Robotic-arm assisted partial knee arthroplasty: a single Centre experience. Acta Biomed. 2017;88:54–9.

51. Illgen RL, Bukowski BR, Abiola R, Anderson P, Chughtai M, Khlopas A, Mont MA. Robotic-assisted total hip arthroplasty: outcomes at minimum two-year follow-up. Surg Technol Int. 2017;30:365.

52. Domb BG, Bitar El YF, Sadik AY, Stake CE, Botser IB. Comparison of robotic-assisted and conventional Acetabular cup placement in THA: a matched-pair controlled study. Clin Orthop Relat Res. 2014;472:329–36.

53. Elson L, Dounchis J, Illgren R, Marchand R. A multicenter evaluation of acetabular cup positioning in robotic-arm assisted total hip arthroplasty. th Annual CAOS Meeting, 2013.

54. Nawabi DH, Conditt MA, Ranawat AS, Dunbar NJ, Jones J, Banks S, Padgett DE. Haptically guided

robotic technology in total hip arthroplasty: a cadaveric investigation. Proc Inst Mech Eng H J Eng Med. 2013;227:302–9.

55. Jerabek SA, Carroll KM, Marratt JD, Mayman DJ, Padgett DE. Accuracy of cup positioning and achieving desired hip length and offset following robotic THA. th Annual CAOS Meeting; 2014.

56. Suarez-Ahedo C, Gui C, Martin TJ, Chandrasekaran S, Lodhia P, Domb BG. Robotic-arm assisted total hip arthroplasty results in smaller acetabular cup size in relation to the femoral head size: a matched-pair controlled study. Hip Int. 2017;27:147–52.

57. Bukowski B, Abiola R, Illgren R. Outcomes after primary total hip arthroplasty: manual compared with robotic assisted techniques. th Annual Advances in Arthroplasty; 2014.

58. Khlopas A, Chughtai M, Hampp EL, et al. Robotic-arm assisted total knee arthroplasty demonstrated soft tissue protection. Surg Technol Int. 2017;30:441–6.

59. Wolf A, Jaramaz B, Lisien B, DiGioia AM. MBARS: mini bone-attached robotic system for joint arthroplasty. Int J Med Rob Comput Assisted Surg. 2005;1:101–21.

60. Kube CR, Parker CAC, Wang T, Zhang H. Biologically inspired collective robotics. Recent developments in biologically inspired computing. https://doi. org/10.4018/9781591403128.ch015.

61. Song S, Mor A, Jaramaz B. HyBAR: hybrid bone-attached robot for joint arthroplasty. Int J Med Rob Comput Assisted Surg. 2009;5:223–31.

62. Conditt MA, Roche MW. Minimally invasive robotic-arm-guided unicompartmental knee arthroplasty. J Bone Joint Surg Am. 2009;91(Suppl 1):63–8.

63. Liow MHL, Xia Z, Wong MK, Tay KJ, Yeo SJ, Chin PL. Robot-assisted total knee arthroplasty accurately restores the joint line and mechanical axis. A prospective randomised study. J Arthroplast. 2014;29:2373–7.

64. Yildirim G, Fernandez-Madrid I, Schwarzkopf R, Walker P, Karia R. Comparison of robot surgery modular and Total knee arthroplasty kinematics. J Knee Surg. 2014;27:157–64.

65. Plate JF, Mofidi A, Mannava S, Smith BP, Lang JE, Poehling GG, Conditt MA, Jinnah RH. Achieving accurate ligament balancing using robotic-assisted unicompartmental knee arthroplasty. Adv Orthop. 2013;2013:1–6.

66. Illgren R. Robotically assisted total hip arthroplasty improves clinical outcome compared with manual technique. rd Annual Course Advances in Arthroplasty.

General Concepts in Robotics in Orthopedics

3

Alexander H. Jinnah, T. David Luo,
Johannes F. Plate, and Riyaz H. Jinnah

The history of robotic hardware in the operating room is a relatively short one, with the first robotic system introduced into the medical field in 1985 [1, 2]. This system, the PUMA 560, was designed for increased accuracy for needle placement in a computerized tomography (CT)-guided brain biopsy. Surgical use of robotics has continued to expand and evolve, being embraced by several surgical specialties, including urology, gastroenterology, oncology, and gynecology [2, 3]. Orthopedic surgery joined this technological surge in the mid-1980s with the development and introduction of the ROBODOC (Curexo Technology Corporation, Fremont, CA, originally by Integrated Surgical Systems), led by Hap Paul and William Bargar [4]. This new technology was introduced with the intent of improving the accuracy of femoral bone preparation and anatomic placement of the femoral component in a cementless primary total hip arthroplasty (THA) by using a CT-based, computer-aided robotic milling device [5]. This technology was first used in human subjects in 1992 and was soon adapted for use in primary total knee arthroplasty (TKA) and revision THA procedures [5]. Despite some promising outcomes [6], the usage of the ROBODOC was limited due to early-generation technical complications related to the device [7].

Following the introduction of the ROBODOC, several passive and semiautonomous systems began to emerge [3]. Semiautonomous systems require surgeon involvement; however, they will not deviate from the planned operative procedure. Initially, these systems used three-dimensional (3D) CT scans and preoperative planning to provide real-time feedback intraoperatively in order to enhance the surgeon's control, thus increasing operative safety [8]. The active constraint robot (ACROBOT) (Imperial College, London, UK) was the first semiautonomous system to become available. Initial trials of this device performed by Justin Cobb and colleagues [9] showed consistent and accurate placement of implants in unicondylar knee arthroplasty (UKA) that were superior to the conventional manual technique. Following the promising results seen with the ACROBOT, the MAKO robotic arm (Stryker, Mahwah, NJ, USA) received approval for use by the US Food and Drug Administration (FDA) in 2008. Encouraging results with these semiautonomous systems in UKA have been demonstrated due in part to the greater precision in bone resection and more consistent soft tissue balancing [10, 11]. The success of these systems has led to fur-

A. H. Jinnah · T. D. Luo · J. F. Plate
Department of Orthopaedic Surgery, Wake Forest School of Medicine, Winston Salem, NC, USA

R. H. Jinnah (✉)
Department of Orthopaedic Surgery, Wake Forest School of Medicine, Winston Salem, NC, USA

Department of Orthopaedic Surgery, Southeastern Regional Medical Center, Lumberton, NC, USA
e-mail: rjinnah@wakehealth.edu

© Springer Nature Switzerland AG 2019
J. H. Lonner (ed.), *Robotics in Knee and Hip Arthroplasty*,
https://doi.org/10.1007/978-3-030-16593-2_3

ther interest and expansion of these systems to also include image-free techniques (NAVIO, Smith and Nephew Memphis, TN; OMNIBotics, OMNIlife Science, Inc.; Raynham, MA). Passive systems have also been developed, which involve assisting in preoperative planning, simulation, and intraoperative guidance. These systems are also known as "navigation" systems, and the main distinction, when compared to semiautonomous and active systems, is that the surgeon has complete control of the entire procedure with the computer-aided navigation providing guidance [3]. These systems create 3D visualization of the patient's anatomy in order to allow detailed preoperative planning. The goal of this chapter is to provide an updated and comprehensive comparison of current robotic systems available within the orthopedic armamentarium.

Technology Platform Types

Image-Guided Versus Image-Free Surgical Planning

Current robotic systems require the creation of a three-dimensional plan derived from a process of mapping the anatomy of the joint surfaces, with or without a preoperative CT scan. In image-guided systems, a preoperative CT scan (or MRI in some navigation systems) of the involved joint and limb is obtained. In knee arthroplasty cases, the protocol involves a scan of the patient's hip, knee, and ankle to gather the patient-specific data on limb alignment (mechanical axis) and anatomic features of the knee. The software converts the CT scan data into segmented slices, which creates the three-dimensional patient-specific bone model for surgeon templating prior to surgery. It then allows manipulation and coordination of the collected bone surface data to model the limb and accurately plan the implant size, alignment, and corresponding volume and orientation of bone resection. In the case of THA, the software utilizes the virtual 3D images to plan bone resection depth, optimal component size and alignment, leg length and offset restoration, and volumetric bone removal. The preoperative

plan is then correlated to the patient's anatomy which is registered intraoperatively by surface mapping after arthrotomy [8]. The virtual plan is then carried out by surgical manipulation of the robotic tool. Despite the benefits of being able to virtually plan the surgery preoperatively, the downsides of a preoperative CT scan include the increased (and often unreimbursed) cost of the imaging study, patient inconvenience to obtain the study at certified centers, and risk of radiation exposure [8, 12–14].

Alternatively, imageless systems rely entirely on intraoperative registration of the anatomical surfaces and kinematics after arthrotomy to create a 3D virtual model, develop a surgical plan, and define boundaries beyond which the bone cutting tools should not remove surface tissue. Specialized CT or MRI scans are unnecessary. Thus, while imageless systems address the disadvantages presented by the image-based system because no preoperative imaging is used, this then creates potential disadvantages. A true preoperative plan that allows the determination of implant size, position, and alignment cannot be performed. Furthermore, the intraoperative registration relies on the surgeon's accuracy of inputting the correct data points, which is subject to human error [8]. Despite these potential disadvantages, cadaveric and early clinical studies discussed above demonstrate that the imageless system results in comparably accurate prosthesis placement [15, 16].

Autonomous, Semiautonomous, and Passive Robotic Systems

There are three broad categories of robotic systems used in orthopedic surgery, including autonomous, semiautonomous, and passive systems. Passive systems provide a virtual road map for surgery but do not provide constraints against inadvertent bone and hard surface preparation. Both autonomous and semiautonomous systems incorporate safeguards against removal of bone beyond the 3D plan; they differ in the method and extent of surgeon direction and control in the process of bone removal.

Autonomous Systems

Autonomous robotic systems have the capability of completing an operation without surgeon input, other than establishing and determining the plan of resection, positioning, and sizing. The surgeon performs the initial dissection and approach to set up the robotic system [17, 18]. The robot then performs the remaining operation independently with surgeon oversight; however, the surgeon controls an emergency switch in case of a desire to pause the procedure or to adjust the plan or if there is an impending or actual mishap. Autonomous robots had fallen out of favor due to concerns over nerve and other soft tissue injury, among other complications, although currently there is a resurgence in enthusiasm for autonomous robotics and redoubled efforts to refine techniques and protocols [17, 18]. Examples of autonomous robotic systems include ROBODOC [now TSolution One] (Curexo Technology Corporation, Fremont, CA) (Fig. 3.1) and CASPAR (Ortho-Maquet/URS, Schwerin, Germany), both of which rely on CT imaging for preoperative planning. Initial studies on anthropomorphic phantoms demonstrated high geometric accuracy of both the ROBODOC and CASPAR systems [8, 19–30]. These systems have a predictable learning curve, as evident in the longer operative time and greater blood loss [21, 26–28], but each had greater precision with mechanical axis alignment compared to conventional techniques [27–29]. Disadvantages and limitations of the autonomous systems included additional time for preoperative planning and registration, aborted procedures contributing to longer duration of surgery, lack of surgeon input and intraoperative adjustment, and technical complications [7, 8, 26, 30].

Passive Systems

Unlike autonomous systems, passive systems do not independently perform the operations. They are also known as computer-assisted or navigation systems, which use patient- and instrument-centered reference points to provide the surgeon with perioperative recommendations and guide positioning of the surgical tools [29]. The navigation system is composed of a dynamic reference base attached to the instrument or anatomical

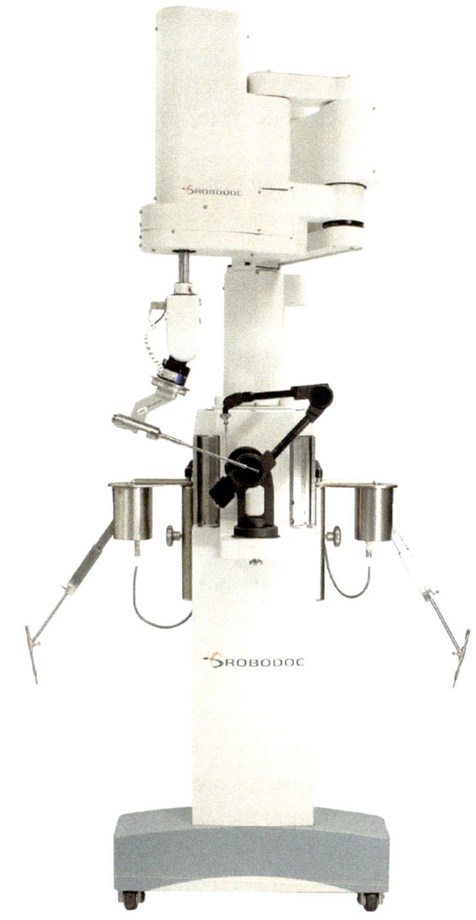

Fig. 3.1 ROBODOC. (Courtesy of Curexo Technology Corporation, THINK Surgical, Inc., Fremont, CA, USA)

landmark that emits or reflects an optical-based medium to the tracker [31]. Passive systems further provide guidance on precise placement of the prostheses [17] and have revolutionized minimally invasive techniques in orthopedic surgery.

Navigation-assisted surgery have been used for performing UKA and TKA to address historical shortcomings associated with component malposition. And while several studies have demonstrated the superior accuracy of navigation for achieving femorotibial mechanical axis and component alignment on postoperative radiographs compared to conventional techniques and reducing outliers compared to jig-based techniques, most studies have shown equivalent functional outcomes and comparable survivorship [32–44]. The use of navigation has further extended to THA, where it has been applied primarily for acetabular component planning, with mixed outcomes in terms of positioning within the targeted "safe zone" [45–51].

Semiautonomous Systems

Semiautonomous robotic systems combine the benefits seen with the passive navigation and the autonomous robotic systems. This is done by using the skills of the surgeon needed for passive navigation and combining these with the control of the robot seen in autonomous systems [17]. Semiautonomous robots, on the one hand, are controlled and manipulated by the surgeon, but the surgeon's control is modulated by the robotic system to limit bone preparation to within a defined volumetric boundary. A feedback loop is established within the system either by haptically constraining the cutting tool or positioning of the cutting blocks or by modulating the exposure or speed of the robotic tool. These safeguards not only optimize precision and reduce error, but they also simplify the surgical procedure. Semiautonomous systems prevent surgeons from deviating from the preoperatively planned bony excision, which has led to an increased accuracy and reduced errors in component placement [8, 15, 52]. Currently, three such systems are in use in the United States for joint arthroplasty. The MAKO robotic arm (Stryker, Mahwah, NJ, USA) (Fig. 3.2) uses a preoperative CT scan to form the predetermined cutting areas for bone preparation and thus is known as an "image-guided" system. The other semiautonomous systems in use are the Navio PFS (Smith & Nephew, Memphis, TN, USA) freehand sculpting robot (Fig. 3.3) and OMNIBOT (OMNIlife Science, Inc.; Raynham, MA) (Fig. 3.4) robotic guide positioner which are "imageless," in that they do not require specialized preoperative imaging for planning or registration [15].

The advantage of semiautonomous robotic systems is that the tools are directly manipulated by the surgeon, which minimizes the learning curve and the potential for inadvertent tissue injury while at the same time facilitating accurate

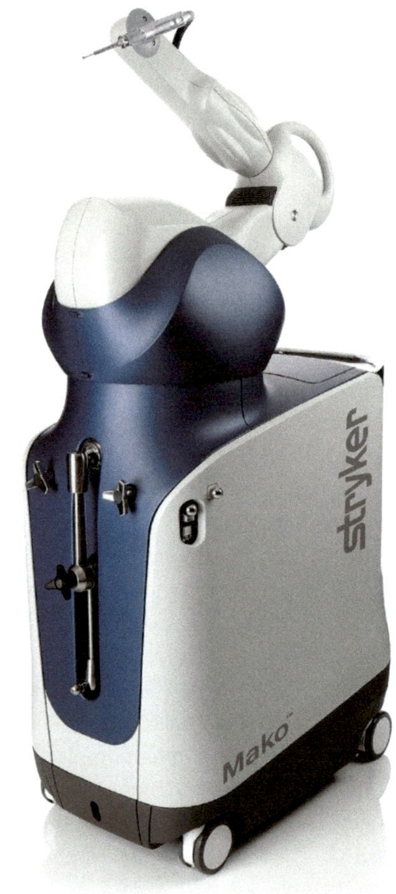

Fig. 3.2 MAKO robotic arm. (Courtesy of Stryker, Mahwah, NJ, USA)

bone preparation even during the early stages of technology adoption [15, 16, 52–63].

Methods of Robotic Restraint

As discussed, the advantage of robotic bone removal is the precision with which surface preparation is accomplished. With current systems, there are essentially two primary methods by which the robotic tools maintain a high level of precision as well as safeguard against inadvertent tissue removal – either by restricting the cutting

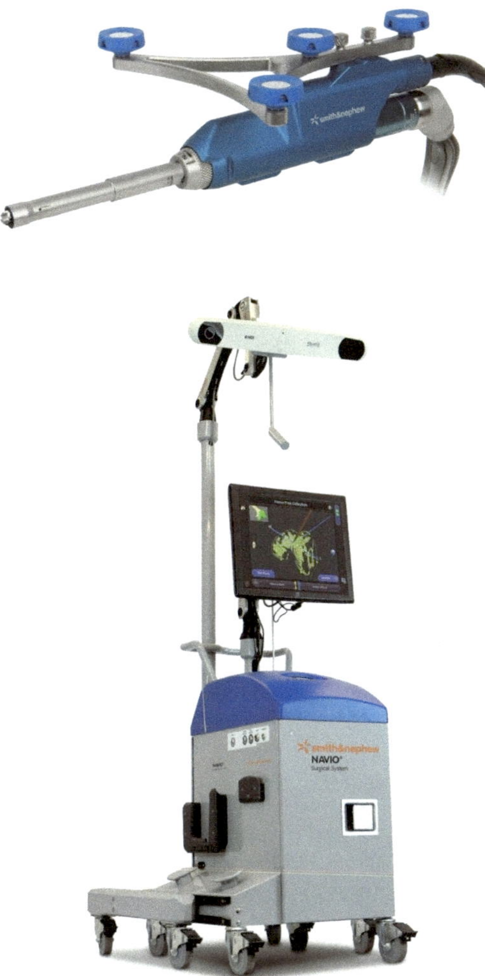

Fig. 3.3 Navio (Courtesy of Smith & Nephew, Memphis TN, USA). (Courtesy of Smith & Nephew, Andover, MA, Memphis TN, USA)

termined cutting zone [4, 5, 7, 8, 11, 17, 21, 29, 30, 54–65]. In the case of OMNIBOT, control comes in the haptic positioning of cutting blocks through which the surgeon uses a conventional saw to prepare the bone. This approach restricts the resection guides but provides no additional safety mechanism to the cutting tool to prevent errant bone preparation. Nonetheless, emerging data shows success with this mechanism of precision in TKA.

Using an alternative method of restraint, the Navio system controls exposure or speed of the robotic burr. In "Exposure Control" setting, the burr continuously rotates, but it is only exposed when it is within the predefined volume of bone to be prepared and retracted within a protective guard when the instrument tip is outside the desired cutting zone [66]. In "Speed Control" setting, the burr will only spin when within the desired cutting zone. The rotating burr is at full power until it approaches the margin of bone being prepared, at which time its speed linearly decreases to zero [66]. Theoretically, the burr speed/exposure control methods will allow more control and minimize errors seen in bony cuts; however, results to date have shown comparable precision to the haptic system [15].

tool or positioning of the cutting blocks by haptic constraint to within a defined region or by modulating the exposure or speed of the robotic tool to within a predetermined 3D surface volume. These safeguards not only optimize precision and reduce error, but they also simplify the surgical procedure. With the MAKO robotic arm and TSolution One (ROBODOC) systems, bone resection is determined initially with a preoperative CT scan and then adjusted intraoperatively if needed [17, 21]. During the procedure, tactile haptic feedback is provided to prevent the robotic arm from moving the high speed burr or saw blade outside the prede-

Soft Tissue Balancing

Finally, soft tissue balancing has been shown to play an important role in knee arthroplasty, to maintain normal knee kinematics and proprioception, and to prevent subsequent wear and instability [67–70]. UKA and TKA outcomes are influenced by lower leg alignment and component rotation, size, and position [71], and intuitively, it makes sense that the use of robotics could help in controlling these multiple variables. However, in both UKA and TKA, precise soft tissue balancing is considered equally, if not more important to successful function and durability. Several current robotic systems incorporate soft tissue balancing algorithms in their planning and procedures, and studies have demonstrated the accuracy of soft tissue balancing associated with robotics in UKA [11] and TKA [28].

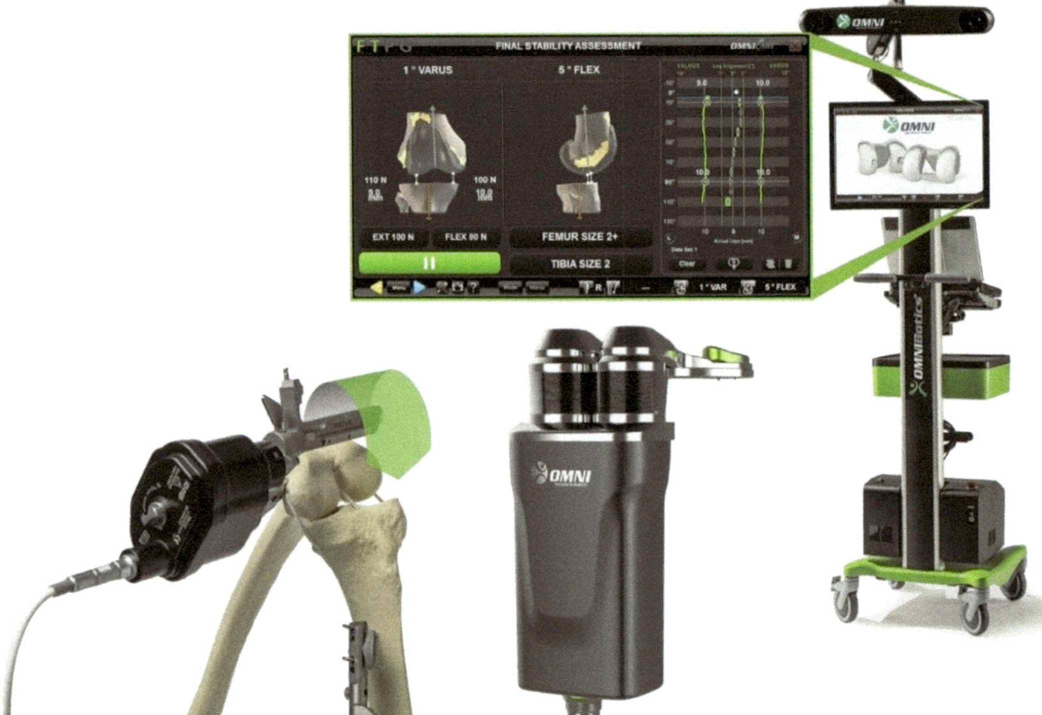

Fig. 3.4 OMNIBotics. (Courtesy of OMNIlife Science, Inc., Raynham, MA, USA)

Limitations of Navigation and Robotic-Assisted Surgery

The use of robotic systems has been shown to increase operative time. They require the placement of optical arrays for registration of bony landmarks. Imageless systems then require tracing of selected anatomic areas to create a 3D image of the operative field. Robotic-assisted systems that are based on preoperative CT scan also require the registration of bony landmarks and surfaces in a similar fashion. In a study comparing robotic and manual UKA systems, the mean operative time with robotic system was increased by 20 minutes, which led to an increase cost of approximately $2466 to $9220 [72]. An unobstructed path between optical arrays and the system's tracker is necessary at all times, and optical instruments need to be held in a certain way to be registered. While this can be cumbersome initially, the learning curve is not steep [16, 63]. The use of robotics is associated with a significant financial investment which may be prohibitive to lower volume surgical centers. Without clear clinical advantages, the cost for these systems may not be justified.

Conclusion

The use of navigation and robotic assistance in orthopedic surgery continues to increase, and their application is expanding. Current applications include UKA, PFA, TKA, THA, and spine surgery, but future development of navigation and robotic-assisted systems may include revision total knee and hip arthroplasty as well as other surgical procedures. There is little doubt that robotic technology is here to stay, and the orthopedic community is beginning to embrace it. Trends are now moving toward miniaturization, and once enough progress is made in this direction, it will become a routine part of our armamentarium. However, long-term clinical outcomes of contemporary robotic systems for UKA and TKA are not available. The survivorship of robotic-assisted UKA using the MAKO robotic arm was 98.9% in 620 patients at 2-year follow-up [73]. The 3-year revision rate for UKAs to TKA using the MAKO robotic system was reported as 5.8% and found to be comparable to conventional UKAs in national registries [74]. Further long-term results are needed to validate the relationship between improved accuracy of component placement and survivorship.

References

1. Kwoh YS, Hou J, Jonckheere EA, et al. A robot with improved absolute positioning accuracy for CT guided stereotactic brain surgery. IEEE Trans Biomed Eng. 1988;35:153–60.
2. Shah J, Vyas A, Vyas D. The history of robotics in surgical specialties. Am J Robot Surg. 2014;1:12–20.
3. Jinnah AH, Multani A, Plate JF, Poehling GG, Jinnah RH. Implementation of robotics in total joint arthroplasty. Robot Surg: Res Rev. 2015;2015:95–103.
4. Paul HA, Bargar WL, Mittlestadt B, et al. Development of a surgical robot for cementless total hip arthroplasty. Clin Orthop Relat Res. 1992:57–66.
5. Bargar WL. Robots in orthopaedic surgery: past, present, and future. Clin Orthop Relat Res. 2007;463:31–6.
6. Digioia AM 3rd, Jaramaz B, Plakseychuk AY, et al. Comparison of a mechanical acetabular alignment guide with computer placement of the socket. J Arthroplast. 2002;17:359–64.
7. Schulz AP, Seide K, Queitsch C, et al. Results of total hip replacement using the Robodoc surgical assistant system: clinical outcome and evaluation of complications for 97 procedures. Int J Med Robot. 2007;3:301–6.
8. Jacofsky DJ, Allen M. Robotics in Arthroplasty: a comprehensive review. J Arthroplast. 2016;31:2353–63.
9. Cobb J, Henckel J, Gomes P, et al. Hands-on robotic unicompartmental knee replacement: a prospective, randomised controlled study of the acrobot system. J Bone Joint Surg Br. 2006;88:188–97.
10. Najarian S, Fallahnezhad M, Afshari E. Advances in medical robotic systems with specific applications in surgery--a review. J Med Eng Technol. 2011;35:19–33.
11. Plate JF, Mofidi A, Mannava S, et al. Achieving accurate ligament balancing using robotic-assisted unicompartmental knee arthroplasty. Adv Orthop. 2013;2013:837167.
12. Ponzio DY, Lonner JH. Preoperative mapping in Unicompartmental knee Arthroplasty using computed tomography scans is associated with radiation exposure and carries high cost. J Arthroplast. 2015;30:964–7.
13. Banerjee S, Cherian JJ, Elmallah RK, et al. Robot-assisted total hip arthroplasty. Expert Rev Med Devices. 2016;13:47–56.
14. Smith-Bindman R, Lipson J, Marcus R, et al. Radiation dose associated with common computed tomography examinations and the associated lifetime attributable risk of cancer. Arch Intern Med. 2009;169:2078–86.
15. Lonner JH, Smith JR, Picard F, et al. High degree of accuracy of a novel image-free handheld robot for unicondylar knee arthroplasty in a cadaveric study. Clin Orthop Relat Res. 2015;473:206–12.
16. Gregori A, Picard F, Bellemans J, et al. Handheld precision sculpting tool for unicondylar knee arthroplasty. A clinical review. 15th EFORT Congress, London, 4–6 June 2014.
17. Lang JE, Mannava S, Floyd AJ, et al. Robotic systems in orthopaedic surgery. J Bone Joint Surg Br. 2011;93:1296–9.
18. Davies BL, Rodriguez y Baena FM, Barrett AR, et al. Robotic control in knee joint replacement surgery. Proc Inst Mech Eng H. 2007;221:71–80.
19. Prymka M, Wu L, Hahne HJ, et al. The dimensional accuracy for preparation of the femoral cavity in HIP arthroplasty. A comparison between manual- and robot-assisted implantation of HIP endoprosthesis stems in cadaver femurs. Arch Orthop Trauma Surg. 2006;126:36–44.
20. Mazoochian F, Pellengahr C, Huber A, et al. Low accuracy of stem implantation in THR using the CASPAR-system: anteversion measurements in 10 hips. Acta Orthop Scand. 2004;75:261–4.
21. Bargar WL, Bauer A, Borner M. Primary and revision total hip replacement using the Robodoc system. Clin Orthop Relat Res. 1998:82–91.
22. Siebel T, Kafer W. Clinical outcome following robotic assisted versus conventional total hip arthroplasty: a controlled and prospective study of seventy-one patients. Z Orthop Ihre Grenzgeb. 2005;143:391–8.
23. Siebert W, Mai S, Kober R, et al. Technique and first clinical results of robot-assisted total knee replacement. Knee. 2002;9:173–80.
24. Nogler M, Polikeit A, Wimmer C, et al. Primary stability of a Robodoc implanted anatomical stem versus manual implantation. Clin Biomech (Bristol, Avon). 2004;19:123–s.
25. Hagio K, Sugano N, Takashina M, et al. Effectiveness of the ROBODOC system in preventing intraoperative pulmonary embolism. Acta Orthop Scand. 2003;74:264–9.
26. Honl M, Dierk O, Gauck C, et al. Comparison of robotic-assisted and manual implantation of a primary total hip replacement. A prospective study. J Bone Joint Surg Am. 2003;85-A:1470–8.
27. Song EK, Seon JK, Park SJ, et al. Simultaneous bilateral total knee arthroplasty with robotic and conventional techniques: a prospective, randomized study. Knee Surg Sports Traumatol Arthrosc. 2011;19:1069–76.
28. Song EK, Seon JK, Yim JH, et al. Robotic-assisted TKA reduces postoperative alignment outliers and

improves gap balance compared to conventional TKA. Clin Orthop Relat Res. 2013;471:118–26.

29. Park SE, Lee CT. Comparison of robotic-assisted and conventional manual implantation of a primary total knee arthroplasty. J Arthroplast. 2007;22:1054–9.

30. Chun YS, Kim KI, Cho YJ, et al. Causes and patterns of aborting a robot-assisted arthroplasty. J Arthroplast. 2011;26:621–5.

31. Zheng G, Nolte LP. Computer-assisted orthopedic surgery: current state and future perspective. Front Surg. 2015;2:66.

32. Jenny JY, Boeri C. Unicompartmental knee prosthesis implantation with a non-image-based navigation system: rationale, technique, case-control comparative study with a conventional instrumented implantation. Knee Surg Sports Traumatol Arthrosc. 2003;11:40–5.

33. Manzotti A, Cerveri P, Pullen C, et al. Computer-assisted unicompartmental knee arthroplasty using dedicated software versus a conventional technique. Int Orthop. 2014;38:457–63.

34. Jung KA, Kim SJ, Lee SC, et al. Accuracy of implantation during computer-assisted minimally invasive Oxford unicompartmental knee arthroplasty: a comparison with a conventional instrumented technique. Knee. 2010;17:387–91.

35. Keene G, Simpson D, Kalairajah Y. Limb alignment in computer-assisted minimally-invasive unicompartmental knee replacement. J Bone Joint Surg Br. 2006;88:44–8.

36. Rosenberger RE, Fink C, Quirbach S, et al. The immediate effect of navigation on implant accuracy in primary mini-invasive unicompartmental knee arthroplasty. Knee Surg Sports Traumatol Arthrosc. 2008;16:1133–40.

37. Chowdhry M, Khakha RS, Norris M, et al. Improved survival of computer-assisted Unicompartmental knee Arthroplasty: 252 cases with a minimum follow-up of 5 years. J Arthroplast. 2017;32:1132–6.

38. Bauwens K, Matthes G, Wich M, et al. Navigated total knee replacement. A meta-analysis. J Bone Joint Surg Am. 2007;89:261–9.

39. Fu Y, Wang M, Liu Y, et al. Alignment outcomes in navigated total knee arthroplasty: a meta-analysis. Knee Surg Sports Traumatol Arthrosc. 2012;20:1075–82.

40. Hetaimish BM, Khan MM, Simunovic N, et al. Meta-analysis of navigation vs conventional total knee arthroplasty. J Arthroplast. 2012;27:1177–82.

41. Rebal BA, Babatunde OM, Lee JH, et al. Imageless computer navigation in total knee arthroplasty provides superior short term functional outcomes: a meta-analysis. J Arthroplast. 2014;29:938–44.

42. Gholson JJ, Duchman KR, Otero JE, et al. Computer navigated total knee arthroplasty: rates of adoption and early complications. J Arthroplasty. 2017; 32:2113–9.

43. Biasca N, Wirth S, Bungartz M. Mechanical accuracy of navigated minimally invasive total knee arthroplasty (MIS TKA). Knee. 2009;16:22–9.

44. Khakha RS, Chowdhry M, Norris M, et al. Five-year follow-up of minimally invasive computer assisted total knee arthroplasty (MICATKA) versus conventional computer assisted total knee arthroplasty (CATKA) - a population matched study. Knee. 2014;21:944–8.

45. Chang JD, Kim IS, Bhardwaj AM, et al. The evolution of computer-assisted Total hip Arthroplasty and relevant applications. Hip Pelvis. 2017;29:1–14.

46. Nogler M, Kessler O, Prassl A, et al. Reduced variability of acetabular cup positioning with use of an imageless navigation system. Clin Orthop Relat Res. 2004:159–63.

47. Gandhi R, Marchie A, Farrokhyar F, et al. Computer navigation in total hip replacement: a meta-analysis. Int Orthop. 2009;33:593–7.

48. Moskal JT, Capps SG. Acetabular component positioning in total hip arthroplasty: an evidence-based analysis. J Arthroplast. 2011;26:1432–7.

49. Xu K, Li YM, Zhang HF, et al. Computer navigation in total hip arthroplasty: a meta-analysis of randomized controlled trials. Int J Surg. 2014;12:528–33.

50. Liu Z, Gao Y, Cai L. Imageless navigation versus traditional method in total hip arthroplasty: a meta-analysis. Int J Surg. 2015;21:122–7.

51. Li YL, Jia J, Wu Q, et al. Evidence-based computer-navigated total hip arthroplasty: an updated analysis of randomized controlled trials. Eur J Orthop Surg Traumatol. 2014;24:531–8.

52. Bell SW, Anthony I, Jones B, et al. Improved accuracy of component positioning with robotic-assisted Unicompartmental knee Arthroplasty: data from a prospective, randomized controlled study. J Bone Joint Surg Am. 2016;98:627–35.

53. Citak M, Suero EM, Citak M, et al. Unicompartmental knee arthroplasty: is robotic technology more accurate than conventional technique? Knee. 2013;20:268–71.

54. Nawabi DH, Conditt MA, Ranawat AS, et al. Haptically guided robotic technology in total hip arthroplasty: a cadaveric investigation. Proc Inst Mech Eng H. 2013;227:302–9.

55. Mofidi A, Plate JF, Lu B, et al. Assessment of accuracy of robotically assisted unicompartmental arthroplasty. Knee Surg Sports Traumatol Arthrosc. 2014;22:1918–25.

56. Dunbar NJ, Roche MW, Park BH, et al. Accuracy of dynamic tactile-guided unicompartmental knee arthroplasty. J Arthroplast 2012;27:803–808 e1.

57. Sinha RK. Outcomes of robotic arm-assisted unicompartmental knee arthroplasty. Am J Orthop (Belle Mead NJ). 2009;38:20–2.

58. Pearle AD, O'Loughlin PF, Kendoff DO. Robot-assisted unicompartmental knee arthroplasty. J Arthroplast. 2010;25:230–7.

59. Kanawade V, Dorr LD, Banks SA, et al. Precision of robotic guided instrumentation for acetabular component positioning. J Arthroplast. 2015;30:392–7.

60. Lonner JH, John TK, Conditt MA. Robotic arm-assisted UKA improves tibial component alignment: a pilot study. Clin Orthop Relat Res. 2010;468:141–6.

61. Domb BG, El Bitar YF, Sadik AY, et al. Comparison of robotic-assisted and conventional acetabular cup

placement in THA: a matched-pair controlled study. Clin Orthop Relat Res. 2014;472:329–36.

62. Lonner JH. Indications for unicompartmental knee arthroplasty and rationale for robotic arm-assisted technology. Am J Orthop (Belle Mead NJ). 2009;38:3–6.

63. Wallace D, Gregori A, Picard F, et al. The learning curve of a novel handheld robotic system for unicondylar knee arthroplasty. International Society of Computer Assisted Orthopaedic Surgery, Milan, 14–18 June 2014.

64. Coon TM. Integrating robotic technology into the operating room. Am J Orthop (Belle Mead NJ). 2009;38:7–9.

65. Hamilton WG, Ammeen D, Engh CA Jr, et al. Learning curve with minimally invasive unicompartmental knee arthroplasty. J Arthroplast. 2010;25:735–40.

66. Smith JR, Riches PE, Rowe PJ. Accuracy of a freehand sculpting tool for unicondylar knee replacement. Int J Med Robot. 2014;10:162–9.

67. Wasielewski RC, Galante JO, Leighty RM, et al. Wear patterns on retrieved polyethylene tibial inserts and their relationship to technical considerations during total knee arthroplasty. Clin Orthop Relat Res. 1994:31–43.

68. Attfield SF, Wilton TJ, Pratt DJ, et al. Soft-tissue balance and recovery of proprioception after total knee replacement. J Bone Joint Surg Br. 1996;78: 540–5.

69. Pagnano MW, Hanssen AD, Lewallen DG, et al. Flexion instability after primary posterior cruciate retaining total knee arthroplasty. Clin Orthop Relat Res. 1998:39–46.

70. Whiteside LA. Making your next unicompartmental knee arthroplasty last: three keys to success. J Arthroplast. 2005;20:2–3.

71. Babazadeh S, Stoney JD, Lim K, et al. The relevance of ligament balancing in total knee arthroplasty: how important is it? A systematic review of the literature. Orthop Rev (Pavia). 2009;1:e26.

72. Hansen DC, Kusuma SK, Palmer RM, et al. Robotic guidance does not improve component position or short-term outcome in medial unicompartmental knee arthroplasty. J Arthroplast. 2014;29:1784–9.

73. Conditt MA, Coon T, Roche M, Pearle A, Borus T, Buechel F, Dounchis J. Two year survivorship of robotically guided Unicompartmental knee Arthroplasty. J Bone Joint Surg Br. 2013;95:294.

74. Plate JF, Augart MA, Seyler TM, et al. Obesity has no effect on outcomes following unicompartmental knee arthroplasty. Knee Surg Sports Traumatol Arthrosc. 2015; 25:645–51.

Learning Curve for Robot- and Computer-Assisted Knee and Hip Arthroplasty

4

Jason P. Zlotnicki and Michael J. O'Malley

Advances in robotic technology over the past several decades have allowed for the conversion of real-time data into precise actions aimed at the successful completion of any number of tasks. These technologies have recently infiltrated orthopaedic surgery, with the goal of producing improved (and more importantly, repeatable) operative results and maximizing patient outcomes [1]. The use of robotic-assisted surgery in hip and knee arthroplasty has increased over the past decade as interest and literature support have grown.

Total hip and knee arthroplasty are two of the most successful and cost-effective surgical procedures performed in orthopaedics [2, 3]. Despite great success, total joint arthroplasty is accompanied by significant risks and costs to the healthcare system [2, 4]. Hip and knee arthroplasty lend themselves well to robotic-assisted technology as they are technically demanding procedures that rely on appropriate component position and joint balance for optimal success. Several studies have shown poor outcomes and decreased implant survival if components are placed outside of appropriate alignment [5–7]. Robotic-assisted technology has improved alignment and decreased the presence of postoperative outliers in the positioning of hip and knee components [8–13]. Surgeons and healthcare systems are concerned by a potential learning curve while implementing robotic-assisted technology effectively and in a cost-efficient manner. This chapter aims to highlight what technologies are being used and early data discussing the learning curve for robotic technologies in unicompartmental knee arthroplasty (UKA), total knee arthroplasty (TKA) and total hip arthroplasty (THA).

Robotic Technology in Arthroplasty

In order to interpret the learning curve for the use of robotic technology in arthroplasty, one must have a basic understanding of the concepts and necessary surgical procedural steps. A thorough discussion of robotic technologies is beyond the scope of this chapter, but a surgeon who seeks to learn this technology must understand the process by which the robot receives information and subsequently what action the robot will perform. Robotic systems can be broadly categorized based on the amount of involvement that is required of the operating surgeon: passive, autonomous or semi-autonomous. Passive systems require continuous and direct action of the surgeon and minimal work by the robot; this is more consistent with navigation. In contrary, autonomous systems function independent of surgeon involvement.

J. P. Zlotnicki
Department of Orthopaedic Surgery, University of Pittsburgh, Pittsburgh, PA, USA

M. J. O'Malley (✉)
Department of Orthopaedic Surgery, University of Pittsburgh Medical Center, Pittsburgh, PA, USA

© Springer Nature Switzerland AG 2019
J. H. Lonner (ed.), *Robotics in Knee and Hip Arthroplasty*,
https://doi.org/10.1007/978-3-030-16593-2_4

Semi-autonomous systems are the most common in use today and share characteristics of each, requiring surgeon involvement while providing real-time feedback to augment the surgeon's control. Semi-autonomous robotic systems provide actual restraints for surgical resection such that the operator cannot operate (cut, burr, etc.) outside the preset parameters. These hard stops prevent aberrant resection and likewise component malposition and soft tissue damage. The perceived benefit of these robotic processes is that operative technique is solely based on real-time quantitative data and therefore should be more accurate as well as repeatable [14, 15].

All robotic systems require the entry, or registration of data, either via virtual mapping with coordinate systems (imageless) or based on three-dimensional preoperative imaging (i.e. MRI or CT scan). Regardless, specific anatomical reference points must be registered such that the robot can assign a relationship between the instrumentation (cutting tool) and the patient anatomy. Once registration is complete, implant planning commences. This entails determining the implant position based on bony references and ligament balance. Once the plan is finalized, bone preparation (cutting phase) ensues. Each robotic system performs this task differently. Some use a fixed robotic arm that prevents aberrant resection, while others use a protective guide or automatically cease operation when the cutting tool is moved outside of the designated cutting field. Lastly, once the bone is prepared, trialing and component implantation commence. These steps have a time element.

The learning of these robotic systems is not limited to the surgeon. The operating room staff must become familiar with the registration process and proper execution of the preoperative plan in order to maximize efficiency [16]. For inexperienced surgeons and staff, these steps include learning the robotic system set-up, positioning and orientation. These steps are an opportunity for the introduction of error and/or increased operative time, both of which may affect the final surgical outcome.

There are reports of difficulties associated with the early stages of robotic technology adoption. Despite the improvement in component positioning and the elimination of outliers [17], increased operative time, heat generation with robot bone-milling and inability for surgeon intervention once the program was initiated were significant drawbacks [15]. With clinical case reports demonstrating a high rate of technical complications (pin loosening, computer interface difficulty, etc.) and aborted robotic surgeries, significant room for improvement in technical application was realized [18]. These early studies clearly identified targets for improvement to optimize the technology and further ease the learning curve for implementation.

The Learning Curve for Robotic-Assisted Arthroplasty

The implementation of robotics in UKA and TKA aims to reduce variability and increase the reliability of successful outcomes. Several studies have documented improved component positioning, increased accuracy and decreased variability or outliers with robotic-assisted systems compared to conventional techniques [13, 19, 20]. Therefore, in an attempt to optimize their surgical outcomes, surgeons and healthcare systems have invested in robotic systems.

A learning curve can be defined as an improvement in performance over time with increased experience. Performance might be measured by time, alignment, component position, complication rate, patient outcome or a number of other metrics. A learning curve for robotic-assisted UKA and TKA has been demonstrated and varies depending on specific outcome of study. Overall, several studies have reported a modest learning curve that can be overcome without an increase in the risk of complications during this introductory period [21–23].

Wallace et al. recently reported a learning curve of 8 surgeries using a handheld robotic-assist system with the primary performance outcome being time. In this study 5 surgeons participated by completing 15 cases each. The average total surgical time from all surgeons across their 15 cases was 56.8 minutes (range:

27–102 minutes). The average improvement over the 15 cases was 46 minutes from slowest to quickest surgical times [21]. The greatest improvement in performance was noted during the cutting phase with an average decrease of 31 minutes, while the other phases (e.g. landmark registration, condyle mapping) had an observed trend towards decreased times.

In a similar study using a handheld robot-assist device, 11 surgeons each performed a minimum of 10 cases (range 10–30). Measured parameters included (1) time for anatomic registration and implant planning, (2) cutting time and (3) time from tracker attachment to termination of bone cutting. The goal was to determine how many cases were needed to achieve 95 percent of learning. The authors determined the learning curve to be eight cases. Improvement was noted in all phases of surgery including total surgical time (Fig. 4.1), cutting time (Fig. 4.2) and mapping/implant time components (Fig. 4.3) of the procedure. Again, the greatest improvement was noted in cutting phase [24].

There have been few studies on the learning curve in total knee arthroplasty. A recent study by Sodhi et al. analysed operative times for two experienced arthroplasty surgeons who had no prior robotic experience. The mean operative times for their first 20 robotic-assisted were significantly greater than that recorded for their last 20 cases (99 vs. 81 minutes, $p < 0.05$). In addition, comparison of their last 20 robotic-assisted case operative times to 20 random manual TKAs yielded no significant differences in operative times (84 vs. 81 minutes, $p > 0.05$) [25]. A recent systematic review by Khlopas et al. evaluating a total of 40 studies reported that robotic-assisted TKA may improve patient satisfaction and outcomes with an anticipated learning curve of roughly 15 cases [26].

Robotics may lessen the effect of surgeon experience on certain performance outcomes.

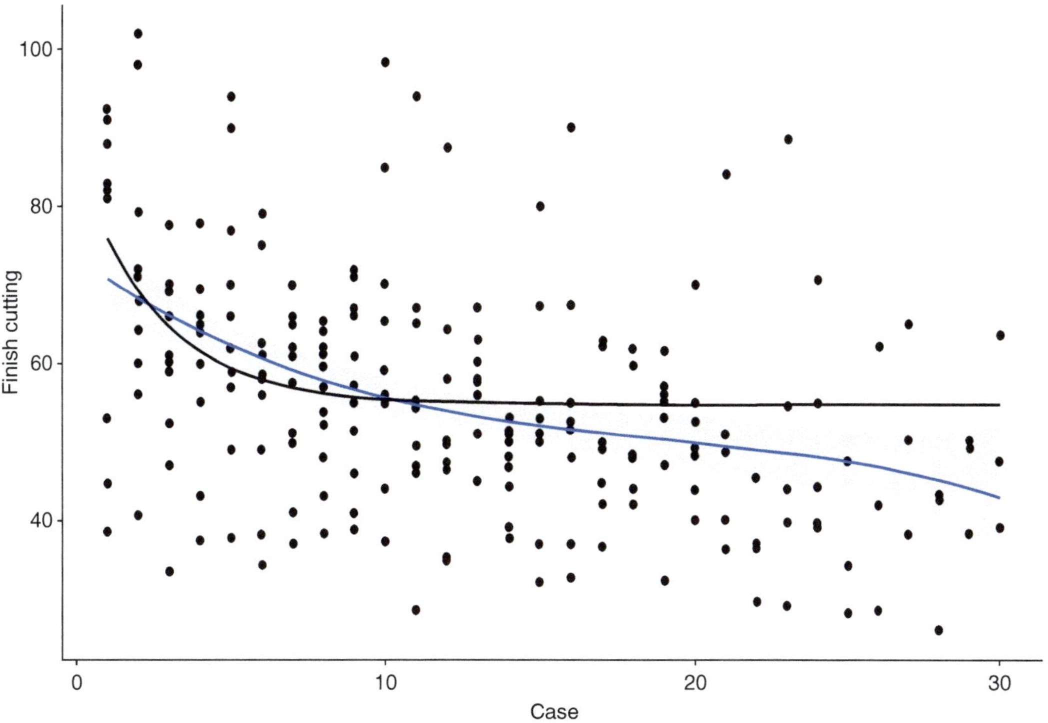

Fig. 4.1 Learning curve surgical time – the learning curve for surgical time (tracker placement to implant trialing) indicates that it takes approximately 8 cases (95% CI 6–11) to achieve 95% of total learning, with a mean decrease in operative time of 28 minutes

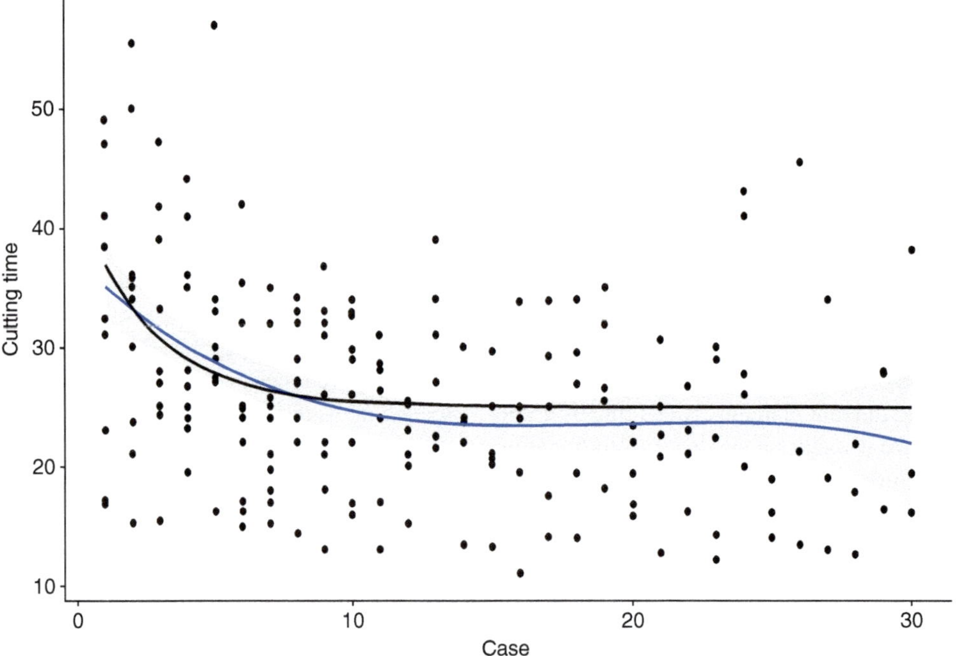

Fig. 4.2 Learning curve cutting time – as a major component of total surgical time, cutting time with robotic technology demonstrated the greatest time reduction during the learning curve with an average improvement from 42 to 25 minutes

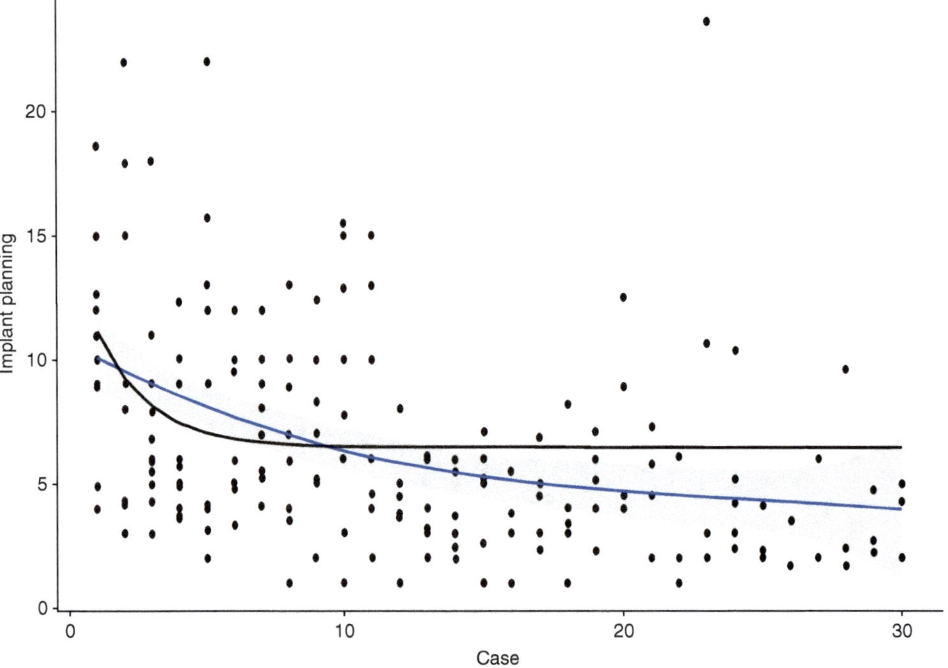

Fig. 4.3 Learning curve implant planning time – as a component of total surgical time, implant planning time (including anatomic point registration and implant planning) demonstrated a decrease during the learning curve from 14 to 6 minutes

Simons et al. sought to evaluate the technological learning curve of an imageless handheld robotic system. In this study, five surgical trainees each performed five robotic-assisted UKA on saw bones. Time to complete each phase of surgery as well as component alignment was evaluated. The average total surgical time for the five orthopaedic trainees decreased significantly ($p < 0.001$) from 85 minutes to 48 minutes after only five surgeries [23]. Most phases of the operation demonstrated a significant decrease in operative time with the gained experience of increasing number of surgeries performed (all $p < 0.05$); most significant was the cutting phase, decreasing from 41 to 23 minutes ($p < 0.001$). In addition, the translational and rotational accuracy of the implants was accurate with the initial surgery and did not vary significantly with surgery number, which suggests that accurate placement can be ensured even during the initial stages of robotic technology adoption. This concept of proper alignment during the learning curve has been observed in other studies as well. Karia et al. randomized 16 inexperienced surgeons to perform 3 UKAs with either conventional instrumentation or a semi-autonomous robot. Mean procedure time decreased for both groups; however, the authors found that accuracy of component position was much greater in the robotic-assisted group. The conventional group component position remained inaccurate over the three attempts [27]. In another study, Coon et al. demonstrated a significant reduction in tourniquet time over the learning curve period while excellent radiographic results were produced. Comparing the first 36 robotic arm patients with their last 45 manually instrumented patients, in age- and sex-matched groups, the accuracy of the tibial slope was improved, and varus alignment was 3.2 degrees better ($p < 0.05$) with less variability in the robotic arm group [16]. The ability to successfully reproduce appropriate component position and alignment, even during the initial period, is a proposed benefit of implementing robotic technology.

Robotic-assisted technology is finding a presence in hip arthroplasty as well, and as such there are concerns over performance during the learning curve. In one of the first and few studies to directly assess the learning curve of robotic-assisted THA, Redmond et al. demonstrated that a learning curve indeed exists. In this study, the first 105 robotically assisted THAs performed by a single surgeon were divided into 3 equal groups based on timing in his learning curve. Outcome measures included component position, operative time and intraoperative technical problems or complications. The authors reported that operating time decreased on average by approximately 13 minutes when comparing the first 35 cases to the subsequent groups ($p = 0.02$). The risk of having an acetabular outlier after the first 35 cases also significantly decreased ($p = 0.02$). There was no difference in intraoperative complications between groups [28]. Some studies suggest that more immediate improvements are noted when compared to conventional techniques. In a recent study by Kamara et al., immediate beneficial effect was noted within the first 100 cases for fluoroscopic and robotic technique, with 76% of manual (conventional) THAs being within the target zone for cup position compared to 84% fluoroscopic guided and 97% robotic-assisted ($p < 0.01$) [12].

Conclusion

With the implementation of a new technology and a new clinical paradigm, a learning curve will undoubtedly exist with the utilization of robotic technology in patient care. However, robotic-assisted arthroplasty has consistently demonstrated a modest learning curve of decreasing surgical time and improved efficiency during which fundamental aspects such as component position and mechanical alignment are optimized and maintained. A modest learning curve is necessary as the robotic technology must be used efficiently enough to justify the cost of implementing the technology. Robotic-assisted arthroplasty is gaining in popularity and use, and as such further studies are warranted to determine if clinical and patient outcomes improve with the use of these technologies.

References

1. Lang JE, Mannava S, Floyd AJ, Goddard MS, Smith BP, Mofidi A, Seyler TM, Jinnah RH. Robotic systems in orthopaedic surgery. J Bone Joint Surg Br. 2011;93(10):1296–9.

2. Bumpass DB, Nunley RM. Assessing the value of a total joint replacement. Curr Rev Musculoskelet Med. 2012;5(4):274–82.

3. Learmonth ID, Young C, Rorabeck C. The operation of the century: total hip replacement. Lancet. 2007;370(9597):1508–19.

4. Kurtz S, Mowat F, Ong K, Chan N, Lau E, Halpern M. Prevalence of primary and revision total hip and knee arthroplasty in the United States from 1990 through 2002. J Bone Joint Surg Am. 2005;87(7):1487–97.

5. Liu HX, Shang P, Ying XZ, Zhang Y. Shorter survival rate in varus-aligned knees after total knee arthroplasty. Knee Surg Sports Traumatol Arthrosc. 2016;24(8):2663–71.

6. Li Z, Esposito CI, Koch CN, Lee YY, Padgett DE, Wright TM. Polyethylene Damage Increases With varus Implant Alignment in Posterior-stabilized and Constrained Condylar Knee Arthroplasty. Clin Orthop Relat Res. 2017;475(12):2981–91.

7. Ritter MA, Davis KE, Davis P, Farris A, Malinzak RA, Berend ME, Meding JB. Preoperative malalignment increases risk of failure after total knee arthroplasty. J Bone Joint Surg Am. 2013;95(2):126–31.

8. Lonner JH, Smith JR, Picard F, Hamlin B, Rowe PJ, Riches PE. High degree of accuracy of a novel image-free handheld robot for unicondylar knee arthroplasty in a cadaveric study. Clin Orthop Relat Res. 2015;473(1):206–12.

9. Moon YW, Ha CW, Do KH, Kim CY, Han JH, Na SE, Lee CH, Kim JG, Park YS. Comparison of robot-assisted and conventional total knee arthroplasty: a controlled cadaver study using multiparameter quantitative three-dimensional CT assessment of alignment. Comput Aided Surg. 2012;17(2):86–95.

10. Cheng T, Zhao S, Peng X, Zhang X. Does computer-assisted surgery improve postoperative leg alignment and implant positioning following total knee arthroplasty? A meta-analysis of randomized controlled trials? Knee Surg Sports Traumatol Arthrosc. 2012;20(7):1307–22.

11. Domb BG, El Bitar YF, Sadik AY, Stake CE, Botser IB. Comparison of robotic-assisted and conventional acetabular cup placement in THA: a matched-pair controlled study. Clin Orthop Relat Res. 2014;472(1):329–36.

12. Kamara E, Robinson J, Bas MA, Rodriguez JA, Hepinstall MS. Adoption of robotic vs fluoroscopic guidance in total hip arthroplasty: is acetabular positioning improved in the learning curve? J Arthroplast. 2017 Jan;32(1):125–30.

13. Song EK, Seon JK, Yim JH, Netravali NA, Bargar WL. Robotic-assisted TKA reduces postoperative alignment outliers and improves gap balance compared to conventional TKA. Clin Orthop Relat Res. 2013 Jan;471(1):118–26.

14. Netravali NA, Shen F, Park Y, Bargar WL. A perspective on robotic assistance for knee arthroplasty. Adv Orthop. https://doi.org/10.1155/2013/970703. 2013 Epub 2013 Apr 30.

15. Jacofsky DJ, Allen M. Robotics in Arthroplasty: a comprehensive review. J Arthroplast. 2016;31(10):2353–63.

16. Coon TM. Integrating robotic technology into the operating room. Am J Orthop. 2009;38(2):7–9.

17. Park SE, Lee CT. Comparison of robotic-assisted and conventional manual implantation of a primary total knee arthroplasty. J Arthroplast. 2007;22(7):1054–9.

18. Schulz AP, Seide K, Queitsch C, von Haugwitz A, Meiners J, Kienast B, Tarabolsi M, Kammal M, Jürgens C. Results of total hip replacement using the Robodoc surgical assistant system: clinical outcome and evaluation of complications for 97 procedures. Int J Med Robot. 2007;3(4):301–6.

19. Liow MH, Xia Z, Wong MK, Tay KJ, Yeo SJ, Chin PL. Robot-assisted total knee arthroplasty accurately restores the joint line and mechanical axis. A prospective randomised study. J Arthroplast. 2014;29(12):2373–7.

20. Alcelik IA, Blomfield MI, Diana G, Gibbon AJ, Carrington N, Burr S. A comparison of short-term outcomes of minimally invasive computer-assisted vs minimally invasive conventional instrumentation for primary total knee arthroplasty: a systematic review and meta-analysis. J Arthroplasty. 2016;31(2):410–8.

21. Wallace D, Gregori A, Picard, Frederic & Bellemans, Johan & Lonner, Jess & Marquez, Raul & McWee (Smith, Julie & Simone, Adam & Jaramaz, Branislav. The learning curve of a novel handheld robotic system for unicondylar knee arthroplasty. J Bone and Joint Surg – British. 2014;96-B:13.

22. Jinnah R, Horowitz S, Lippencott C, Conditt M. Learning curve of robotically assisted UKA. In: International meeting on early intervention for knee arthritis (IMUKA), 56th Annual Meeting of the Orthopaedic Research Society; 2009.

23. Simons M, Riches P. The learning curve of robotically-assisted unicondylar knee arthroplasty. Bone Joint J. 2014;96(SUPP 11):152.

24. O'Malley M, Gregori A, Picard F, Jaramaz B, Lonner J. The learning curve of an image-free handheld robotic system for unicompartmental knee arthroplasty. Poster presented at AAOS 2017 annual meeting, San Diego, 14–18 Mar 2017.

25. Sodhi N, Khlopas A, Piuzzi NS, Sultan AA, Marchand RC, Malkani AL, Mont MA. The learning curve

associated with robotic total knee arthroplasty. J Knee Surg. 2018;31(1):17–21.

26. Khlopas A, Sodhi N, Sultan AA, Chughtai M, Molloy RM, Mont MA. Robotic arm assisted total knee arthroplasty. J Arthroplast. 2018; https://doi.org/10.1016/j.arth.2018.01.060.

27. Karia M, Masjedi M, Andrews B, Jaffry Z, Cobb J. Robotic assistance enables inexperienced surgeons to perform unicompartmental knee arthroplasties on dry bone models with accuracy superior to conventional methods. Adv Orthop. 2013. https://doi.org/10.1155/2013/481039. Epub 2013 Jun 19.

28. Redmond JM, Gupta A, Hammarstedt JE, Petrakos AE, Finch NA, Domb BG. The learning curve associated with robotic-assisted total hip arthroplasty. J Arthroplast. 2015;30(1):50–4.

Perioperative Protocols to Facilitate Early Discharge and Rapid Recovery After Robotic Surgery

5

Michael J. Feldstein and Jess H. Lonner

As robotic surgical innovations advance, the ancillary technologies that support the procedures themselves evolve concurrently. Facilitating the various processes around robotic surgery requires attention to several perioperative elements in order to optimize success and improve recovery. Appropriate preoperative planning to help with execution of the surgery, to optimize the patient physically and medically, and to set patient expectations will ensure a smooth transition toward early discharge and full recovery. Self-directed home exercise regimens, to support or supplant formal physical therapy, as well as multimodal pain management to limit narcotic consumption – both inhospital and at home – will assist in maximizing clinical results and patient satisfaction. Web-based rehabilitation, augmented by burgeoning technologies, promises to offer improved results at a lower cost and greater ease for patients. Finally, it is important to prepare the clinic, hospital, and staff accordingly for the transition to rapid recovery and early discharge after robotic surgery.

M. J. Feldstein
Department of Orthopaedic Surgery, Kaiser
Permanente, San Francisco, CA, USA

J. H. Lonner (✉)
Department of Orthopaedic Surgery,
Rothman Orthopaedic Institute, Sidney Kimmel
Medical College, Thomas Jefferson University,
Philadelphia, PA, USA
e-mail: jess.lonner@rothmanortho.com

Preoperative Planning

Preoperative planning is an essential step in all orthopedic surgical procedures, and robotic assistance in joint arthroplasty or spine surgery is no exception. In fact, depending on the system, the use of robotics often requires additional preoperative planning (such as advanced imaging) to ensure that the robotic system can be properly utilized to reach the desired endpoint. In this section, we will outline the essential steps in perioperative planning for robotic-assisted knee and hip arthroplasty surgery that can facilitate the experience through the entire episode of care. Specific details of surgery-related planning for each system will be reviewed in other individual chapters.

The first step in preoperative planning is confirming that the particular surgery is indeed indicated and will address the patient's particular pathology. A thorough history and physical examination is indispensable. It is important to know if there have been any prior surgeries or trauma that may interfere with the planned incision or with the placement of pins that are required by some robotic systems to hold fiducials that allow registration of the bony anatomy. Quality preoperative imaging is essential, and it is important to know whether additional imaging will be required for the given robotic system. For instance, some robotic systems require a preoperative CT scan using specialized protocols that must be specifically uploaded and calibrated

© Springer Nature Switzerland AG 2019
J. H. Lonner (ed.), *Robotics in Knee and Hip Arthroplasty*,
https://doi.org/10.1007/978-3-030-16593-2_5

at particular imaging centers in coordination with the robotics company. Those scans have to be pre-approved by the insurers and arrangements made in advance to have the patients go specifically to those sites. Advanced planning is important so that three-dimensional segmented virtual models can be built from those images and the surgery planned. The additional radiation exposure [1, 2] imparted by the use of CT scan should be discussed with patients beforehand. For some patients who are being considered for partial knee replacement, it may be prudent to obtain a preoperative MRI to rule out pathology in other compartments if in doubt regarding the optimal procedure. This is especially important for robotic-assisted partial knee replacement, because the setup and planning for robotic-assisted partial knee replacement differ substantially from the setup for a total knee replacement, and if pathology were found in the other compartments intraoperatively, it would add time to switch from a robotic unicompartmental knee setup to either a standard or robotic-assisted total knee setup. As more systems become available that allow for robotic unicompartmental (UKA), patellofemoral (PFA), total knee (TKA), and bi-cruciate retaining total knee surgery (BiKA), the intraoperative interchangeability between procedures will undoubtedly become easier, and this point may become moot. Additionally, while several available systems have capacity for both TKA and partial knee arthroplasties, many hospitals may only have software and hardware loaded on their robot for either TKA or partial knee arthroplasty, but not both, further challenging interchangeability between procedures based on intraoperative findings or unforeseen circumstances.

During the preoperative clinical visits, it is important to set the patient's expectations regarding the surgical process and outcomes, including limitations and possible complications. The role of robotics in the surgery should be outlined to the patient clearly. Educating patients on the rationale and potential utility of the robot is important for aligning patient expectations. Some patients may have unrealistic expectations regarding the role of the robot during surgery and how it will affect their outcome. On the other hand, other patients may have a misguided notion about a robot taking control of the surgery, and these concerns should be addressed and assuaged early in the process.

Planning your OR day and workflow around robotic surgery is another important factor. When first starting it is prudent to plan the robotic cases with additional time allotted due to the anticipated learning curve, as the OR team and robotics representative will need ample time for setup and the surgeon will require a natural ramp-up period before which surgical efficiencies are realized. The role of the representative in the execution of a smooth robotic-assisted surgery should not be underestimated. The representative should coordinate with the OR staff to make sure that the robot is stored and maintained properly. In some circumstances, the robot is brought in to the hospital or outpatient surgery facility specifically for a given OR day, while in others it will reside there. In either situation, the representative will ensure that the robot is setup and fully operational. A suitable OR suite should be chosen that will accommodate the size of the robot, have adequate power supply, and allow adequate space for any accessory sensors that may be needed for registration. Having select OR staff that are designated as the robotics team that goes through formalized training and assists frequently during these cases will optimize system and room setup, surgical efficiencies, and the overall perioperative experience.

While some surgeons may be concerned that robotic surgery may decrease OR efficiency and add to operative time, with the proper room setup, team training, and communication, robotic surgery can be accomplished efficiently. The extra initial preparation often encountered after technology adoption should not discourage the use of robotics, but instead should be considered an essential part of maximizing the utility of robotic assistance to ensure a seamless surgical experience and optimal results.

Perioperative Management and Advanced Planning

For the majority of patients, robotic UKA, PFA, and BiKA are performed on an outpatient basis, either at a surgery center or hospital. Increasingly, total joint surgery and some spine surgeries are being performed with the expectation that patients can be discharged on the day of surgery or sometime the next day. Early discharge of course cannot be performed without appropriate expectation management; coordination with an identified caregiver; advanced planning with the facility and practice navigator to evaluate perioperative risk and plan discharge and postoperative services; and provision of prescriptions in advance of surgery for postoperative venous thromboembolism prophylaxis, antibiotics, and pain medications as well as physical therapy [3].

Preemptive analgesia, intraoperative fluid management, minimization of intraoperative sedation, low-dose spinal anesthesia with bupivacaine (or general anesthesia with laryngeal mask airway to reduce the risk of urinary retention in men), and perioperative nausea control are critical to secure safe and early discharge. Standard-risk patients are typically discharged within 2–6 hours after partial knee arthroplasty; higher-risk patients or those undergoing total joint arthroplasty can often be discharged by 23 hours; even when patients are admitted overnight depending on circumstances, advanced preparation is critical. Patients are encouraged to ambulate immediately with in-facility supervision and after discharge, using crutches, walker, or a cane, with immediate range of motion exercises administered via an interactive web-based program or simple preprinted handout. Formal outpatient physical therapy should be commenced within 2–5 days of surgery, although some surgeons prefer to wait several weeks to determine if formal PT is necessary. Transition from walker/crutches to a cane and then weaning from all ambulatory aids can be considered once the patient recovers adequate balance and strength.

Effective postoperative pain management is one of the most important factors contributing to safe early discharge to home and successful overall outcomes after surgery. Patients whose pain is well-controlled are more likely to engage in their rehabilitation and resume independent unassisted ambulation. While perioperative protocols are re-evaluated periodically and may evolve over time, one particular protocol, which has been used successfully for the past few years for both TKA and partial knee arthroplasty in the senior surgeon's practice, includes the following, unless contraindicated due to allergy, medical comorbidity, age-related issues, or drug intolerances or interactions:

1. **Preoperative Patient Preparation**
   (a) One preoperative consultation with a physical therapist is prescribed for gait training with the use of a cane, crutch, and walker on level ground and on stairs and to work with the patient on the methods of getting into and out of a car or other tasks.
   (b) Patients are given access to a web-based interactive rehabilitation program (FORCE Therapeutics) (Figs. 5.1 and 5.2) in order to initiate an account and begin a tutorial so that web-based exercises can begin as soon as the day of surgery or early the next day.
   (c) Prescriptions are given preoperatively for postoperative physical therapy, walker, crutches, and cane, a commode if needed, and, in the case of knee arthroplasty, a cryotherapy pack.
   (d) Additionally, preoperatively prescriptions are given for the postoperative medications which may be needed after discharge, including multimodal pain medications, antiemetics, thromboprophylaxis agents, and antibiotics (for outpatient surgery) [see below].

2. **Perioperative Management of Pain and Nausea: Antibiotic Prophylaxis**
   (a) Medications to be given on the morning of surgery, preoperatively:

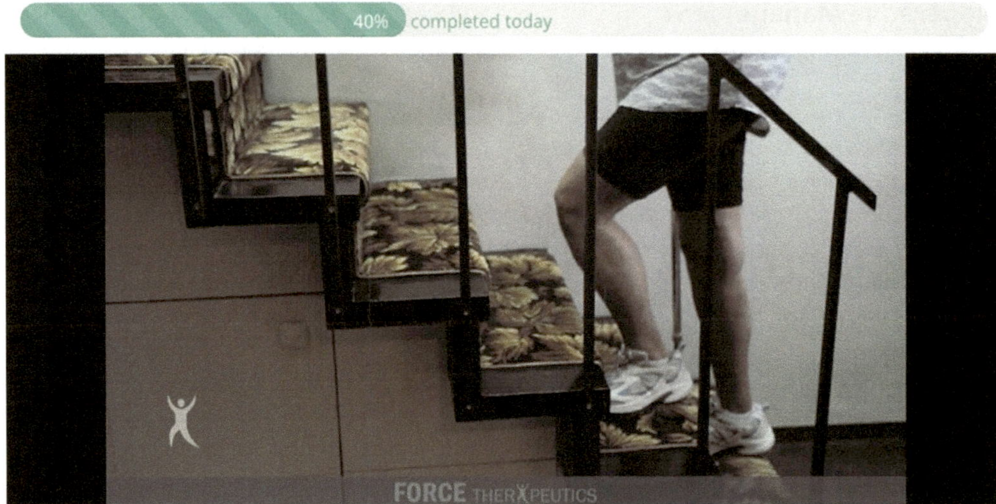

Fig. 5.1 FORCE Therapeutics web-based therapy platform helps patients perform therapy at home, in some cases supplanting the need for a physical therapist. (Courtesy of FORCE Therapeutics)

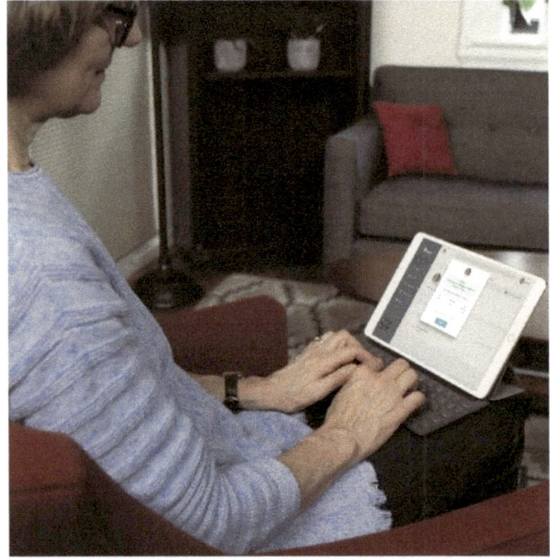

Fig. 5.2 This is an example of a patient interfacing with the FORCE Therapeutics mobile app in the comfort of their own home. (Courtesy of FORCE Therapeutics)

    (i) Acetaminophen 975 mg po
    (ii) Gabapentin 300 mg po
    (iii) Celecoxib 200 mg po
(b) Anesthesia:
    (i) Either low-dose bupivacaine spinal or LMA (reduces urinary retention in men).
    (ii) Indwelling catheters, epidural anesthesia, and postoperative patient-controlled anesthesia are avoided.
(c) Preop antibiotics:
    (i) Keflex or clindamycin or vancomycin
(d) Regional analgesia current choices:
    (i) TKA/UKA/PFA – adductor canal block – single injection [4–8]
    (ii) Peri-incisional injections
      – The composition of the injection does not have clear evidence and is at the discretion of the attending.

(a) Selection of ropivacaine or bupivacaine may vary by surgeon, including %, volume, and plain vs. with epinephrine.
  (i) Current preference: 40 cc of 0.5% ropivacaine without epinephrine (15 cc injected into adductor canal; 25 cc pericapsular injection) (in the case of knee arthroplasty)
  (b) Liposomal bupivacaine is not supported.
(e) Blood loss management:
  (i) Tranexamic acid 1 gm IV administered during surgery (unless patient considered high risk [history of coronary artery disease, peripheral vascular disease, ischemic stroke or VTE]) [9–13]
(f) Additional intraoperative medications for nausea prevention:
  (i) Decadron 4 mg IV
  (ii) Zofran 4 mg IV
(g) Fluid management:
  (i) Adequate hydration per anesthesia
(h) In-facility standing orders for pain management:
  (i) IV – Toradol 15–30 mg IV q6h (age dependent)
  (ii) Oral
    – Tylenol 975 mg q6h
    – Neurontin 300 mg q 8 h
    – Celecoxib 200 mg BID
(i) In-facility PRN orders for pain management:
  (i) Mild/moderate – tramadol 50 mg po q6h
  (ii) Moderate/severe
    – Toradol is first choice (see above for dose).
    – Oxycodone 5–10 mg po q4h.
(j) Other in-facility post-op medications:
  (i) Zofran 4–8 mg IV for nausea (prn)
3. **Post-discharge Medicine Management**
  (a) Standing medications (for 2–4 weeks):
    (i) Tylenol 650 mg PO q6h
    (ii) Neurontin 300 mg PO tid
    (iii) Celecoxib 200 mg BID

– Modify use of NSAIDs in patients with peptic ulcer disease or intolerance, renal insufficiency
  (iv) Protein pump inhibitor Protonix 40 mg po QD for 4 weeks
(b) PRN medications:
  (i) Pain
    – Mild/moderate pain
      (a) Tramadol 50 mg PO q6h
    – Moderate/severe pain
      (a) Oxycodone 10 mg po q4h
  (ii) Nausea
    – Zofran 4 mg 1–2 pills PO every 6–8 hrs as needed for nausea
(c) Post-op antibiotics for outpatient surgeries:
  (i) Keflex 500 mg 1 po Q8 h (3 pills)
  (ii) Or Cipro 500 mg po Q8 h for PCN allergic patients (3 pills)
(d) Venous thromboembolism (VTE) prophylaxis:
  (i) ASA 81 mg plain po BID (325 mg enteric coated BID if patient is already on that preop) starting on the evening of surgery [14].
  (ii) Anticoagulants other than ASA (low molecular weight heparin, Xarelto, Eliquis, etc.) can be used as indicated in patients considered to be at higher risk for VTE, starting 1 day after surgery [15, 16].

Physical Therapy

Physical therapy is an important aspect of recovery after joint arthroplasty, and to facilitate outpatient robotic surgery, a modern and efficient physical therapy plan should be implemented. Given reduced hospital stays after surgery, physical therapists may be relied on to identify concerning findings such as wound drainage or irritation, swelling, and unusual levels of pain that must be conveyed to the care team. Streamlined and technologically up-to-date physical therapy programs are now available to augment or enhance therapy and, in many cases, may supplant formal PT altogether. Indeed, the role of the physical therapist may be changing as new technologies are introduced such as robotics [17], wearable motion tracking [18–20], video game interfaces [21–23], and web-based rehabilitation platforms [24–26]. It is important to note that new technologies will work as force multipliers allowing physical therapists to treat more patients, more effectively while utilizing fewer resources. This increase in efficiency could positively impact outcomes for the patient at a lower cost [27].

Web-Based Rehabilitation

The trend toward outpatient and short-stay arthroplasty has been an improvement for caregivers and patients alike. However, it has shifted the rehabilitation burden from the inpatient setting to the outpatient and home setting. The increased usage of home health physical therapy to act as a bridge to outpatient therapy has added cost to the outpatient portion of arthroplasty, and burgeoning technologies, especially web-based rehabilitation, are helping ease the cost and man power burden associated with outpatient and in-home therapy [25]. Automating the physical therapy process and reducing the human capital burden has potential for major cost savings for the episode of care, which can offset to an extent the increased cost of robotic surgery and may even lead to better results by tracking patients at home more closely. Furthermore, the ideal physical therapy program, both pre- and post-op, is still unknown. Data collection from technologically enhanced therapy programs may help surgeons and clinicians optimize therapy programs in general and for each individual patient.

Web-based rehabilitation (Figs. 5.1, 5.2, and 5.3) offers the convenience of accessing rehabilitation protocols anywhere that an Internet connection is available [28–30]. Web-based rehabilitation is inherently superior to simple computer-aided rehabilitation that may involve watching video tutorials or even interacting with a video game interface because web-based rehabilitation allows for feedback, tracking, and accountability. Several technologies are being developed to help improve the efficacy and adherence to web-based physical therapy protocols. These technologies include messaging, phone and video calls, reminders and automated surveys, games with avatars [31, 32], and a combination of sensors and tracking devices [33–35] to provide feedback to patients and providers (Figs. 5.4, 5.5, and 5.6). Providers can track how their patients are doing and therapies can be tailored and customized depending on a patient's progress [36]. Several randomized clinical studies have found that compared to formal outpatient PT, self-directed web-based therapy in inclined patients produces comparable functional outcomes and improvements in knee motion after both total and unicompartmental knee arthroplasty, although in both groups there remains a subset of patients who will still benefit from formal PT to obtain optimal outcomes [25, 37].

There may be a future where web-based therapies employ robotic assistance [38] to help patients reach range of motion, gait, and strengthening goals. Although the technology has not yet matured, augmenting robotic surgery with web-based rehabilitation makes intuitive sense to optimize outcomes while reducing cost. Further integration with wearable devices and sensors will increase the interactive potential of the modality [18, 20]. Research and development of web-/mobile-based platforms (Tracpatch, El Dorado Hills, Ca. USA; Muvr Labs, San Francisco, Ca. USA; SWORD Health [20], Porto, Portugal) augmented with wearable devices is helping to further advance the technology (Figs. 5.7, 5.8, 5.9, and 5.10). The usability and utility of wearables for medical applications remain a burgeoning area, and more work must be done for the technology to mature. Patients who seek out robotic-assisted surgery are likely to be computer savvy and will be more amenable to adopting new technologies such as web-based rehabilitation than luddites who may prefer more traditional surgical techniques and rehabilitation protocols. Currently these systems are being actively researched, and the ideal combination of interface, sensors, and feedback to most effectively motivate patients throughout their recovery remains elusive.

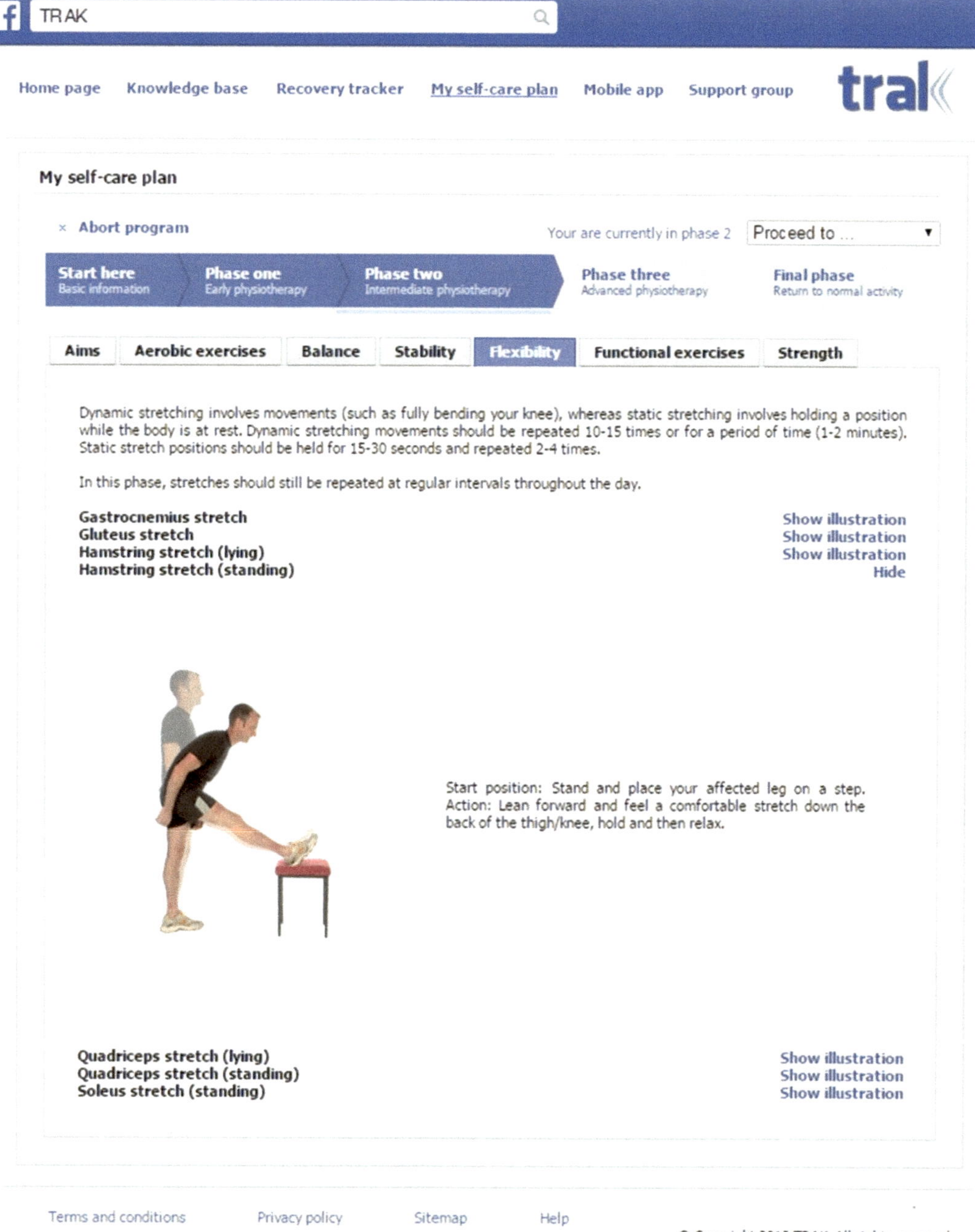

Fig. 5.3 TRAK Web interface is another web-based platform that originated out of the university setting in the UK to research web-based physical therapy. (From [26], with permission)

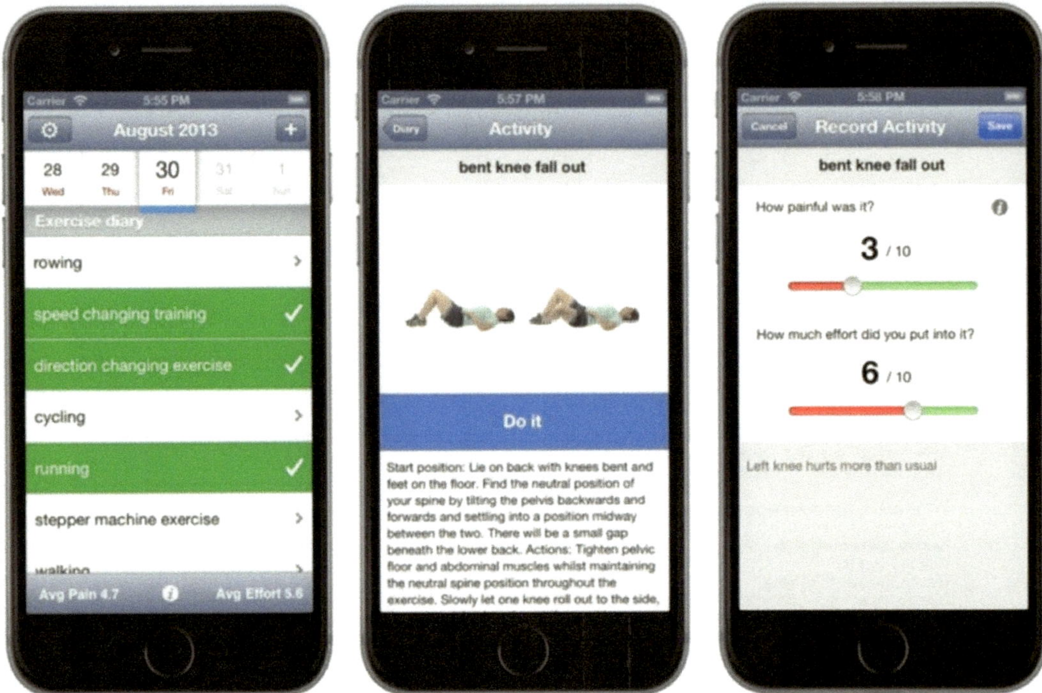

Fig. 5.4 TRAK also has a mobile interface. (From [26], with permission)

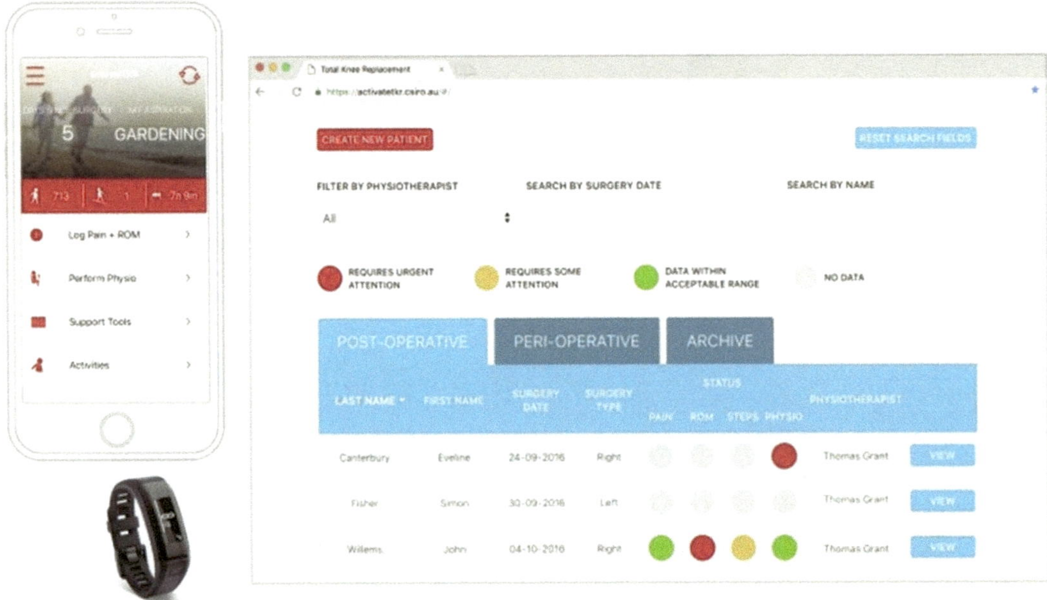

Fig. 5.5 Some web-based platforms have attempted to use sensors within smartphones as the wearable device or off the shelf commercially available wearable devices as in this case. (From [24], with permission)

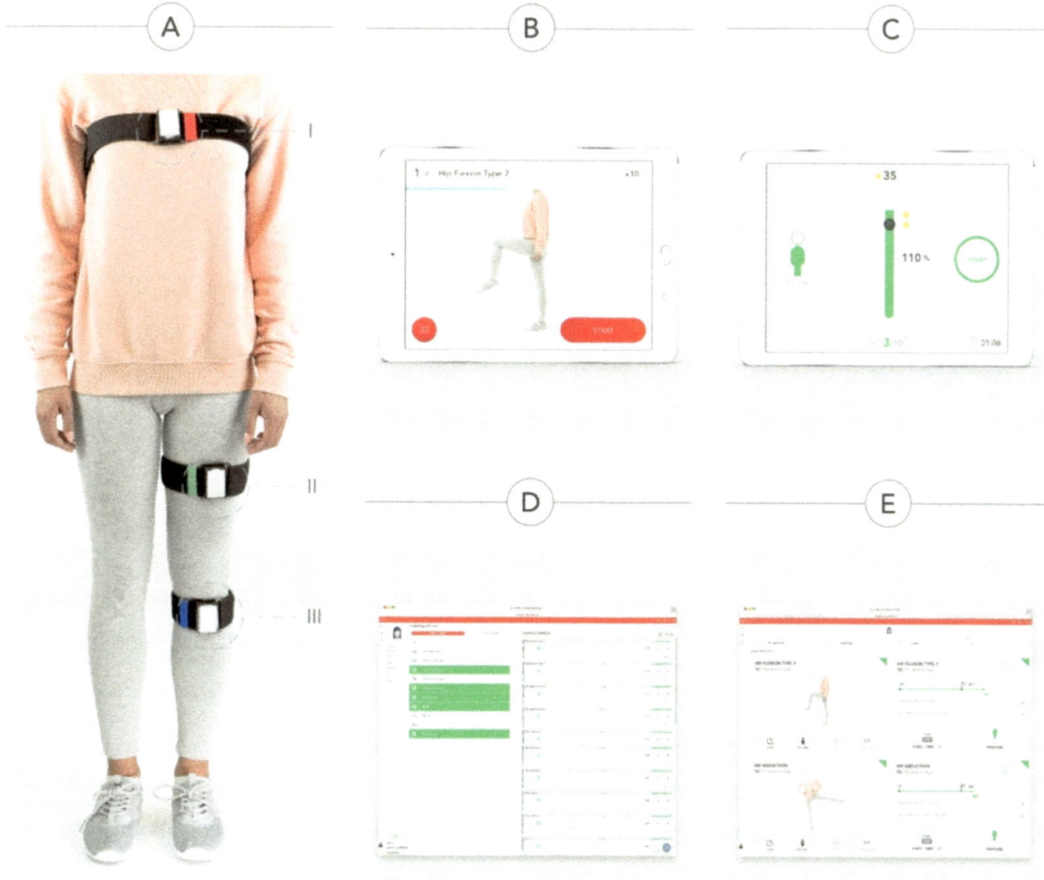

Fig. 5.6 Several companies are now working on combination web/mobile rehabilitation interfaces with custom wearable inertial measurement units (IMUs). This is an example from SWORD Health, Porto Portugal. (From [20], with permission)

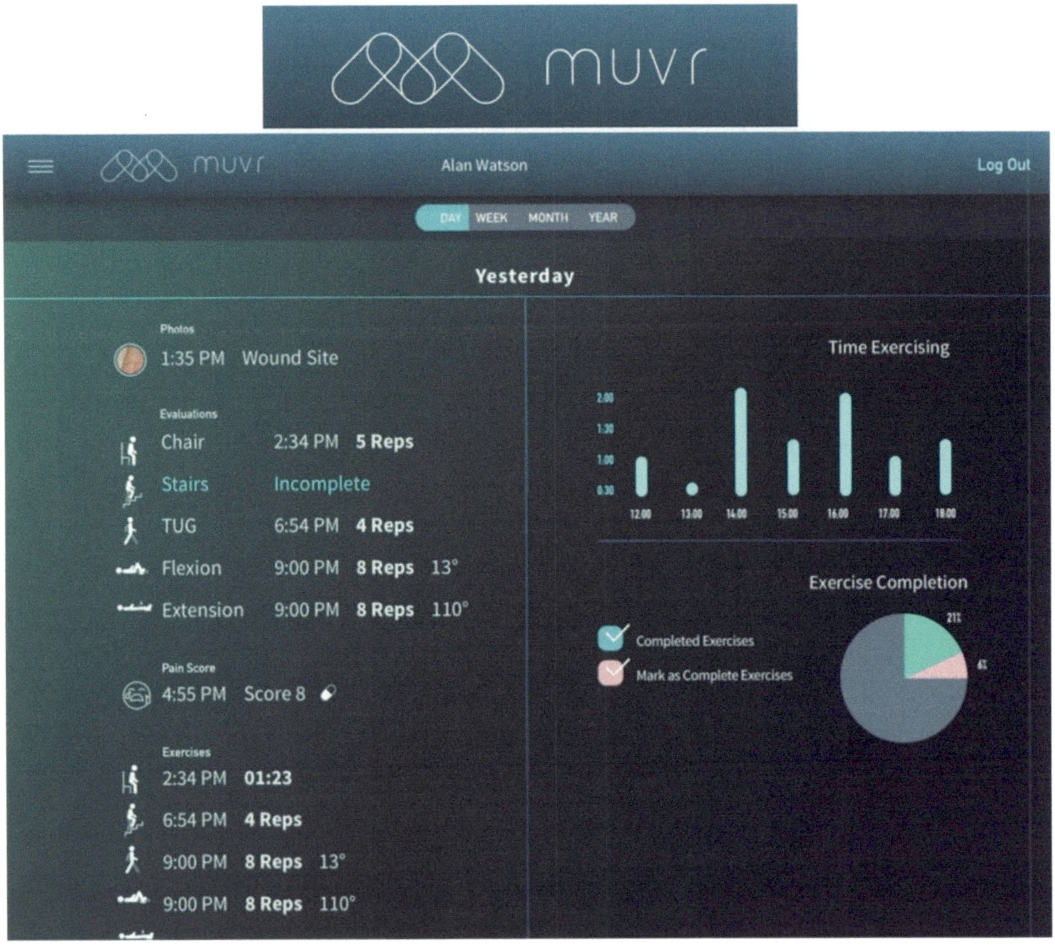

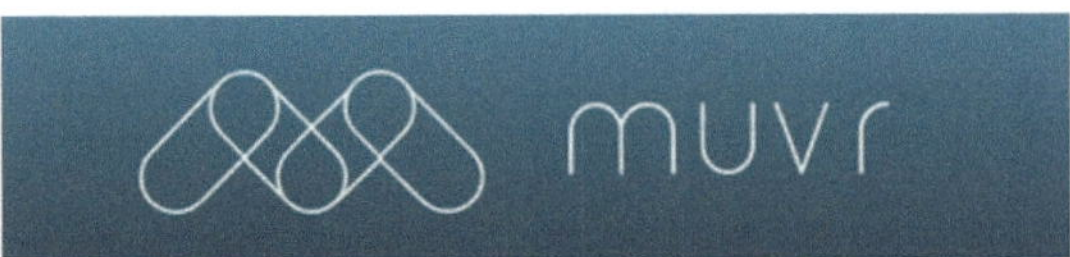

Fig. 5.7 Muvr Labs is developing a web/mobile interface with wearable IMUs. Muvr Web interface with dashboard. (Courtesy of Muvr Labs, San Francisco, CA, USA)

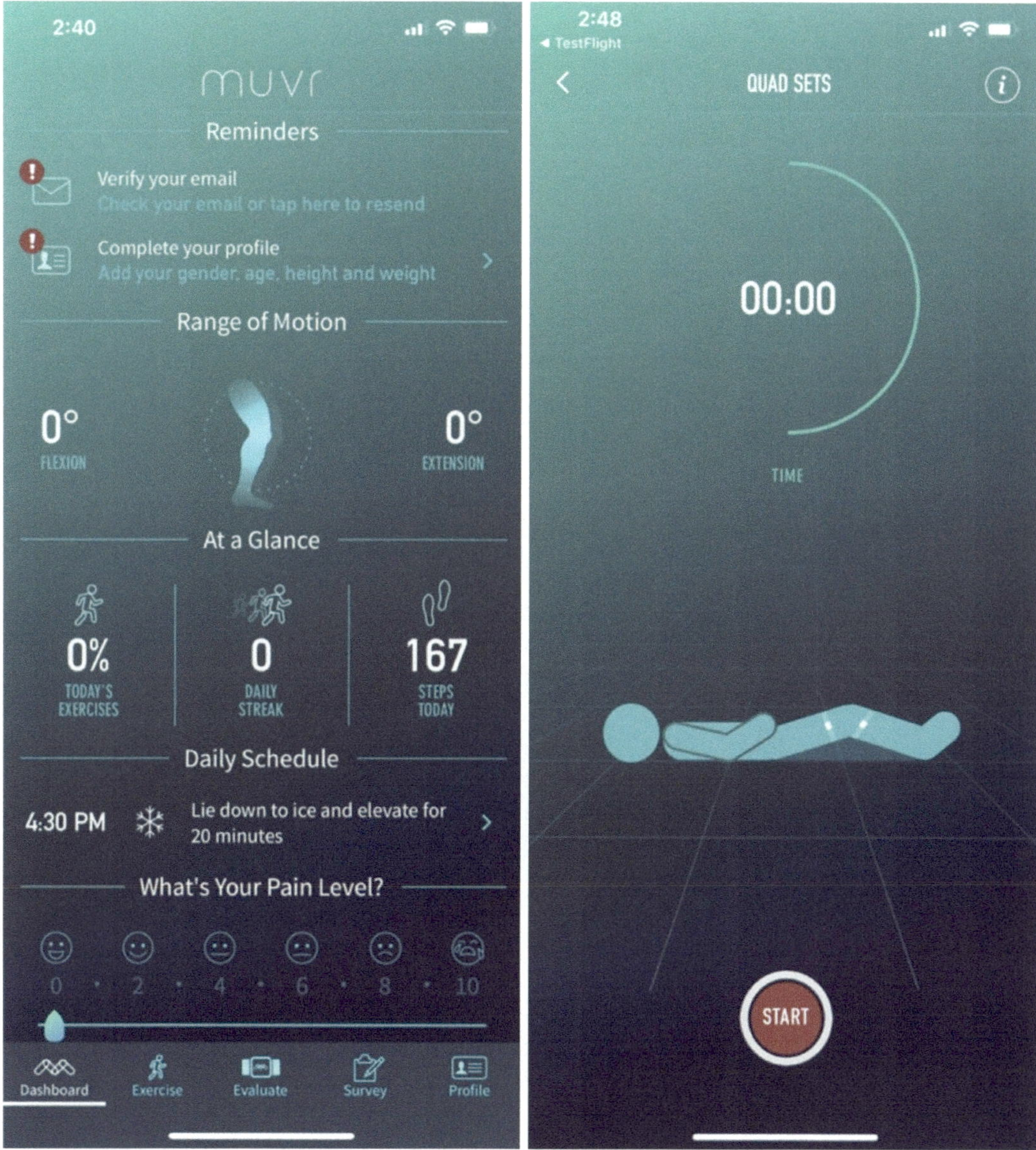

Fig. 5.8 Muvr mobile interface. (Courtesy of Muvr Labs, San Francisco, CA, USA)

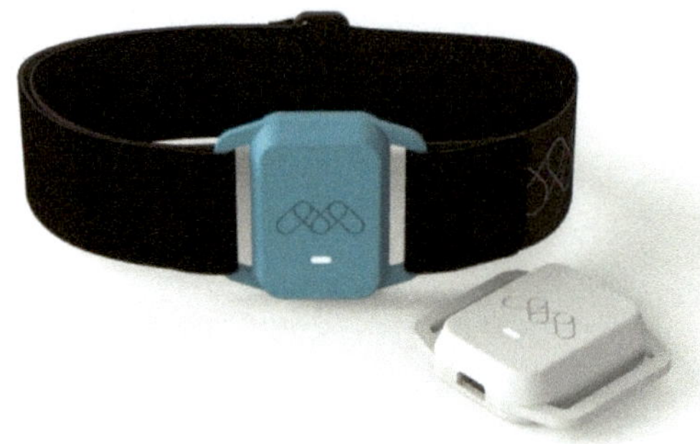

Fig. 5.9 Muvr custom wearable inertial measurement unit with autocalibration. (Courtesy of Muvr Labs, San Francisco, CA, USA)

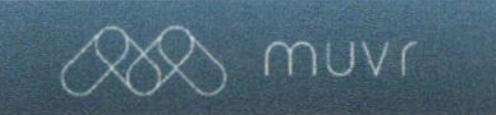

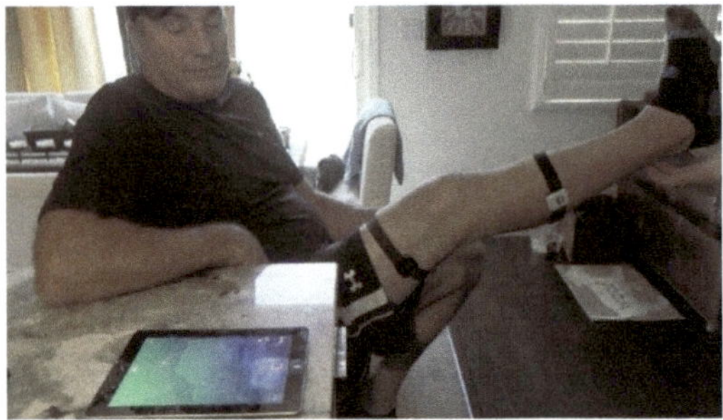

Fig. 5.10 Patient using the Muvr device and mobile app. (Courtesy of Muvr Labs, San Francisco, CA, USA)

Conclusion

In conclusion, outpatient and short-stay robotic surgery has matured and has a promising and exciting future. New robotic systems are precise and increasingly more efficient, making adoption more widespread. With the proper preoperative planning and perioperative management, recovery from robotic surgery can be optimized. Advanced preparations, multimodal pain management strategies, and rethinking physical therapy protocols that take advantage of wearable sensors and interactive systems such as web-based rehabilitation are further augmenting the surgical advances seen with robotics.

References

1. Urish KL, Conditt M, Roche M, Rubash HE. Robotic total knee Arthroplasty: surgical assistant for a customized normal kinematic knee. Orthopedics. 2016;39:e822–7. https://doi.org/10.3928/01477447-20160623-13.
2. Jacofsky DJ, Allen M. Robotics in arthroplasty: a comprehensive review. J Arthroplast. 2016;31:2353–63. https://doi.org/10.1016/j.arth.2016.05.026.
3. Lonner JH. Robotically assisted unicompartmental knee arthroplasty with a handheld image-free sculpting tool. Oper Tech Orthop. 2015;47:29–40. https://doi.org/10.1053/j.oto.2015.03.001.
4. Jenstrup MT, Jæger P, Lund J, et al. Effects of adductor-canal-blockade on pain and ambulation after total knee arthroplasty: a randomized study. Acta Anaesthesiol Scand. 2012;56:357–64. https://doi.org/10.1111/j.1399-6576.2011.02621.x.
5. Hanson NA, Allen CJ, Hostetter LS, et al. Continuous ultrasound-guided Adductor Canal block for Total knee Arthroplasty. Surv Anesthesiol. 2015;59:52–3. https://doi.org/10.1097/SA.0000000000000114.
6. Chan EY, Fransen M, Parker DA, et al. Femoral nerve blocks for acute postoperative pain after knee replacement surgery. Cochrane Database Syst Rev. 2014. https://doi.org/10.1002/14651858.CD009941.pub2.
7. Shah NA, Jain NP, Panchal KA. Adductor canal blockade following total knee arthroplasty-continuous or single shot technique? Role in postoperative analgesia, ambulation ability and early functional recovery: a randomized controlled trial. J Arthroplast. 2015;30:1476–81. https://doi.org/10.1016/j.arth.2015.03.006.
8. Parvizi J, Miller AG, Gandhi K. Multimodal pain management after total joint arthroplasty. J Bone Jt Surg – Ser A. 2011;93:1075–84. https://doi.org/10.2106/JBJS.J.01095.
9. Jain RK, Porat MD, Klingenstein GG, et al. The AAHKS clinical research award: liposomal bupivacaine and periarticular injection are not superior to single-shot intra-articular injection for pain control in Total knee Arthroplasty. J Arthroplast. 2016;31:22–5.
10. Schroer WC, Diesfeld PG, LeMarr AR, et al. Does extended-release liposomal bupivacaine better control pain than bupivacaine after total knee arthroplasty (TKA)? A prospective, randomized clinical trial. J Arthroplast. 2015;30:64–7. https://doi.org/10.1016/j.arth.2015.01.059.
11. Bramlett K, Onel E, Viscusi ER, Jones K. A randomized, double-blind, dose-ranging study comparing wound infiltration of DepoFoam bupivacaine, an extended-release liposomal bupivacaine, to bupivacaine HCl for postsurgical analgesia in total knee arthroplasty. Knee. 2012;19:530–6. https://doi.org/10.1016/j.knee.2011.12.004.

12. Bagsby DT, Ireland PH, Meneghini RM. Liposomal bupivacaine versus traditional periarticular injection for pain control after total knee arthroplasty. J Arthroplast. 2014;29:1687–90. https://doi.org/10.1016/j.arth.2014.03.034.

13. Collis PN, Hunter AM, Vaughn MDD, et al. Periarticular injection after total knee arthroplasty using liposomal bupivacaine vs a modified ranawat suspension: a prospective, randomized study. J Arthroplast. 2016;31:633–6. https://doi.org/10.1016/j.arth.2015.09.025.

14. Parvizi J, Huang R, Restrepo C, et al. Low-dose aspirin is effective chemoprophylaxis against clinically important venous thromboembolism following total joint arthroplasty a preliminary analysis. J Bone Jt Surg – Am. 2017;99:91–8. https://doi.org/10.2106/JBJS.16.00147.

15. Nam D, Nunley RM, Johnson SR, et al. The effectiveness of a risk stratification protocol for thromboembolism prophylaxis after hip and knee arthroplasty. J Arthroplast. 2015. https://doi.org/10.1016/j.arth.2015.12.007.

16. Parvizi J, Huang R, Raphael IJ, et al. Symptomatic pulmonary embolus after joint arthroplasty: stratification of risk factors. Clin Orthop Relat Res. 2014;472:903–12. https://doi.org/10.1007/s11999-013-3358-z.

17. Yoshikawa K, Mutsuzaki H, Sano A, et al. Training with hybrid assistive limb for walking function after total knee arthroplasty. J Orthop Surg Res. 2018;13:1–10. https://doi.org/10.1186/s13018-018-0875-1.

18. Toogood PA, Abdel MP, Spear JA, et al. The monitoring of activity at home after total hip arthroplasty. Bone Jt J. 2016;98-B:1450–4. https://doi.org/10.1302/0301-620X.98B11.BJJ-2016-0194.R1.

19. Chiang CY, Chen KH, Liu KC, et al. Data collection and analysis using wearable sensors for monitoring knee range of motion after total knee arthroplasty. Sensors (Switzerland). 2017. https://doi.org/10.3390/s17020418.

20. Correia FD, Nogueira A, Magalhães I, et al. Home-based rehabilitation with a novel digital biofeedback system versus conventional in-person rehabilitation after total knee replacement: a feasibility study. Sci Rep. 2018;8:1–12. https://doi.org/10.1038/s41598-018-29668-0.

21. Fung V, Ho A, Shaffer J, et al. Use of Nintendo Wii fit™ in the rehabilitation of outpatients following total knee replacement: a preliminary randomised controlled trial. Physiother (United Kingdom). 2012;98:183–8. https://doi.org/10.1016/j.physio.2012.04.001.

22. Bonnechere B, Jansen B, Salvia P, et al. Validity and reliability of the Nintendo Wii balance board for assessment of standing balance. Gait Posture. 1991. https://doi.org/10.1016/0167-9457(91)90046-z.

23. Oh J, Kuenze C, Jacopetti M, et al. Validity of the Microsoft Kinect™ in assessing spatiotemporal and lower extremity kinematics during stair ascent and descent in healthy young individuals. Med Eng Phys. 2018. https://doi.org/10.1016/j.medengphy.2018.07.011.

24. Hussain MS, Li J, Brindal E, et al Supporting the delivery of total knee replacements care for both patients and their clinicians with a mobile app and web-based tool: randomized controlled trial protocol. JMIR Res Protoc. 2017. https://doi.org/10.2196/resprot.6498.

25. Fillingham YA, Darrith B, Lonner JH, et al. Formal physical therapy may not be necessary after unicompartmental knee arthroplasty: a randomized clinical trial. J Arthroplast. 2018;33:S93–S99.e3. https://doi.org/10.1016/j.arth.2018.02.049.

26. Spasić I, Button K, Divoli A, et al. TRAK app suite: a web-based intervention for delivering standard care for the rehabilitation of knee conditions. JMIR Res Protoc. 2015;4:e122. https://doi.org/10.2196/resprot.4091.

27. Jiang S, Xiang J, Gao X, et al. The comparison of telerehabilitation and face-to-face rehabilitation after total knee arthroplasty: a systematic review and meta-analysis. J Telemed Telecare. 2018;24:257–62. https://doi.org/10.1177/1357633X16686748.

28. Russell TG, Buttrum P, Wootton R, G a J. Internet-based outpatient telerehabilitation for patients following total knee arthroplasty: a randomized controlled trial. J Bone Joint Surg Am. 2011;93:113–20. https://doi.org/10.2106/JBJS.I.01375.

29. Shukla H, Nair SR, Thakker D. Role of telerehabilitation in patients following total knee arthroplasty: evidence from a systematic literature review and meta-analysis. J Telemed Telecare. 2016;23:339–46. https://doi.org/10.1177/1357633X16628996.

30. Nelson MJ, Crossley KM, Bourke MG, Russell TG. Telerehabilitation feasibility in Total joint replacement. Int J Telerehabil. 2017;9:31–8. https://doi.org/10.5195/ijt.2017.6235.

31. Chughtai M, Kelly JJ, Newman JM, et al. The role of virtual rehabilitation in total and unicompartmental knee arthroplasty. J Knee Surg. 2019;32:105–10. https://doi.org/10.1055/s-0038-1637018.

32. Gonzalez-Franco M, Gilroy S, Moore JO. Empowering patients to perform physical therapy at home. In: 2014 36th annual international conference of the IEEE engineering in medicine and biology society, EMBC 2014: IEEE; 2014. p. 6308–11.

33. Bahadori S, Immins T, Wainwright TW. A review of wearable motion tracking systems used in rehabilitation following hip and knee replacement. J Rehabil Assist Technol Eng. 2018;5:205566831877181. https://doi.org/10.1177/2055668318771816.

34. Kwasnicki RM, Ali R, Jordan SJ, et al. A wearable mobility assessment device for total knee replacement: A longitudinal feasibility study. Int J Surg. 2015. https://doi.org/10.1016/j.ijsu.2015.04.032.

35. Lin JFS, Kulić D. Human pose recovery using wireless inertial measurement units. Physiol Meas. 2012;33:2099–115. https://doi.org/10.1088/0967-3334/33/12/2099.

36. Lam AWK, Varona-Marin D, Li Y, et al. Automated rehabilitation system: movement measurement and feedback for patients and physiotherapists in the rehabilitation clinic. Human-Computer Interact. 2016;31:294–334. https://doi.org/10.1080/07370024. 2015.1093419.

37. Fleischman AN, Crizer MP, Tarabichi M, Smith S, Rothman RH, Lonner JH, Chen AF. 2018 John N. Insall Award: Recovery of knee flexion with unsupervised home exercise is not inferior to outpatient physical therapy after TKA: a randomized trial. Clin Orthop. 2019;477:60–9.

38. Meng W, Liu Q, Zhou Z, et al. Recent development of mechanisms and control strategies for robot-assisted lower limb rehabilitation. Mechatronics. 2015. https://doi.org/10.1016/j.mechatronics.2015.04.005.

Richard Southgate and Derek Ward

The primary goal of total joint arthroplasty (TJA) and partial knee arthroplasty (PKA) is to alleviate pain to maximize functionality and improve quality of life. However, surgery is associated with significant short-term pain. Failure to control postoperative pain results in decreased patient satisfaction, prolonged hospital stays, and increased healthcare costs [1]. Developments in postoperative pain management have moved the standard of care away from strictly narcotic regimens to multimodal techniques, with increasing use of regional and spinal anesthesia along with combinations of nonnarcotic drugs. The ultimate goal of opioid-sparing multimodal analgesia is to maintain adequate pain relief while avoiding side effects from any single medication [2]. For the most part, we see no need for alterations in perioperative anesthetic or pain management protocols, whether or not robotic assistance is utilized; however, if robotic usage lengthens substantially one's surgical times, such as early in a surgeon's learning curve, longer-acting anesthetics may be necessary. This chapter provides an overall summary of perioperative anesthetic and analgesic options. Individualized protocols will vary among clinicians, depending on experiences, preferences, formulary restrictions, and emerging data.

Medication Types and Options

Opioid medications, administered via oral (PO), intravenous (IV), or patient-controlled anesthesia (PCA) route, were traditional mainstays of postoperative pain treatment following TJA. Examples of opioid medications include oxycodone, hydrocodone, hydromorphone, morphine, and fentanyl. These are effective pain relievers but have numerous side effects such as nausea/vomiting, ileus, sedation, respiratory depression, pruritus, withdrawal, and addiction. These medications continue to have a role in post-TJA analgesia; however, other classes of medications are now used on a scheduled basis to prevent pain and decrease narcotic usage. Tramadol, available in both PO and IV formulations, is a synthetic opioid which works by binding to the mu opioid receptor as well as inhibiting reuptake of serotonin and norepinephrine. Tramadol is thought to have a more favorable side effect profile than other opioids and carry less risk of addiction with long-term use; however, there are no conclusive studies demonstrating the latter.

Acetaminophen/paracetamol is an effective adjunct in pain control and has a favorable safety profile. Although the medication is widely used,

R. Southgate
Department of Orthopaedic Surgery, Division of Adult Reconstruction, University of California, San Francisco, CA, USA

D. Ward (✉)
Department of Orthopaedic Surgery, University of California, San Francisco, CA, USA

© Springer Nature Switzerland AG 2019
J. H. Lonner (ed.), *Robotics in Knee and Hip Arthroplasty*,
https://doi.org/10.1007/978-3-030-16593-2_6

its exact mechanism is unknown; it is thought to be a centrally acting cyclooxygenase inhibitor. Commonly given orally, this route is subject to delayed absorption; intravenous acetaminophen is a recent addition and as effective as some weaker narcotics or ketorolac. Cost issues may prevent adoption of the IV formulation [3].

Nonsteroidal anti-inflammatory drugs (NSAIDs) such as ibuprofen, aspirin, and meloxicam are often available in PO and IV formulations. This class of medications inhibits cyclooxygenase, which leads to decreased production of prostaglandins, resulting in analgesia and decreased inflammation. There are two isozymes of cyclooxygenase: COX-1 and COX-2. COX-1 is constitutively active in many tissues including gastric mucosa and kidneys, so nonselective COX inhibitors carry the risk of gastric ulcers and renal insufficiency. Selective COX-2 inhibitors such as celecoxib (Celebrex) focus on COX-2 isozyme found in areas of increased inflammation, thereby resulting in reduced risk for gastric ulcers and less platelet dysfunction than nonselective COX inhibitors. While there has been an increased risk of cardiovascular events associated with COX-2 inhibitors, doses of celecoxib up to 400 mg per day have not been shown to increase this risk [2]. The use of scheduled celecoxib 200 mg twice daily for 6 weeks has been shown to reduce pain up to 12 weeks and increase flexion up to 1 year; additionally those taking celecoxib also took far fewer narcotics than those taking placebo [4]. Ketorolac is another NSAID which deserves special mention. Available in both PO and IV formulation, this is the most potent NSAID with near-opioid levels of pain control. Unfortunately, it can only be prescribed for a course of less than 5 days to avoid side effects such as impaired renal function.

Neuromodulators such as gabapentin and pregabalin are centrally acting medications that affect signaling of gamma-aminobutyric acid (GABA) receptors, resulting in reduced central sensitization at the level of the spinal cord and brain. Pregabalin is more potent than gabapentin, requiring a lower dose to achieve the same effect. Although the use of gabapentin and pregabalin for acute pain prevention is considered off-label use, there is evidence that they are effective. A 14-day taper of gabapentin has been shown to reduce opioid use and improve knee flexion at 30 days as well as decrease the chance of the patient developing chronic neuropathic pain [5]. There is some concern over the side effects of sedation and confusion with these medications.

Preoperative Evaluation and Mitigation

With the preoperative history and physical, an accurate medication history is important, especially with regard to the patient's average daily dose of narcotics. Patients who have been taking opioids on a chronic basis should be counseled that pain control is going to be more difficult. Attempts should be made to work with the patient's primary care or pain management physician to decrease their narcotic use prior to surgery, as this can affect postoperative pain medication requirements as well as outcomes [6]. Elective surgery can be justifiably delayed to accommodate reduction of narcotics to maximize outcomes and minimize complications.

Clinicians should inquire about allergies, reactions, and sensitivities to previous medications. These include gastrointestinal bleeding/upset to nonsteroidal anti-inflammatories, allergies to sulfa-containing medications which preclude the use of celecoxib, and prior nausea/vomiting with specific types of narcotics. A thorough medical history is important as certain medications are contraindicated with conditions such as renal failure or cardiac disease.

Preemptive Analgesia

As part of a multimodal analgesia regimen, preoperative medications can be given to prevent sensitization of nociceptors and pain fibers secondary to surgery. Normal pain fiber sensitization results in hypersensitivity to innocuous stimuli during the postoperative period, prevention of which can both decrease the amount of postoperative pain and decrease the risk of chronic neuropathic pain [7]. Options for preoperative analgesia include acetaminophen, narcotics, nonsteroidal anti-inflammatories, and gabapentinoids, with any of these in combination. Pre-treating pain leads to lower doses of anesthetic agents which are safer and allow for quicker recovery.

Regional Anesthesia

Regional anesthesia has contributed significantly to the improvement of multimodal pain strategies. If given preoperatively it can help decrease the amount of anesthesia required by the patient. Other benefits include shorter length of stay, decreased opioid consumption, and earlier participation in therapy. Potential drawbacks include the need for specialized anesthesia skills, complications related to the administration of the block, and variable failure rates ranging from 0% to 67% [2, 8]. Additionally, femoral nerve blocks are associated with quadriceps motor weakness, which can result in falls. Although rare, peripheral nerve injury and/or dysesthesias can occur if the medication is administered into the nerve or nerve sheath. Severe side effects such as cardiac arrest, death, or seizure can occur if the medication is administered intravenously [9].

Appropriate choice of peripheral nerve blockade around the hip and knee requires understanding of the related anatomy. Sensory innervation around the knee consists of the femoral nerve (anterior cutaneous innervation), posterior cutaneous nerve of the thigh (posterior), obturator nerve (medial), and lateral femoral cutaneous nerve (lateral). With a femoral nerve block, local anesthetic is introduced into the femoral canal, which results in anesthesia in the distribution of the femoral nerve as well as lateral femoral cutaneous and obturator nerves. The effect is both sensory and motor. The sensory distribution affected by a femoral nerve block includes the anterior, lateral, and medial thigh as well as the anterior shin. A key aspect of femoral nerve blocks is associated quadriceps weakness, which

requires a knee immobilizer to prevent falls with early ambulation. The risk of falling after a femoral nerve block is reported to be 1.6–7%, while the risk of reoperation in one study was found to be 0.4% [10]

Adductor canal blocks target sensory nerves in the adductor canal with rare motor weakness. The sensory nerves include the saphenous nerve, the articular branch of the obturator nerve, and the medial retinacular nerve, providing blockade to the anteromedial knee (from the superior pole of the patella) and medial lower leg. Adductor canal blocks also involve the motor nerve to the vastus medialis, but this is of little functional consequence. Since quadriceps function is spared, there is no concern for weakness. No large-scale clinical trials have been performed comparing adductor canal blocks to femoral nerve blocks; however, smaller trials have shown equivalent pain relief with improved postoperative mobility with the former [11–13].

Other types of peripheral nerve blockade used mostly for hip procedures include lumbar plexus block, fascia iliaca block, and sciatic nerve block. The lumbar plexus block (psoas compartment block) and fascia iliaca block both have similar sensory and motor blockade as a femoral nerve block, whereas the sciatic nerve block covers posterior aspect of the hip and knee and entire lower limb below the knee (motor and sensory) except the medial leg and foot (covered by the saphenous nerve). The skin overlying the posterior aspect of thigh is innervated by posterior cutaneous nerve of the thigh which originates more proximally in the sacral plexus.

Regional anesthesia can be delivered as a single shot or continuously via insertion of a catheter. Since local anesthetics wear off in a matter of hours, insertion of a catheter at the time of administering the blockade can help prolong anesthesia. The risks of continuous catheters are relatively low, and the main contraindication is active infection in the area receiving the peripheral nerve blockade. Multiple regional anesthesia strategies demonstrate efficacy; however, specifics will depend on hospital resources, anesthesia skill set, and perioperative work flow.

Intraoperative Anesthesia

When performing hip and knee arthroplasty, the anesthetic options include general anesthesia, neuraxial anesthesia (spinal/epidural), or combination general/neuraxial. Overall the literature supports an increased safety profile and improved outcomes with neuraxial anesthesia. Multiple reports (including several large database studies) had been published showing neuraxial anesthesia is associated with decreased mortality, surgical site infections, transfusion rates, length of stay, cost, and surgical times [14–16]. Notably, the benefits of spinal anesthesia may be greatest in less healthy patients with higher American Society of Anesthesiologist scores.

Neuraxial anesthesia involves delivery of a local anesthetic with or without narcotic to either the spinal or epidural space. Similar to peripheral nerve blockade, this can be given as a single shot or a continuous infusion via catheter. Methods to extend a single-shot neuraxial anesthetic include following the injection with an epinephrine wash to elicit vasoconstriction or adding long-acting narcotics to the cocktail. The risks of neuraxial anesthesia are quite low, with a reported complication rate of 0.03% and failure rate of 4% [2]. Serious but rare risks include spinal/epidural hematoma or abscess, cauda equina, and meningitis. More common adverse effects include postoperative hypotension and urinary retention (leading to common use of urinary catheters). Urinary retention is rare when spinals are performed with local anesthetic as opposed to opioids, so some surgeons only use catheters in those patients that have risk factors for retention including a history of benign prostatic hypertrophy, renal failure, neurogenic bladder, longer operative time, and age over 67 years [17].

The American Society of Regional Anesthesiologists has developed guidelines for the use of neuraxial anesthesia and chemoprophylaxis, noting that the use of twice-daily dosing for low molecular weight heparin (LMWH) is associated with a greater risk of spinal hematoma formation [18]. Their guidelines stipulate the removal of epidural catheters before any LMWH has been administered and waiting 2 hours after catheter removal to initiate chemoprophylaxis. Low molecular weight heparin may be initiated 6–8 hours after surgery, but the epidural catheter may only be removed 10–12 hours after the last administration of LMWH. If warfarin is used, then the catheters should be removed before the international normalized ratio rises above 1.4. The use of aspirin does not affect timing of removal of epidural catheters.

Periarticular Injections

Surgeon-administered intraoperative analgesia includes periarticular injections, which have been consistently shown to alleviate pain and decrease narcotic usage. The individual formulation of the periarticular injection remains a matter of debate and personal preference, with multiple studies showing efficacy for various mixtures (Table 6.1). Anesthetics that have been studied include formulations of local amide anesthetics, clonidine, ketorolac, corticosteroids, epinephrine, and morphine with or without the addition of antibiotics. Injections are given into the surrounding tissue around the knee joint during surgery, and care should be taken to administer the medication thoroughly into the periarticular structures and periosteum including the posterior capsule. It is important, however, to avoid the central posterior capsule near the neurovascular bundle as well as the far posterolateral aspect of the knee joint to avoid the peroneal nerve.

Particularly controversial is liposomal bupivacaine, with some studies showing benefits and others showing no significant difference in alalgesia when compared to standard formulations. Given the limited evidence of significant benefit of liposomal bupivacaine compared to other modalities and its significant additional cost, its routine use is likely not justified [22–25]. Periarticular infusion through an elastomeric device placed intraoperatively is another option for intra-articular pain control. Studies have shown these devices to be of some efficacy; however, they carry a higher cost, and patient tolerance and management can be an issue [26].

Table 6.1 Periarticular injections

Study	Components	Administration
Busch et al. [19]	400 mg ropivacaine (80 mL of 0.5% ropivacaine at 5 mg/mL) 30 mg ketorolac (1 mL at 30 mg/mL) 0.6 mg of 1:1000 epinephrine (0.6 mL At 1 mg/mL) 5 mg epimorphine (0.5 mL at 10 mg/mL)	Dilute cocktail to a total volume of 100 mL using normal saline. Prior to component implantation, inject 20 mL into posterior capsule and medial and lateral collateral ligaments. During cement curing, inject 20 mL into quadriceps and retinacular tissues. After component implantation, inject 60 mL into fat and subcuticular tissues
Kelley et al. [20]	246.25 mg ropivacaine (49.25 mL of 0.5% ropivacaine at 5 mg/mL) 0.5 mg 1:1000 epinephrine (0.5 mL at 1 mg/mL) 30 mg ketorolac (1 mL at 30 mg/mL) 0.08 mg clonidine (0.8 mL at 1 mg/10 mL)	Dilute cocktail to a total volume of 100 mL using normal saline. Prior to component implantation, inject 9 mL into posterolateral soft tissues and lateral femoral periosteum, 10 mL into posteromedial soft tissues and medial femoral periosteum, and 1 mL into PCL. After component implantation, inject 25 mL into medial meniscus remnant and inferomedial capsule, 25 mL into superomedial capsule, 10 mL into lateral capsule, 10 mL into medial subcutaneous tissues, and 10 mL into lateral subcutaneous tissues
Parvataneni et al. [21]	200–400 mg bupivacaine (40 mL of 0.5% bupivacaine [200 mg] at 5 mg/mL or 53 mL of 0.75% bupivacaine [400 mg] at 7.5 mg/mL) 4–10 mg morphine sulfate (0.421 mL at 10 mg/mL) 0.3 mg of 1:1000 epinephrine (0.3 mL at 1 mg/mL) 40 mg methylprednisolone acetate (1 mL at 40 mg/mL) (contraindicated in diabetic or immune-compromised patients) 750 mg cefuroxime (substitute vancomycin if patient has penicillin allergy)	Dilute cocktail to a total volume of 60 mL using normal saline. After components cemented, but before liner is inserted, inject 15 mL into posterior capsule and posteromedial and posterolateral structures. After liner is inserted and knee is reduced, inject remaining 45 mL into extensor mechanism, synovium, capsule, pes anserinus, anteromedial capsule, periosteum, iliotibial band, and collateral ligaments and origins

The comparisons of various periarticular injections and regional anesthesia make distinct conclusions difficult given the variability in the literature; however, there is sound evidence that periarticular injections have benefit when compared to standard narcotic-based regimens without regional anesthesia. The low cost and potential benefit of most periarticular injections likely justify their routine use.

Postoperative Medications

Multimodal postoperative pain control begins with scheduled nonnarcotic medications including acetaminophen, celecoxib or other nonsteroidal anti-inflammatories, gabapentinoids with scheduled and as-needed opioids, tramadol, and ketorolac. Although patient-controlled analgesia (PCA) machines were previously the standard of care at many institutions, there is concern that these increase the overall use of narcotics and associated side effects while negatively affecting length of stay; therefore, PCA is rarely utilized after joint arthroplasty. Medications to decrease the side effects of opioids are also an important adjunct, including antiemetics and constipation mitigation. Multimodal postoperative regimens result in improved pain control and patient satisfaction while decreasing narcotic use and length of stay [8, 27, 28].

While a standard multimodal pain management protocol is able to provide adequate analgesia for most patients, there are some patients who need increased doses of pain medications. The first step should be to increase the dose of short-acting narcotics. Some may consider long-acting narcotics in certain situations. There are patients whose pain needs exceed the expertise of the orthopedic surgeon, and consultation of the anesthesia pain service is beneficial in these situations. The pain service should be preemptively consulted in patients identified preoperatively who consume high doses of narcotics on a daily basis (>100 mg oral morphine equivalents) and have a history of substance abuse disorder or those who are on methadone or buprenorphine.

Opioid Addiction Epidemic

The United States is in the midst of a national epidemic of nontherapeutic opioid use. Opioid-related deaths occur with greater frequency than suicide or motor vehicle collisions. With the introduction of pain as the fifth vital sign and growing emphasis of controlling a patient's pain as an integral part of patient satisfaction, physicians have up until recently been incentivized to prescribe more narcotics. In many instances, this is a patient's first step into addiction. Orthopedic surgeons write 7.7% of all opioid prescriptions in the United States, placing them as the third highest prescribers of narcotics among all physicians [29]. While our patients are likely to be in pain in the postoperative period or following an acute injury, it is important that orthopedic surgeons prescribe opioid medications for as short of a duration as possible. In the setting of elective surgery such as arthroplasty, patients should be informed ahead of time that they are only going to receive narcotics for a defined period following surgery and that the surgeon will not continue to provide them with such medications after they have recovered from their procedure. Additionally, patients should be advised preoperatively that the alternative nonnarcotic multimodal pain management regimens should reduce the need for narcotics.

Current Protocol

While pain management strategies vary across centers, the current protocol at our institution is as follows. Preemptive preoperative medications for all patients unless contraindicated are acetaminophen 1000 mg PO, celecoxib 400 mg PO, and gabapentin 600 mg PO administered in preoperative suite within 1–2 hours of surgical incision. Patients undergoing total knee replacement receive an adductor canal catheter that is dosed with ropivacaine pre- and intraoperatively, infused postoperatively, and removed on the morning of postoperative day 1. We also use the periarticular "cocktail" described by Kelley et al. (Table 6.1) for total knee and total hip patients [20].

All total joint and partial knee arthroplasty recipients receive a short-acting spinal anesthetic. Postoperatively all patients receive around-the-clock acetaminophen (1000 mg every 6–8 hours), gabapentin (600 mg at bedtime), and celecoxib (200 mg twice daily) with oxycodone PO (5–10 mg every 4 hours) as needed. Hydromorphone is available for IV breakthrough pain but is not needed in most patients. Patients may also receive up to 4 doses of ketorolac (15 mg IV every 6 hours) if needed for additional pain control. Long-acting narcotics are avoided. Patients are discharged on the same multimodal regimen of acetaminophen, celecoxib, gabapentin, and oxycodone.

Summary

Hip and knee arthroplasty are among the most successful procedures in medicine for restoring function and decreasing pain. Significant improvements in perioperative pain control with a multimodal pain strategy can maximize functional gain while decreasing complications and minimizing narcotic side effects. Treating pain involves frank conversations with the patient and their family as well as coordination with all members of the team from the orthopedic surgeon and anesthesiologist to the nursing and physiotherapy staff. The modern arthroplasty surgeon should employ a combination of preemptive, perioperative, and regional modalities to take a global approach toward pain management.

References

1. Joshi GP, Ogunnaike BO. Consequences of inadequate postoperative pain relief and chronic persistent postoperative pain. Anesthesiol Clin North Am. 2005;23:21–36. https://doi.org/10.1016/j.atc.2004.11.013.
2. Moucha CS, Weiser MC, Levin EJ. Current strategies in anesthesia and analgesia for total knee arthroplasty. J Am Acad Orthop Surg. 2016;24(2):60–73. https://doi.org/10.5435/JAAOS-D-14-00259.
3. Yeh YC, Reddy P. Clinical and economic evidence for intravenous acetaminophen. Pharmacotherapy. 2012;32:559–79. https://doi.org/10.1002/j.1875-9114.2011.01085.x.
4. Schroer WC, Diesfeld PJ, LeMarr AR, Reedy ME. Benefits of prolonged postoperative cyclooxygenase-2 inhibitor administration on total knee arthroplasty recovery: a double-blind, placebo-controlled study. J Arthroplast. 2011;26:2–7. https://doi.org/10.1016/j.arth.2011.04.007.
5. Buvanendran A, Kroin JS, Della Valle CJ, Kari M, Moric M, Tuman KJ. Perioperative oral pregabalin reduces chronic pain after total knee arthroplasty: a prospective, randomized, controlled trial. Anesth Analg. 2010;110:199–207. https://doi.org/10.1213/ANE.0b013e3181c4273a.
6. Nguyen L-CL, Sing DC, Bozic KJ. Preoperative reduction of opioid use before total joint arthroplasty. J Arthroplast. 2016;31:282–7. https://doi.org/10.1016/j.arth.2016.01.068.
7. Woolf CJ. Central sensitization: implications for the diagnosis and treatment of pain. Pain. 2012;152:1–31. https://doi.org/10.1016/j.pain.2010.09.030.Central.
8. Hebl JR, Dilger JA, Byer DE, Kopp SL, Stevens SR, Pagnano MW, et al. A pre-emptive multimodal pathway featuring peripheral nerve block improves perioperative outcomes after major orthopedic surgery. Reg Anesth Pain Med. 2008;33:510–7. https://doi.org/10.1016/j.rapm.2008.04.008.
9. Ben-David B. Complications of regional anesthesia: an overview. Anesthesiol Clin North Am. 2002;20:665–7, ix
10. Sharma S, Iorio R, Specht LM, Davies-Lepie S, Healy WL. Complications of femoral nerve block for total knee arthroplasty. Clin Orthop Relat Res. 2010;468:135–40. https://doi.org/10.1007/s11999-009-1025-1.
11. Patterson ME, Bland KS, Thomas LC, Elliott CE, Soberon JR, Nossaman BD, et al. The adductor canal block provides effective analgesia similar to a femoral nerve block in patients undergoing total knee arthroplasty: a retrospective study. J Clin Anesth. 2015;27:39–44. https://doi.org/10.1016/j.jclinane.2014.08.005.
12. Kim DH, Lin Y, Goytizolo EA, Kahn RL, Maalouf DB, Manohar A, et al. Adductor canal block versus femoral nerve block for total knee arthroplasty: a prospective, randomized, controlled trial. Anesthesiology. 2014;120:540–50. https://doi.org/10.1097/ALN.0000000000000119.
13. Ludwigson JL, Tillmans SD, Galgon RE, Chambers TA, Heiner JP, Schroeder KM. A comparison of single shot adductor canal block versus femoral nerve catheter for total knee arthroplasty. J Arthroplast. 2015;30:68–71. https://doi.org/10.1016/j.arth.2015.03.044.
14. Pugely AJ, Martin CT, Gao Y, Mendoza-Lattes S, Callaghan JJ. Differences in short-term complications between spinal and general anesthesia for primary total knee arthroplasty. J Bone Joint Surg Am. 2013;95:193–9. https://doi.org/10.2106/JBJS.K.01682.
15. Basques BA, Toy JO, Bohl DD, Golinvaux NS, Grauer JN. General compared with spinal anesthesia for total hip arthroplasty. J Bone Joint Surg Am. 2015;97:455–61. https://doi.org/10.2106/jbjs.n.00662.
16. Parvizi J, Bloomfield MR. Multimodal pain management in orthopedics: implications for joint arthroplasty surgery. Orthopedics. 2013;36:7–14. https://doi.org/10.3928/01477447-20130122-51.
17. Miller AG, McKenzie J, Greenky M, Shaw E, Gandhi K, Hozack WJ, et al. Spinal anesthesia: should everyone receive a urinary catheter?: a randomized, prospective study of patients undergoing total hip arthroplasty. J Bone Joint Surg Am. 2013;95:1498–503. https://doi.org/10.2106/JBJS.K.01671.
18. Horlocker TT, Wedel DJ, Rowlingson JC, Enneking FK, Kopp SL, Benzon HT, et al. Regional anesthesia in the patient receiving antithrombotic or thrombolytic therapy: American Society of Regional Anesthesia and Pain Medicine Evidence-Based Guidelines (Third Edition). Reg Anesth Pain Med. 2010;35:64–101. https://doi.org/10.1097/AAP.0b013e3181c15c70.
19. Busch CA, Shore BJ, Bhandari R, Ganapathy S, MacDonald SJ, Bourne RB, et al. Efficacy of periarticular multimodal drug injection in total knee arthroplasty. A randomized trial. J Bone Joint Surg Am. 2006;88:959–63. https://doi.org/10.2106/JBJS.E.00344.
20. Kelley TC, Adams MJ, Mulliken BD, Dalury DF. Efficacy of multimodal perioperative analgesia protocol with periarticular medication injection in total knee arthroplasty: a randomized, double-blinded study. J Arthroplasty. 2013;28:1274–7. https://doi.org/10.1016/j.arth.2013.03.008.
21. Parvataneni HK, Shah VP, Howard H, Cole N, Ranawat AS, Ranawat CS. Controlling pain after total hip and knee arthroplasty using a multimodal protocol with local periarticular injections: a prospective randomized study. J Arthroplasty. 2007;22:33–8. https://doi.org/10.1016/j.arth.2007.03.034.
22. Schroer WC, Diesfeld PG, LeMarr AR, Morton DJ, Reedy ME. Does extended-release liposomal bupivacaine better control pain than Bupivacaine after total

knee Arthroplasty (TKA)? A prospective, randomized clinical trial. J Arthroplast. 2015;30:64–7. https://doi.org/10.1016/j.arth.2015.01.059.

23. Bagsby DT, Ireland PH, Meneghini RM. Liposomal bupivacaine versus traditional periarticular injection for pain control after total knee arthroplasty. J Arthroplast. 2014;29:1687–90. https://doi.org/10.1016/j.arth.2014.03.034.

24. Whiteside LA, Arima J. The anteroposterior axis for femoral rotational alignment in valgus total knee arthroplasty. Clin Orthop Relat Res. 1995;(321):168–72.

25. Alijanipour P, Tan TL, Matthews CN, Viola JR, Purtill JJ, Rothman RH, et al. Periarticular injection of liposomal bupivacaine offers no benefit over standard bupivacaine in total knee arthroplasty: a prospective, randomized, controlled trial. J Arthroplast. 2016;32(2):628–34. https://doi.org/10.1016/j.arth.2016.07.023.

26. Pagnano MW. Intra-articular infusion with bupivacaine decreased pain and opioid consumption after total knee arthroplasty. J Bone Joint Surg Am. 2013;95A:940. https://doi.org/10.2106/JBJS.9510.ebo195.

27. Duellman TJ, Gaffigan C, Milbrandt JC, Allan DG. Multi-modal, pre-emptive analgesia decreases the length of hospital stay following total joint arthroplasty. Orthopedics. 2009;32:167.

28. Parvizi J, Miller AG, Gandhi K. Multimodal pain management after total joint arthroplasty. J Bone Joint Surg Am. 2011;93:1075–84. https://doi.org/10.2106/JBJS.J.01095.

29. Morris B. The opioid epidemic: impact on orthopaedic surgery. J Am Acad Orthop Surg. 2015;23:267–71. https://doi.org/10.5435/JAAOS-D-14-00163.

Cost-Effectiveness Analysis of Robotic Arthroplasty

7

Kevin K. Chen, Kelvin Y. Kim,
Jonathan M. Vigdorchik, Patrick A. Meere,
Joseph A. Bosco, and Richard Iorio

Throughout modern history, there has been a trend toward automation as technology advances to replace human labor. Machines have consistently proven to be an efficient, cost-effective, and valuable addition to the productivity of the human labor force [1]. Similarly, the introduction of robotic systems into orthopedic surgery has been touted as a promising opportunity to improve surgical and clinical outcomes. For nearly 20 years, robotic-assisted orthopedic surgeries have been performed [2]. Since then, the field of robotic surgery has rapidly expanded to include multiple systems. It is now utilized in various procedures with the goal of limiting human error and maximizing the ability to restore proper joint alignment and kinematics while providing optimal component positioning [2, 3].

The use of robotic systems in orthopedic surgery has primarily focused on total knee arthroplasty (TKA), total hip arthroplasty (THA), unicompartmental knee arthroplasty (UKA), with lesser but expanding use in patellofemoral arthroplasty (PFA), and spinal procedures. Early reports on surgical outcomes have been favorable, specifically with respect to more accurate and precise alignment, implant positioning, and improved gap balancing compared to conventional techniques [4–6]. However, given the relatively recent introduction of these procedures, there is limited data on long-term clinical outcomes to justify their associated economic burden. As healthcare systems continue to emphasize the delivery of value-based care through quality improvement and expenditure reductions, the margins for inefficiencies and sub-optimal quality of care continue to narrow. Thus, the utilization of cost-effectiveness analysis to evaluate the value of these novel technologies before they can be accepted as alternatives to traditional techniques is necessary [7, 8].

This chapter will discuss the economic viability of implementing robotic-assisted technology for THA, TKA, and UKA procedures. Emphasis will be placed on the costs of purchasing and operating the systems, the increasing demand for these procedures, and the clinical and cost-effectiveness outcomes associated with each robotic system.

K. K. Chen · K. Y. Kim · J. M. Vigdorchik
P. A. Meere · J. A. Bosco
Department of Orthopaedic Surgery, NYU Langone
Medical Center, Hospital for Joint Diseases,
New York, NY, USA

R. Iorio (✉)
Department of Orthopaedic Surgery, Brigham and
Women's Hospital, Boston, MA, USA
e-mail: Richard.Iorio@nyumc.org

© Springer Nature Switzerland AG 2019
J. H. Lonner (ed.), *Robotics in Knee and Hip Arthroplasty*,
https://doi.org/10.1007/978-3-030-16593-2_7

Types of Robotic Systems

Robotic arthroplasty systems can broadly be divided into active, semi-active, and passive control systems based on the degree of surgeon control over the robot. These systems are currently limited to primary joint arthroplasty procedures, with ongoing development to expand to revision arthroplasty. Passive robotic systems are under the full control of the surgeon while active systems can perform a procedure without any surgeon involvement. Semi-active systems are a combination of the two in which the surgeon is in total control of the robotic tool but is restricted by a restrictive feedback system. These systems prevent the robot from making bony cuts beyond a set of predetermined boundaries, thus protecting vulnerable and important soft tissue structures immediately adjacent to the joint (specifically the neurovascular bundles and support ligaments). Reliable spatial awareness allows for less dependence on direct visualization and consequently smaller soft tissue exposure with corollary potential rehabilitation advantage. Semi-active systems include *Mako* (Mako Stryker, Mahwah, New Jersey, USA), *Navio* (Smith & Nephew, Memphis, TN, USA), and *Omni* (OmniLife Science, Raynham, Mass), while *TSolutioin One* robots (THINK Surgical, Fremont, CA, USA) are fully autonomous, active systems. A summary of the surgical capabilities and pricing requirements of each of these systems is illustrated in Table 7.1.

Table 7.1 Robot-specific fees and capabilities of various robotic arthroplasty systems

	Mako	Navio	TSolution One	Omni
Robot-specific fees				
Capital investment	Yes	Yes	Yes	No
Service/maintenance contract	Yes	Yes	Yes	No
Preoperative CT scan required?	Yes	No	Yes	No
Closed platform?	Yes	No	No	Yes
Capabilities				
THA	Yes	No	Yes	Yes
TKA	Yes	Yes	No	Yes
UKA	Yes	Yes	No	No

THA total hip arthroplasty, *TKA* total knee arthroplasty, *UKA* unicompartmental knee arthroplasty

Direct Costs of the Robotic Systems

The costs associated with purchasing and operating robotic systems include the (1) robot tool itself and operational costs, (2) disposables, (3) preoperative imaging and scans (with some robotic systems), and (4) implants. As with all medical technologies, these expenses vary widely between each robotic system based on the unique manufacturer's license agreements, hospital volume, and negotiated pricing. In order to assess the economic feasibility of the various robotic systems, a discussion of these list prices is useful.

The price of the various robotic systems is reported to be between $400,000 and $1.2 million [9, 10]. The annual maintenance agreement, which is required in most systems, is listed between $40,000 and $150,000 per robot. Another significant and costly yearly cost is the software upgrade, which may be included in the annual maintenance agreement. In some cases, discounted pricing may be negotiated if multiple systems are purchased, but this again varies by institution. Alternative payment models may also be offered, whereby systems are leased with a per-case pricing model instead of charging an upfront capital investment for the robotic equipment. In those circumstances, there may be no charge to use or maintain the robot; instead, costs are generated through charges of the company-specific implants and the disposables used during the case [9, 11].

Disposable costs include charges for intraoperative equipment used in each case such as drapes, pins, burs, saw blades, robotic-assist kits, and battery packs. Although traditional techniques have their own disposable costs, the per-case cost attributed to robotic-assisted cases are greater. Prices vary slightly between robotic systems and types of procedures (THA, TKA, UKA) but are estimated to cost between $750 and $1300 per case for all four robotic systems listed [9].

In order for proper calibration of the navigation system and implant placement planning and preparation, some robotic systems require an additional preoperative CT scan of the lower extremity. A lower extremity CT scan without contrast is approximately $260 [12]. These imaging modalities are required for every *Mako* and *TSolution One* procedure. Conversely, *Navio* and *Omni* are imageless systems that do not require any preoperative imaging. Instead they rely on intraoperative morphing technology, whereby a 3-D model of the knee in space can be created by manual registration of key joint surfaces and bony landmarks. It should be noted that although imageless modeling may save costs and patient travel time, it may add intraoperative time for morphing computation and implant templating.

The price of the implants makes up a significant portion of the overall hospital cost of any joint replacement procedure. In a 2012 report by Robinson et al., implants accounted for 12.71–87.07% of the total cost of a primary TKA procedures and 14.96–87.24% of a primary THA. This wide range in implant price range is explained in part by variances in geographical location, prices charged by different manufacturers, and negotiations with hospitals [13].

Implant choice in robotic-assisted procedures is often limited by whether or not a robotic system utilizes an "open" or "closed" platform. Though in principle all systems have the theoretical capacity to make generic cuts that might satisfy leg alignment and joint line obliquity requirements, the implant-customized pre-cut templating is restricted and proprietary. Closed platforms limit the surgeon to these specific, proprietary implant types. Open platforms, however, permit the surgeon to use multiple implant companies and designs depending on the surgeon's preference. Having an open platform allows the surgeon to choose implant systems that they may be more comfortable with while also providing variability in the cost of the implants. As with any market, a lack of variability can lead to decreased competition and increased pricing. It is not surprising, therefore, that robotic systems with closed platforms tend to have a greater proportion of their overall hospital cost dedicated to implants when compared to open platform systems. Open platform systems, such as *Navio* and *THINK,* provide per-case cost savings by allowing physicians to choose from a competitively priced implant market.

Direct Cost Comparison per Case to Traditional TJA

A cost analysis was performed to compare the increase in cost associated with the various robotic platforms to traditional techniques. The prices for each robotic system's fixed contractual costs, such as capital investment fees and manufacturer's maintenance agreements, as well as procedural costs, including disposable costs and imaging requirements, were individually assessed in this analysis. First, the fixed contractual costs were divided by estimated annual case volumes (100 or 300 cases) along with theoretical robotic life spans (5 or 10 years), providing us with the fixed contractual cost per case. Next, the procedural costs of a robotic TJA were subtracted from those of a traditional TJA to determine the projected increase in procedural costs per case. The fixed contractual costs per case were then added to the projected increase in procedural costs to ascertain the total increased direct costs per case. Finally, we converted this direct cost into a percentage relative to a traditional TJA by dividing this value by the average total cost of a traditional, non-robotic case (Table 7.2).

Using this method, we found that *Mako* adds roughly 12.2% and 6.1%, respectively, to the cost of each case if 100 and 300 cases are performed annually, assuming a 5-year robotic life span (Table 7.2). Under the same price model, *THINK* surgical, *Navio*, and *Omni* procedures add 13.9%, 6.1%, and 2.3%, respectively, per case when 100 cases are performed on a robot given a 5-year life span and 6.6%, 3.5%, and 2.3%, respectively, when 300 cases are performed. These analyses,

Table 7.2 Percentage increase in cost by annual case volume and robotic life span relative to traditional TJA based upon capital investment, maintenance fees, disposable cost, and imaging requirements

Estimated robotic lifetime	Annual case volume	Mako	Navio	TSolution One	Omni
5	100	12.19%	6.10%	13.90%	2.25%
	300	6.05%	3.53%	6.61%	2.25%
10	100	9.19%	4.82%	10.04%	2.25%
	300	5.05%	3.11%	5.33%	2.25%

***Implant pricing was not factored into this model

however, do not account for implant pricing variability, which can affect the overall value of these procedures significantly.

Institutional Data

At our institution, over 800 robotic procedures have been performed since 2012 with 2 of the 4 mentioned robotic systems (*Mako* and *Navio*). In the calendar year from April 2016 to April 2017, 199 Stryker *Mako* procedures were performed (TKA and THA). In this same time period, 29 *Smith & Nephew Navio* TKAs were performed and 25 Navio UKAs were used with various implants.

Surgical and Clinical Outcomes

As the use of robotics has become integrated more commonly into the practices of orthopedic surgeons over the past few decades, the body of literature reporting the radiographic outcomes associated with these techniques has grown substantially. To justify the large capital fees, service costs, and institution-wide learning curves associated with the integration of these technologies, incremental cost savings measured through clinical improvements, such as revision rates, implant durability, length of stay, and patient satisfaction, among other quality metrics, must be assessed. Once long-term outcomes are available, a better assessment of the cost-effectiveness of these techniques can be made.

THA, TKA, and UKA Procedures

Provided here is a brief overview of the short-term surgical and clinical outcomes associated with the use of robotics in THA, TKA, and UKA procedures followed by a review of their cost-effectiveness.

Total Knee Arthroplasty

Robotic-assisted TKA has produced improved accuracy with respect to leg alignment and flexion/extension gap balancing while significantly

reducing outliers compared to traditional methods [14–19]. When assessing implant placement specifically, improvements in both accuracy and precision have been achieved along the coronal femoral, sagittal femoral, and sagittal tibial angles, consistently measuring within 1 degree of error compared with manual techniques [14, 15, 20, 21].

These surgical findings, however, have not always translated into clinical benefits. A study comparing the *Robodoc* system and conventional techniques by Park and Lee [21] showed no differences in clinical outcome with respect to postoperative range of motion and patient-reported outcome (PRO) scores measured using the Knee Society Score over a 4-year follow-up period [21]. Other randomized control trials have found a similar lack of differences in PRO scores measured by the Hospital for Special Surgery (HSS) score and Western Ontario and McMaster University Arthritis Index (WOMAC) at both 1-year and 3-year follow-up periods [15, 17].

Total Hip Arthroplasty

In an early large multicentered randomized clinical trial comparing 65 *Robodoc*-assisted cementless THAs to 62 manual THA procedures, significant improvements in fit, fill, and alignment were achieved [22]. Since then, robotic-assisted techniques have demonstrated up to a sixfold increase in accuracy with respect to anteversion, inclination, offset, and desired leg length when compared to manual THA [23–25]. Robotic-assisted THA has also shown improvements with respect to short-term clinical outcomes. Patients have experienced improved complication rates including a significantly lower prevalence of dislocations when compared to manual THA [5]. Patient-reported outcome (PRO) data has also demonstrated improved activity levels, pain levels, level of deformity, and range of motion [26].

Unicompartmental Knee Arthroplasty

The first 57 UKAs using the *Navio* system achieved postoperative mechanical alignment within 1 degree of the intraoperative plan in 91% of cases. Robotic-assisted *Mako* UKAs have shown similar success in recreating the posterior tibial slope and achieving coronal-tibial alignment significantly more accurately and with less variability than manual techniques [27–29]. Moreover, *Mako*-assisted tibial and femoral component alignment has proven to be more accurate and precise when measured in all planes [30, 31]. Clinically, studies that have investigated robotic UKA outcomes with respect to patient satisfaction, postoperative pain, functionality, and revision rates have all demonstrated advantageous results [32]. A multicenter study by Conditt et al. showed that 93% of patients who underwent robotic-assisted UKA were either very satisfied or satisfied with their procedure at 2-year follow-up [33]. The same study showed that cumulative revision rates (1.1%) were lower than previous reports of 4.5% in manual UKAs.

Cost-Effectiveness

There is a paucity of data regarding major cost drivers throughout the postoperative stages of joint arthroplasty such as revisions and readmissions. The data is further limited by the fact that the majority of the literature available assesses first-generation robotic platforms. Among TKA procedures, robotic techniques have been reported to have a 5% lower rate of readmission than conventional techniques [9]. Extrapolating this data, we can calculate differences in cost with respect to robotic and traditional TKA by factoring in the average cost of a typical revision TKA. This cost was then converted into a percentage increase by comparing it to the cost of an average primary TKA (Table 7.3). This amounts

Table 7.3 Percentage cost difference for robotic-assisted procedures

% Cost Difference due to:	THA	UKA	TKA
Revision rate	+20.88%	−5.39%	–
Minimum 90-day readmission rate	−0.53%	–	−4.01%
Total	+20.35%	−5.39%	−4.01%

***Costs reported as % increase or decrease from traditional primary procedure

to a 4.0% decrease in the overall cost of a primary TKA when using robotic instrumentation (Table 7.3).

In a study comparatively evaluating robotic and traditional THA, the rate of revision was 12.3% higher in the robotic cohort [34]. Conversely, another study reported a slightly decreased rate of postoperative complications resulting in fewer readmissions with robotic-assisted THA (13.8% vs. 14.5%), albeit not statistically significant [22]. Using a similar methodology as above, robotic-assisted THA was associated with a 20.3% increase in cost when compared to traditional THA.

The difference in revision rate between robotic and traditional UKAs has been reported to be 3.4% [10], potentially resulting in a cost savings of 5.39% per UKA (Table 7.3) when robotic-assisted instrumentation is utilized. Approximately 80% of UKAs that require revision receive a TKA [35] incurring a cost of roughly $49,360 per revision [36]. As a result, with respect to revision rates, robotic-assisted UKAs may save institutions approximately $170,000 dollars annually assuming a case volume of 100 UKAs.

Surgical Limitations of Robotic-Assisted Techniques

Robotic-assisted procedures are associated with specific complications not observed in manual procedures. These include fractures during pin placement, as well as mechanical and hardware failures that necessitate conversion to a manual procedure. Rates of complications have been reported to be as high as 22%, the majority arising from technical or mechanical errors [37]. Robotic procedures have also demonstrated significantly longer operating times largely due to a steep learning curve as well as the time needed to prepare and calibrate the robotic system intraoperatively. Not only are longer operating times associated with substantial financial expenditures, they also increase the risk of superficial and deep infection, additional sources of avoidable expenses [38]. Altogether, as more longitudinal data becomes available, these limitations must be considered carefully when judging the overall value of these procedures.

Case Volume and Robotic Lifetime

One requirement to justify the use of robotic systems in arthroplasty procedures is an adequate demand for such procedures. As the "baby-boomer" population continues to age, the prevalence of osteoarthritis and the demand for lower extremity arthroplasty procedures have substantially increased. The demand for THA and TKA is projected to reach 4 million procedures by 2030 [7]. Furthermore, there are approximately 45,000 UKA procedures performed in the United States annually, and this number continues to increase at a rate of 32.5% per year [8]. Previous studies have projected that based on the incremental cost savings, which take into account the clinical benefits of the procedures, associated with robotic-assisted UKA and TKA procedures, returns on investments may occur after just 2 years, given caseloads of 50 and 20 after 1 year and 70 and 30 after 2 years, respectively [39]. A Markov decision analysis performed on patients undergoing *Mako* UKAs determined that its incremental cost-effectiveness ratio (ICER) was $47,180 per quality-adjusted life year (QALY). Based on previous studies that have identified $50,000 as the lowest threshold of willingness to pay (WTP) for a QALY, robotic UKAs were identified as cost-effective. However, in their analysis, Moschetti et al. point out that these values can only be achieved in high-volume centers that perform greater than 94 robotic UKA cases annually while maintaining a 2-year failure rate below 1.2%. Although most institutions do not currently meet these case volume thresholds, platforms such as the *Navio*, which requires significantly lower capital fees (almost 50% lower) and affords more variability in implant pricing, may serve as an alternative for institutions with smaller cases performed. In a very low-volume situation, the Omni model, with no capital expense, becomes more attractive.

With the exception of *Omni* robots, there is a direct inverse relationship between case volume and percentage increase in cost. As demonstrated by prior studies, high-volume institutions have a much greater opportunity to profit from the incremental cost savings of each robotic case [37, 39]. These case volumes are not currently the norm for most institutions. However, as the popularity of robotic-assisted procedures increases and surgeon familiarity improves, these thresholds will gradually become more attainable. Furthermore, if improved surgical and clinical outcomes continue to accompany these procedures, costs may be increasingly offset by higher reimbursement rates. Given the impact that case volumes have on determining the value of robotic systems, those that are capable of multiple types of procedures (THA, TKA, and UKA) are expected to be economically more advantageous. This removes the need to invest in separate robotic systems for each procedure type while also distributing the fixed contractual costs over a greater case volume.

Finally, the life span of the robot itself is paramount to the long-term practicality of these procedures. If a new capital investment is required every 10 years rather than 5 years, it would significantly alter the number of procedures needed to create a return on investment. This is apparent considering an institution that performs 100 procedures annually adds a hypothetical cost of 9% per case over a 10-year period when using Mako systems but as much as 12% per case over a 5-year estimated robotic life span (Table 7.2).

Conclusion

The economic practicality of implementing a novel technique with large upfront costs and uncertain long-term clinical improvements must be examined closely. This issue is magnified by the fact that traditional joint arthroplasty is already considered a highly successful and expensive procedure [35]. As the goal of patient care continues to evolve to optimize clinical outcomes in an economically responsible manner, opportunities exist to improve upon traditional techniques.

Given the costly capital fees and annual contracts of robotic systems, value relies on an inverse relationship between case volume and cost-per-case pricing. Since fixed contractual costs are distributed equally among the number of cases performed, the more robotic-assisted cases an institution is capable of performing, the lower the economic burden will be on each case. Moreover, as surgeons gain more experience with these techniques, and patients become more comfortable with this novel concept, increased case volumes can be expected to follow. Preliminary literature has presented mostly favorable short-term clinical outcomes with decreased revision rates in UKA and decreased readmission rates following robotic THA and TKA. In order for robotic techniques to remain viable, long-term outcome assessment will need to continue to support current short-term findings.

Other unknowns remain including the modifications that payment models will undergo as companies adapt to growing competition within this field. These changes may facilitate the development of more economically feasible pricing arrangements. For example, *Omni* does not require any capital investment or an annual maintenance fee but instead relies on per-case charges such as implants and disposables. Thus, smaller institutions that cannot maintain large case volumes or cannot afford the initial capital fees may consider *Omni* as a more viable option compared to other systems. Furthermore, uncertainties exist as to whether companies will decide to reduce restrictions on implant compatibility with their robotic systems. As implant pricing can play a large role in the total cost of arthroplasty, the ability to choose from a wider range of implants is potentially an area for significant cost savings. Thus, open platform systems including *THINK* and *Navio* may help mitigate the overall cost of these robotic-assisted procedures by providing the opportunity for reduced implant pricing. Closed systems such as Omni and Mako may offer wider ranges of implants in order to decrease per-case costs for robotic-assisted arthroplasty. The increase of value-based implant availability and the decrease in perceived benefit of high-priced implants in the US marketplace make implant choice a critical feature of robotic-assisted systems.

Overall, there is optimism surrounding the concept of robotic-assisted procedures becoming a standard technique in joint arthroplasty. However, in a cost-effective, performance-based healthcare environment, clinicians must thoroughly consider all aspects of these techniques to ensure that patient care is delivered in a value-based manner.

References

1. Bohn RE. From art to science in manufacturing: the evolution of technical knowledge. Found Trends Technol Informat Oper Manag. 2005;1(2):1–82.
2. Jacofsky DJ, Allen M. Robotics in arthroplasty: a comprehensive review. J Arthroplast. 2016;31(10):2353–63. https://doi.org/10.1016/j.arth.2016.05.026.
3. Bargar WL. Robots in orthopaedic surgery: past, present, and future. Clin Orthop Relat Res. 2007;463:31–6. http://www.ncbi.nlm.nih.gov/pubmed/17960673. Accessed 24 Apr 2017.
4. Bell SW, Anthony I, Jones B, MacLean A, Rowe P, Blyth M. Improved accuracy of component positioning with robotic-assisted unicompartmental knee arthroplasty: data from a prospective, randomized controlled study. J Bone Joint Surg Am. 2016;98(8):627–35. https://doi.org/10.2106/JBJS.15.00664.
5. Elson L, Dounchis J, Illgen R, et al. Precision of acetabular cup placement in robotic integrated total hip arthroplasty. Hip Int. 2015;25(6):531–6. https://doi.org/10.5301/hipint.5000289.
6. Keene G, Simpson D, Kalairajah Y. Limb alignment in computer-assisted minimally-invasive unicompartmental knee replacement. J Bone Joint Surg Br. 2006;88(1):44–8. https://doi.org/10.1302/0301-620X.88B1.16266.
7. Kurtz S, Ong K, Lau E, Mowat F, Halpern M. Projections of primary and revision hip and knee arthroplasty in the United States from 2005 to 2030. J Bone Joint Surg Am. 2007;89(4):780–5. https://doi.org/10.2106/JBJS.F.00222.
8. Riddle DL, Jiranek WA, McGlynn FJ. Yearly incidence of unicompartmental knee arthroplasty in the United States. J Arthroplast. 2008;23(3):408–12. https://doi.org/10.1016/j.arth.2007.04.012.
9. Frost and Sullivan. Comprehensive Care for Joint Replacement (CJR) ROI model – comparative analysis of robot assisted versus conventional surgical technique; 2017.
10. Mako Surgical Corp. Makoplasty Financial Summary; 2017. http://www.makosurgical.com/.
11. Argenson J-NA, Blanc G, Aubaniac J-M, et al. Modern unicompartmental knee arthroplasty with cement: a concise follow-up, at a mean of twenty years, of a previous report. J Bone Joint Surg Am. 2013;95(10):905–9. https://doi.org/10.2106/JBJS.L.00963.
12. Centers for Medicare and Medicaid Services. No Title. https://www.medicare.gov/coverage/diagnostic-tests.html. Published 2017. Accessed 1 March 2017.
13. Robinson JC, Pozen A, Tseng S, et al. Variability in costs associated with total hip and knee replacement

implants. J Bone Joint Surg Am. 2012;94(18):1693–8. https://doi.org/10.2106/JBJS.K.00355.

14. Banerjee S, Cherian JJ, Elmallah RK, Jauregui JJ, Pierce TP, Mont MA. Robotic-assisted knee arthroplasty. Expert Rev Med Devices. 2015;12(6):727–35. https://doi.org/10.1586/17434440.2015.1086264.

15. Song E-K, Seon J-K, Park S-J, Jung W, Park H-W, Lee GW. Simultaneous bilateral total knee arthroplasty with robotic and conventional techniques: a prospective, randomized study. Knee Surg Sports Traumatol Arthrosc. 2011;19(7):1069–76. https://doi.org/10.1007/s00167-011-1400-9.

16. Bellemans J, Vandenneucker H, Vanlauwe J. Robot-assisted total knee arthroplasty. Clin Orthop Relat Res. 2007;464:111–6. https://doi.org/10.1097/BLO.0b013e318126c0c0.

17. Song E-K, Seon J-K, Yim J-H, Netravali NA, Bargar WL. Robotic-assisted TKA reduces postoperative alignment outliers and improves gap balance compared to conventional TKA. Clin Orthop Relat Res. 2013;471(1):118–26. https://doi.org/10.1007/s11999-012-2407-3.

18. Suero EM, Plaskos C, Dixon PL, Pearle AD. Adjustable cutting blocks improve alignment and surgical time in computer-assisted total knee replacement. Knee Surg Sport Traumatol Arthrosc. 2012;20(9):1736–41. https://doi.org/10.1007/s00167-011-1752-1.

19. Koulalis D, O'Loughlin PF, Plaskos C, Kendoff D, Cross MB, Pearle AD. Sequential versus automated cutting guides in computer-assisted total knee arthroplasty. Knee. 2011;18(6):436–42. https://doi.org/10.1016/j.knee.2010.08.007.

20. Bellemans J, Vandenneucker H, Vanlauwe J. Robot-assisted total knee arthroplasty. Clin Orthop Relat Res. 2007;PAP:111–6. https://doi.org/10.1097/BLO.0b013e318126c0c0.

21. Park SE, Lee CT. Comparison of robotic-assisted and conventional manual implantation of a primary total knee arthroplasty. J Arthroplast. 2007;22(7):1054–9. https://doi.org/10.1016/j.arth.2007.05.036.

22. Bargar WL, Bauer A, Börner M. Primary and revision total hip replacement using the Robodoc system. Clin Orthop Relat Res. 1998;(354):82–91. http://www.ncbi.nlm.nih.gov/pubmed/9755767. Accessed 24 Apr 2017.

23. Domb BG, El Bitar YF, Sadik AY, Stake CE, Botser IB. Comparison of robotic-assisted and conventional acetabular cup placement in THA: a matched-pair controlled study. Clin Orthop Relat Res. 2014;472(1):329–36. https://doi.org/10.1007/s11999-013-3253-7.

24. Nawabi DH, Conditt MA, Ranawat AS, et al. Haptically guided robotic technology in total hip arthroplasty: a cadaveric investigation. Proc Inst Mech Eng H. 2013;227(3):302–9. https://doi.org/10.1177/0954411912468540.

25. Illgren R. Comparison of robotic-assisted and conventional acetabular cup placement in THA: a matched-pair controlled study. In: 43rd annual course: advances in arthroplasty. Cambridge, MA; 2013.

26. Bukowski B, Abiola R, Illgen R. Outcomes after primary total hip manual compared with robotic assisted techniques. In: 44th annual advances in arthroplasty. Cambridge, MA; 2014.

27. Pearle AD, O'Loughlin PF, Kendoff DO. Robot-assisted unicompartmental knee arthroplasty. J Arthroplast. 2010;25(2):230–7. https://doi.org/10.1016/j.arth.2008.09.024.

28. Lonner JH. Indications for unicompartmental knee arthroplasty and rationale for robotic arm-assisted technology. Am J Orthop (Belle Mead NJ). 2009;38(2 Suppl):3–6. http://www.ncbi.nlm.nih.gov/pubmed/19340375. Accessed 24 Apr 2017.

29. Sinha RK. Outcomes of robotic arm-assisted unicompartmental knee arthroplasty. Am J Orthop (Belle Mead NJ). 2009;38(2 Suppl):20–2. http://www.ncbi.nlm.nih.gov/pubmed/19340379. Accessed 29 Aug 2016.

30. Citak M, Suero EM, Citak M, et al. Unicompartmental knee arthroplasty: is robotic technology more accurate than conventional technique? Knee. 2013;20(4):268–71. https://doi.org/10.1016/j.knee.2012.11.001.

31. Lonner JH, John TK, Conditt MA. Robotic arm-assisted UKA improves Tibial component alignment: a pilot study. Clin Orthop Relat Res. 2010;468:141–6. https://doi.org/10.1007/s11999-009-0977-5.

32. Jones B, et al. Accuracy of UKA implant positioning and early clinical outcomes in a RCT comparing robotic assisted and manual surgery. In: 13th annual CAOS meeting. Orlando, FL; 2013.

33. Conditt M, Coon T, Roche M, et al. Two year survivorship of robotically guided unicompartmental knee arthroplasty. Orthop Proc. 2013;95-B(SUPP 34). http://www.bjjprocs.boneandjoint.org.uk/content/95-B/SUPP_34/294. Accessed 12 Apr 2017.

34. Honl M, Dierk O, Gauck C, et al. Comparison of robotic-assisted and manual implantation of a primary total hip replacement. A prospective study. J Bone Joint Surg Am. 2003;85-A(8):1470–8. http://www.ncbi.nlm.nih.gov/pubmed/12925626. Accessed 28 Apr 2017.

35. AOA. Australian Orthopaedic Association National Joint Replacement Registry. https://aoanjrr.sahmri.com/en/annual-reports-2016. Published 2016.

36. Bozic KJ, Kurtz SM, Lau E, et al. The epidemiology of revision total knee arthroplasty in the United States. Clin Orthop Relat Res. 2010;468(1):45–51. https://doi.org/10.1007/s11999-009-0945-0.

37. Moschetti WE, Konopka JF, Rubash HE, Genuario JW. Can robot-assisted unicompartmental knee arthroplasty be cost-effective? A Markov decision analysis. J Arthroplast. 2016;31(4):759–65. https://doi.org/10.1016/j.arth.2015.10.018.

38. Peersman G, Laskin R, Davis J, Peterson MGE, Richart T. Prolonged operative time correlates with increased infection rate after total knee arthroplasty. HSS J. 2006;2(1):70–2. https://doi.org/10.1007/s11420-005-0130-2.

39. Swank ML, Alkire M, Conditt M, Lonner JH. Technology and cost-effectiveness in knee arthroplasty: computer navigation and robotics. Am J Orthop (Belle Mead NJ). 2009;38(2 Suppl):32–6. http://www.ncbi.nlm.nih.gov/pubmed/19340382. Accessed 19 Aug 2016.

Risks and Complications of Autonomous and Semiautonomous Robotics in Joint Arthroplasty

Laura J. Kleeblad and Andrew D. Pearle

Total joint arthroplasty (hip, THA and knee, TKA) and unicompartmental knee arthroplasty (UKA) have been shown to be reliable treatment options for end-stage degenerative disease. Systematic reviews report survivorship rates over 95% for total joint arthroplasty and 92% for UKA at long-term follow-up [1–3]. However, survivorship reported by national registries is lower [4–8]. Over the last two decades, there has been special interest for the surgical variables which can be controlled intraoperatively, in order to increase survivorship rates. Motivated by the desire to improve accuracy, decrease the risk of outliers, and improve component position, robotic systems have been implemented into orthopedic surgery [9–11]. There are many advantages of robot-assisted surgery, allowing a surgeon to control and improve the surgical precision of the procedure. On the contrary, the use of robotic systems in joint arthroplasty is associated with risks and complications related to the system [12, 13]. Several robotic systems are on the market, all with a different combination of features [13]. To date, there are four robotic sys-

tems approved for joint arthroplasty, of which the characteristics are shown in Table 8.1.

The aim of this chapter is to discuss the main risks and complications of robot-assisted surgery, which include radiation exposure, pin-related complications, registration malfunction, soft tissue damage, and longer operating times.

Risks and Complications

Radiation Exposure

Some autonomous as well as semiautonomous systems involve preoperative planning based on an imaging modality. The Robodoc (autonomous) and the MAKO (semiautonomous) system require computed tomography (CT) scans preoperatively to create a three-dimensional (3D) map and define the amount and orientation of bone to be removed. Potential disadvantages of image-based systems include extra costs of the imaging study and risk of radiation exposure during the CT scan [14–16]. The biological effects from radiation depend on the dose as well as the tissue's biological sensitivity. The difference in biological sensitivity is called the effective dose (ED), which is expressed in millisievert (mSv, 1 mSv = 1 mGy). Normally, a single pelvic CT scan corresponds to a radiation dose around 6 mSv and a knee CT to 1 mSv in an adult according to current literature [14]. However, the risk of

L. J. Kleeblad
Department of Orthopedic Surgery, Noordwest Hospital Group, Alkmaar, The Netherlands

A. D. Pearle (✉)
Department of Orthopedic Surgery, Sports Medicine, and Shoulder Service, Hospital for Special Surgery, New York, NY, USA
e-mail: pearlea@hss.edu

© Springer Nature Switzerland AG 2019
J. H. Lonner (ed.), *Robotics in Knee and Hip Arthroplasty*,
https://doi.org/10.1007/978-3-030-16593-2_8

Table 8.1 Current robotic platforms

System	Corporation	Arthroplasty	Preoperative planning	Control	Platform	Bone resection
TSolution One (Robodoc)	Think Surgical, Fremont, CA, USA	TKA, THA (femur)	CT scan	Autonomous	Open	Mill
iBlock	OMNIlife Science, East Taunton, MA, USA	TKA	None	Autonomous	Closed	Saw
MAKO	Stryker Corporation, Mahwah, NJ, USA	UKA, PFA, TKA, THA	CT scan	Semiautonomous, haptic	Closed	Burr, saw
Navio PFS	Smith and Nephew, Memphis, TN, USA	UKA, PFA,TKA	None	Semiautonomous	Open	Burr, saw
ROSA Knee	Zimmer Biomet, Warsaw, IN, USA	TKA	None	Semiautonomous	Closed	Saw

radiation exposure is cumulative during the course of one's life regardless of time intervals between scans, taken into account the annual level of naturally occurring background radiation (3 mSv in the United States) and previously performed imaging studies [17]. An ED of 10 mSv may be associated with an increase in the risk of fatal cancer of approximately 1 in 2000 compared to 1 in 5 natural incidence of fatal cancer in the US population [16, 18]. In other words, for any one person, the risk of radiation-induced cancer is much smaller than the natural risk of cancer. Furthermore, the biological sensitivity of tissue is greater in young adults; therefore, it is necessary to be more cautioned in requesting CT scans [16].

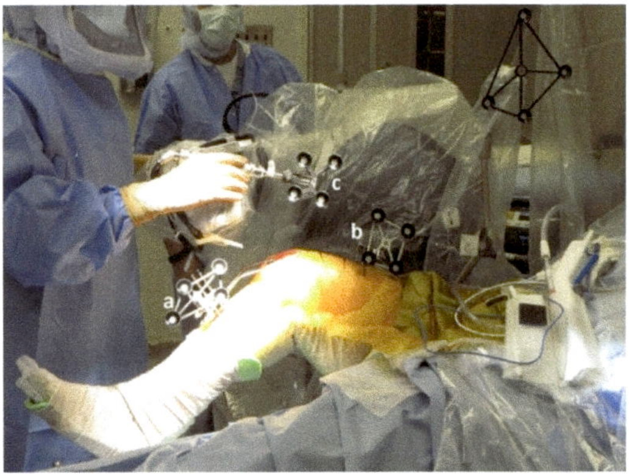

Fig. 8.1 Intraoperative registration of robot-assisted unicompartmental knee arthroplasty surgery using the MAKO (Stryker) system. (**a**) Tibial pins with reference array, (**b**) femoral pins with reference array, and (**c**) robotic semiautonomous arm, which includes the burr, now set up for registration of the arm before the burring starts

Pin-Related Complications

The anatomical surface landmarks are registered through reference arrays, which are attached to the bone using pins (Fig. 8.1). A stable construction allows accurate registration and depending on the system verification of the digitized CT model. However, the application of the bone pins might require an extended surgical approach or some additional skin incisions outside the surgical field. Total hip arthroplasty using the Robodoc system requires a wider exposure of the proximal femur, particularly of the greater trochanter [19, 20]. The comprehensive approach is needed to fit the leg-holder equipment to obtain rigid fixation and facilitate accurate registration and cutting

maneuver. The combination of extended approach and prolonged fixation of the leg in adduction and external rotation may damage the abductor muscles [19]. Bach et al. showed less hip abduction in mid-and terminal stance following robotic THA using a transgluteal approach compared to patients without THA. However, no significant difference was found between robotic and conventional THA patients, indicating that the robotic procedure does not impair hip abductor function more than conventional techniques [19].

Most robotic systems require reference arrays to be attached to both tibia and femur in case of TKA or UKA, allowing anatomical surface landmarks to be registered [11, 21, 22]. Besides

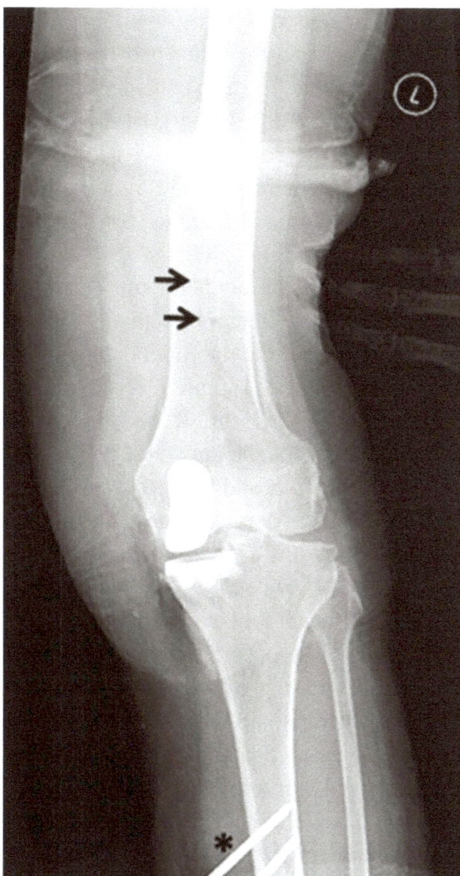
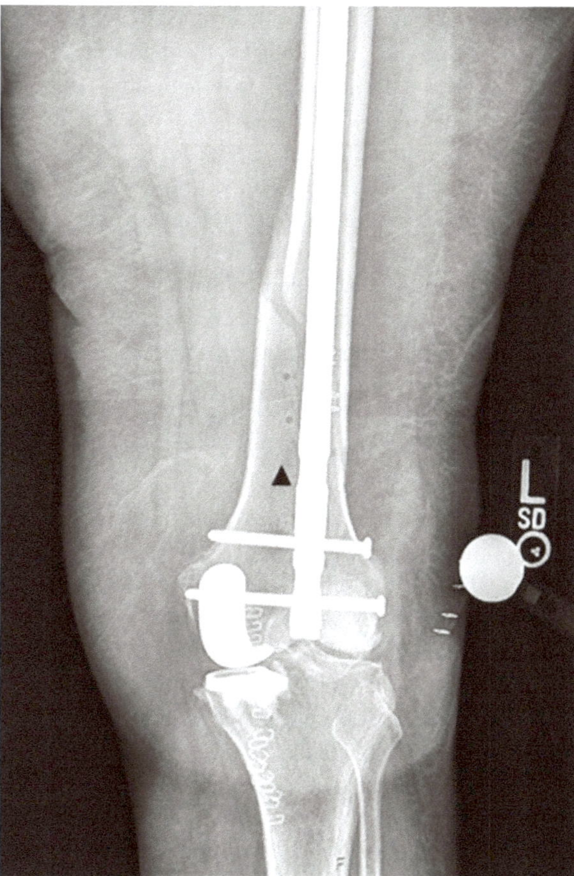

Fig. 8.2 Anteroposterior radiographs of intraoperative femoral shaft fracture during robot-assisted unicompartmental arthroplasty using MAKO (Stryker) system. Left image: Arrows show the pinholes in the center of the fracture and * the metal pins in the tibia. Right picture shows the intramedullary nail postoperative at the triangle

additional incisions, it has also been suggested that the pin tracks could work as a stress riser in the cortical bone, which poses a risk for fracture [23]. The incidence of pin-related fractures is not reported in literature. The senior author of this chapter has performed over 1400 robot-assisted UKAs; in his cohort, one femoral shaft fracture occurred (Fig. 8.2). The pin track-related complications mentioned in literature are mostly pin site infections and skin irritations [9, 24, 25].

Registration Malfunction

The success of robot-assisted surgery relies on the precise registration, which is dependent on the patients' anatomy and the construction of pins, arrays, and markers. Accuracy of registration depends on the technique of landmark pointing and soft tissue thickness as is shown by Hohmann et al. [26]. For example, studies show that body mass index (BMI) greater than 27 kg/m^2 was associated with an increase in acetabular cup position measurement error with an imageless system [25, 27].

The risk of using an image-free system is the lack of true preoperative planning and the inability to verify the anatomic registration landmarks at the time of surgery with the 3D digital map [13]. Therefore, CT-based systems might still have some advantages over the imageless system in patients with abnormal anatomy such as hip dysplasia and post-traumatic deformities or in revision procedures [28].

In the end stage of unicompartmental or tri-compartmental knee osteoarthritis, the deformity of the leg normally increases to more varus or valgus depending on a patient's original mechanical axis. Severely deformed patients are at risk for registration failure, because the primary designated points for surface registration do not exist or are beyond the software ability to be recognized. However, if a surgeon decides that robot-assisted surgery is indicated, it is recommended to use an image-based system to be able to evaluate the deformity preoperatively and create the ability to check the registration intraoperatively.

With the use of open systems (Table 8.1), some specificity and functionality will be sacrificed, although it allows surgeons to utilize the most preferable implant design. The systems contain 3D data for several implants but often lack the depth of design specificity and biomechanical data to optimally predict kinematics for component positioning [13, 15]. Combining open systems with imageless systems, a precise registration of the anatomic landmarks is critical. The clinical significance of system differences remains debated [13].

In the unfortunate case of registration errors, re-registration is needed to fulfill the system requirements and continue the procedure. This will possibly extend the surgical time and might even lead to conversion of the procedure to conventional techniques when the defect cannot be repaired. Bellemans et al. aborted 12% of their TKA patients because of technical difficulties with the recognition of the markers' position leading to continuous error signaling on the screen [21]. Furthermore, Siebert et al. reported that the femoral milling process could not be completed in one patient due to a defective registration marker [24].

Soft Tissue Damage

Unnecessary soft tissue damage is one of the most serious of all risks. Robotic systems track the bone surfaces; however, they are usually unable to track the soft tissue and therefore damage can occur. With regard to THA with the autonomous Robodoc system, the tip of the greater trochanter and the inner part of the gluteal muscles attached to the trochanter could be damaged during milling [12, 29]. Honl and colleagues reported higher rates of postoperative dislocation and revision in their robotic THA patient group compared to the conventional group (18% vs. 4% and 13% vs. 0%, respectively). At revision, the abductor muscles were detached from the greater trochanter in all patients; this implied that the robot damaged the muscles causing them to rupture [30]. According to many authors using the Robodoc system, these complications can be prevented by protecting and retracting the abductors appropriately. Several studies showed no damage of the abductor muscles following THA with the Robodoc system [13, 19, 20, 29].

For TKA, damage to the patellar tendon poses significant problems concerning the extension of the leg and the stability of the prosthetic knee [12, 31]. Concerning robot-assisted medial UKA, the medial collateral ligament is in danger and must be protected carefully during the tibial cut. During robotic lateral UKR, the popliteus tendon is particularly at risk as it drapes over the bone and is not tracked by the robotic system.

Another risk of robotic surgery using an autonomous system (Table 8.1) is the inability for the surgeon to prepare the surfaces, other than having access to a "shutdown" switch [15, 32]. Therefore, it is important to protect the soft tissues surrounding the milling or cutting area while the robotic tool is preparing the bone surfaces (Fig. 8.3).

Robotic systems still lack the ability to make creative decisions or change the pre-programmed plan in case of an unexpected event (e.g., fracture, soft tissue damage). In these cases, the surgeon may need to convert to conventional techniques [13].

Extended Operating Times

With the use of robotic systems, longer operating times are reported by several authors. For most systems, the learning curve is completed

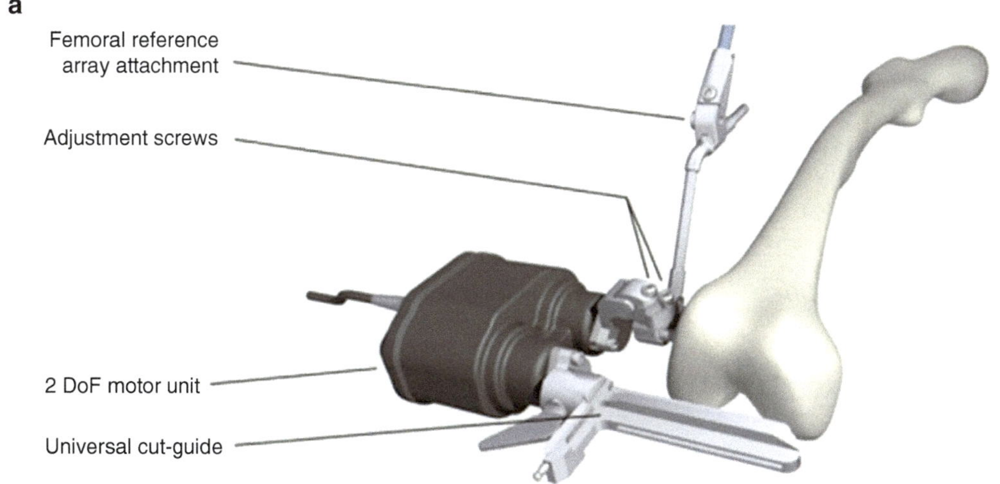

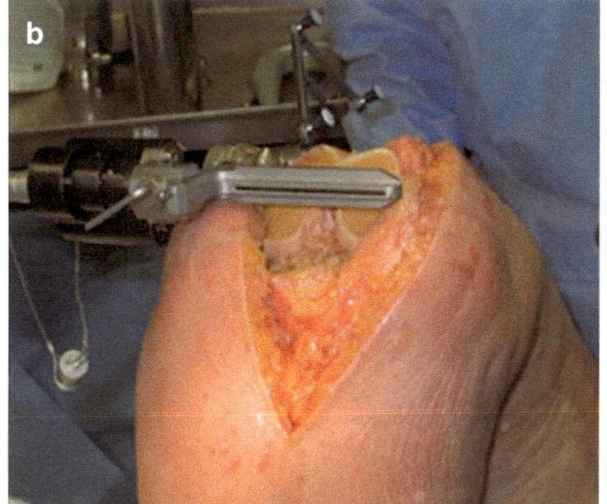

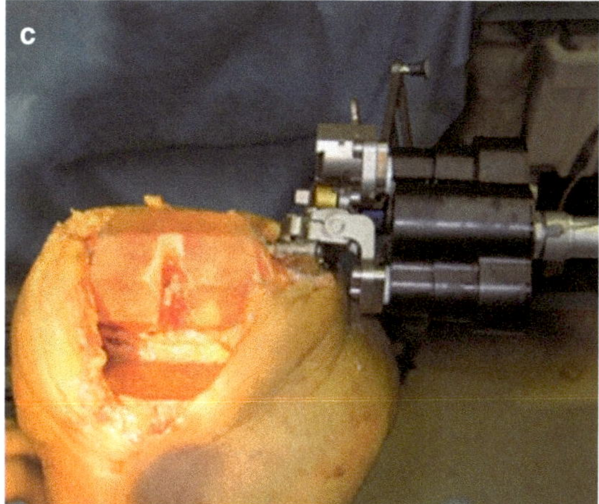

Fig. 8.3 The iBlock® universal cutting guide mounts on the medial aspect of the femur and automatically positions the guide in the sagittal plane for the five femoral cuts, automating implant positioning in the flexion, distoproximal, and anteroposterior directions. Frontal and axial alignment is performed before making any cuts, using the mechanical adjustment screws (**a**) under navigated control. The iBlock was used to make all five femoral cuts in the following sequence: distal, anterior chamfer (**b**), anterior, posterior chamfer, and posterior. The positioning of the two femoral fixation pins relative to the five cuts is illustrated in (**c**). (From Koulalis et al. [22], with permission)

after the first five to eight cases according to current literature [11, 20, 33]. However, even if surgeons are familiar with the systems, the operating times are often longer and more variable when compared to conventional techniques. In many cases, the registration setup, which includes bone pin fixation with the arrays, and the registration process are responsible for the additional surgical time when compared to conventional surgery. In the literature on THA, it has been reported that the average surgical time ranges from 96 to 120 minutes, which is approximately 25 mins longer than conventional THA [29, 33]. The mean operating time for TKA is more variable among the different studies, ranging from 90 to 195 minutes [9, 21, 24]. For UKA, the average operating time is between 56 and 95 minutes [11, 23, 34]. However, no comparative studies have been performed to compare surgical times of robotic TKA or UKA with conventional surgeries. The main concern of the prolonged time for surgery is the risk of deep infection [12]. However, this has not been proven in current studies.

Conclusion

In summary, the main risks of autonomous and semiautonomous robotic systems in joint arthroplasty are radiation exposure, pin-related complications, registration malfunction, soft tissue damage, and extended operating times. Future innovations will likely focus on improving the planning, setup, and registration process during robot-assisted joint arthroplasty.

References

1. van der List JP, McDonald LS, Pearle AD. Systematic review of medial versus lateral survivorship in unicompartmental knee arthroplasty. Knee Elsevier. 2015;22:454–60.
2. Mont MA, Pivec R, Issa K, Kapadia BH, Maheshwari A, Harwin SF. Long-term implant survivorship of cementless total knee arthroplasty: a systematic review of the literature and meta-analysis. J Knee Surg. 2014;27:369–76.
3. Zywiel MG, Sayeed SA, Johnson AJ, Schmalzried TP, Mont MA. Survival of hard-on-hard bearings in total hip arthroplasty: a systematic review. Clin Orthop Relat Res. 2011;469:1536–46.
4. National Joint Registry for England, Wales and Northern Ireland. 12th Annual Report 2015 http://www.njrreports.org.uk/Portals/0/PDFdownloads/NJR12thAnnualReport2015.pdf.
5. Swedish Knee Arthroplasty Register. Annual report 2015 - Swedish knee arthroplasty Register 2015. http://www.myknee.se/pdf/SVK_2015_Eng_1.0.pdf.
6. Norwegian National Advisory Unit on Arthroplasty and Hip Fractures. Norwegian arthroplasty register. Report 2015 http://nrlweb.ihelse.net/Rapporter/Report2015_english.pdf.
7. Australian Orthopaedic Association National Joint Registry. Hip and knee arthroplasty annual report 2015. https://aoanjrr.sahmri.com/documents/10180/217745/HipandKneeArthroplasty.
8. New Zealand Joint Registry. The New Zealand registry annual report [Internet]. 2014. http://nzoa.org.nz/system/files/Web_DH7657_NZJR2014Report_v4_12Nov15.pdf.
9. Song EK, Seon JK, Yim JH, Netravali NA, Bargar WL. Robotic-assisted TKA reduces postoperative alignment outliers and improves gap balance compared to conventional TKA knee. Clin Orthop Relat Res. 2013;471:118–26.
10. Moon Y-W, Ha C, Do K-H, Kim C-Y, Han J-H, Na S-E, et al. Comparison of robot-assisted and conventional total knee arthroplasty: a controlled cadaver study using multiparameter quantitative three-dimensional CT assessment of alignment. Comput Aided Surg. 2012;17:86–95.
11. Pearle AD, O'Loughlin PF, Kendoff DO. Robot-assisted unicompartmental knee arthroplasty. J Arthroplast. 2010;25:230–7.
12. Chun YS, Kim KI, Cho YJ, Kim YH, Yoo MC, Rhyu KH. Causes and patterns of aborting a robot-assisted arthroplasty. J Arthroplasty. Elsevier Inc. 2011;26:621–5.
13. Jacofsky DJ, Allen M. Robotics in arthroplasty: a comprehensive review. J Arthroplast. 2016;31:2353–63.
14. Ponzio DY, Lonner JH. Preoperative mapping in unicompartmental knee arthroplasty using computed tomography scans is associated with radiation exposure and carries high cost. J Arthroplasty Elsevier Inc. 2015;30:964–7.
15. Lonner JH, Moretti VM. The evolution of image-free robotic assistance in unicompartmental knee arthroplasty. Am J Orthop (Belle Mead NJ). 2016;45:249–54.
16. Costello JE, Cecava ND, Tucker JE, Bau JL. CT radiation dose: current controversies and dose reduction strategies. Am J Roentgenol. 2013;201:1283–90.
17. Brenner DJ, Hall EJ. Computed tomography--an increasing source of radiation exposure. N Engl J Med. 2007;357:2277–84.
18. U.S. Food and Drug Administration. Radiation-emitting products: what are the radiation risks from CT? Risk estimates from medical imaging. Last Update. 03/25/2016. http://www.fda.gov/Radiation-EmittingProducts/RadiationEmittingProductsandProcedures/MedicalImaging/MedicalX-Rays/ucm115329.htm.
19. Bach CM, Winter P, Nogler M, Göbel G, Wimmer C, Ogon M. No functional impairment after Robodoc total hip arthroplasty: gait analysis in 25 patients. Acta Orthop Scand. 2002;73:386–91.
20. Schulz AP, Seide K, Queitsch C, von Haugwitz A, Meiners J, Kienast B, et al. Results of total hip replacement using the Robodoc surgical assistant system: clinical outcome and evaluation of complications for 97 procedures. Int J Med Robot. 2007;3:301–6.
21. Bellemans J, Vandenneucker H, Vanlauwe J. Robot-assisted total knee arthroplasty. Clin Orthop Relat Res. 2007;PAP:111–6.
22. Koulalis D, O'Loughlin PF, Plaskos C, Kendoff D, Cross MB, Pearle AD. Sequential versus automated cutting guides in computer-assisted total knee arthroplasty. Knee Elsevier BV. 2011;18:436–42.
23. Lonner JH. Robotically assisted unicompartmental knee arthroplasty with a handheld image-free sculpting tool. Orthop Clin North Am. Elsevier Inc. 2016;47:29–40.
24. Siebert W, Mai S, Kober R, Heeckt PF. Technique and first clinical results of robot-assisted total knee replacement. Knee. 2002;9:173–80.
25. Ryan JA, Jamali AA, Bargar WL. Accuracy of computer navigation for acetabular component placement in THA. Clin Orthop Relat Res. 2010;468:169–77.
26. Hohmann E, Bryant A, Tetsworth K. Anterior pelvic soft tissue thickness influences acetabular cup positioning with imageless navigation. J Arthroplast. 2012;27:945–52.

27. Parratte S, Argenson JN. Validation and usefulness of a computer-assisted cup-positioning system in total hip arthroplasty. A prospective, randomized, controlled study. J Bone Joint Surg Am. 2007;89:494–9.
28. Kalteis T, Handel M, Bäthis H, Perlick L, Tingart M, Grifka J. Imageless navigation for insertion of the acetabular component in total hip arthroplasty: is it as accurate as CT-based navigation? J Bone Joint Surg Br. 2006;88–B:163–7.
29. Bargar WL. Robots in orthopaedic surgery: past, present, and future. Clin Orthop Relat Res. 2007;463:31–6.
30. Honl M, Dierk O, Gauck C, Carrero V, Lampe F, Dries S, et al. Comparison of robotic-assisted and manual implantation of a primary total hip replacement. A prospective study. J Bone Joint Surg Am. 2003;85–A:1470–8.
31. Park SE, Lee CT. Comparison of robotic-assisted and conventional manual implantation of a primary total knee arthroplasty. J Arthroplast. 2007;22:1054–9.
32. Lang JE, Mannava S, Floyd AJ, Goddard MS, Smith BP, Mofidi A, et al. Robotic systems in orthopaedic surgery. J Bone Joint Surg Br. 2011;93:1296–9.
33. Liow MHL, Chin PL, Tay KJD, Chia SL, Lo NN, Yeo SJ. Early experiences with robot-assisted total knee arthroplasty using the digiMatch™ ROBODOC® surgical system. Singap Med J. 2014;55:529–34.
34. Cobb J, Henckel J, Gomes P, Harris S, Jakopec M, Rodriguez F, et al. Hands-on robotic unicompartmental knee replacement: a prospective, randomised controlled study of the acrobot system. J Bone Joint Surg Br. 2006;88:188–97.

Unicompartmental Knee Arthroplasty Technique: Navio

Jess H. Lonner and Christopher P. Bechtel

Unicompartmental knee arthroplasty (UKA) has become an increasingly popular surgical option for patients with arthritis limited to an isolated compartment, offering a tissue-preserving surgical alternative to total knee arthroplasty, with better kinematics, functionality, and satisfaction, less postoperative morbidity, and lower perioperative costs [1, 2]. UKA currently accounts for roughly 8–10% of all knee arthroplasty procedures, and this percentage could potentially increase to more than 20–30% in the future, particularly with increasing use in younger patients [3, 4]. Even without expanding the appropriate surgical indications, a growing interest in outpatient knee arthroplasty procedures and the emerging use of surgery centers for UKA will likely increase training and endorsement of these procedures by a growing volume of surgeons.

Despite reports of excellent outcomes, functionality, and durability from high-volume surgeons [5–9], higher revision rates and decreased survivorship of UKA have been demonstrated among lower-volume surgeons and in nationwide databases and registries [10, 11]. While the etiology of aseptic failure in UKA is multifactorial, component malposition or malalignment and soft tissue imbalance predispose to failure [12, 13]. One study [13] found that 12% of aseptic failures of UKA were due to faulty implantation and inadequate positioning of the components, with half occurring within the first 5 years after implantation. Similarly, an analysis of revision UKA from the Norwegian Arthroplasty Register found that component malalignment and soft tissue imbalance and knee instability are the prevalent modes of failure [12]. Several studies have provided evidence that small errors of more than $2°$ or $3°$ in the coronal plane and excessive tibial slope predispose to mechanical failure in UKA [14–19]. Even in the hands of skilled surgeons, achieving consistently accurate alignment in UKA is difficult using conventional techniques, particularly with minimally invasive approaches [15–18, 20]. Component positioning beyond $2°$ of the desired alignment may occur in as many as 40–60% of cases with conventional techniques [20, 21]. In a study analyzing the results of 221 consecutive UKAs performed through a minimally invasive approach, tibial component alignment had a standard deviation of $±4°$ and a range from $18°$ varus to $6°$ valgus [19]. It is for these reasons that robotic assistance has been advanced for bone preparation and soft tissue balancing during UKA.

Computer navigation was introduced in an effort to reduce the number of outliers and improve the

J. H. Lonner (✉)
Department of Orthopaedic Surgery,
Rothman Orthopaedic Institute, Sidney Kimmel
Medical College, Thomas Jefferson University,
Philadelphia, PA, USA
e-mail: jess.lonner@rothmanortho.com

C. P. Bechtel
Department of Orthopedics, University Hospitals
Westlake Health Center, Westlake, OH, USA

© Springer Nature Switzerland AG 2019
J. H. Lonner (ed.), *Robotics in Knee and Hip Arthroplasty*,
https://doi.org/10.1007/978-3-030-16593-2_9

accuracy of UKA. Even with computer navigation, the incidence of outliers (beyond 2° of the preoperatively planned implant position) may approach 15% resulting from the imprecision with the use of standard cutting guides and conventional methods of bone preparation [20]. Semiautonomous robotic guidance was therefore introduced to not only capitalize on the improvements seen with computer navigation but also to further refine and enhance the accuracy of bone preparation, even with minimally invasive techniques, by better interfacing and integrating the planning and performance of bone preparation [21–33].

Although the emergence of robotics in knee and hip arthroplasty has been gradual, semiautonomous robotic technology is currently being utilized in more than 15% of the UKA cases performed in the United States [34], and those numbers are anticipated to grow substantially to over 35% during the next few years as more surgeons embrace the robotic platforms available, pricing improves, additional robotic options enter the space, and greater utilization expands beyond UKA into total knee arthroplasty (TKA) and other procedures [35]. While this technology has enhanced the precision of the surgery, the challenge facing the robotics sector is producing technologies that are also efficient and economically feasible. Several factors that impeded broader adoption of the first-generation robotic technology, which was largely dependent on preoperative planning with computed tomography (CT) scans, included the high capital and maintenance costs of the first-generation systems; soft tissue complications observed with an autonomous (active) robotic system used for a brief time by several centers for total hip and knee arthroplasty primarily in Asia and Europe; skepticism regarding the importance of optimizing precision in UKA; expense, inconvenience, and delays associated with having to obtain preoperative CT scans for planning and mapping; and concern regarding the radiation exposure with CT-based planning [27, 29, 36, 37].

A newer image-free semiautonomous robotic technology (Navio, Smith & Nephew, Memphis TN) is an alternative to the first-generation autonomous and semiautonomous CT-based systems [26]. This chapter focuses on the specifics of this technology and early data.

Navio System

The Navio system is a handheld image-free robotic sculpting tool available for assistance in UKA, patellofemoral arthroplasty (PFA), and total knee arthroplasty (TKA), having received initial CE mark and US Food and Drug Administration clearances in February and December 2012, respectively (Fig. 9.1a, b). This lightweight robotic tool combines image-free intraoperative registration, planning, and navigation with precise bone preparation and dynamic soft tissue balancing. As a semiautonomous system, it augments the surgeon's movements, with safeguards in place to optimize both accuracy

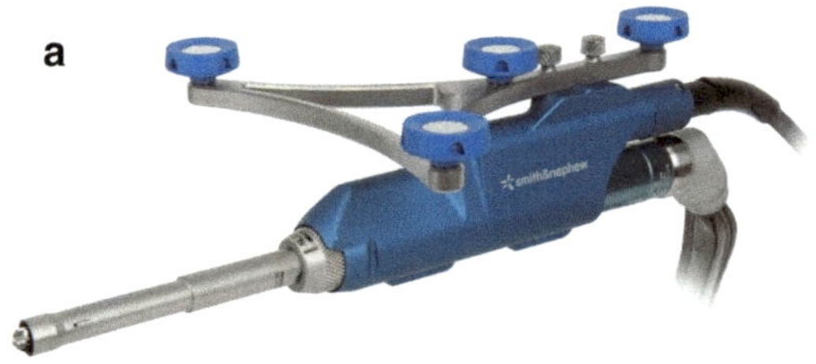

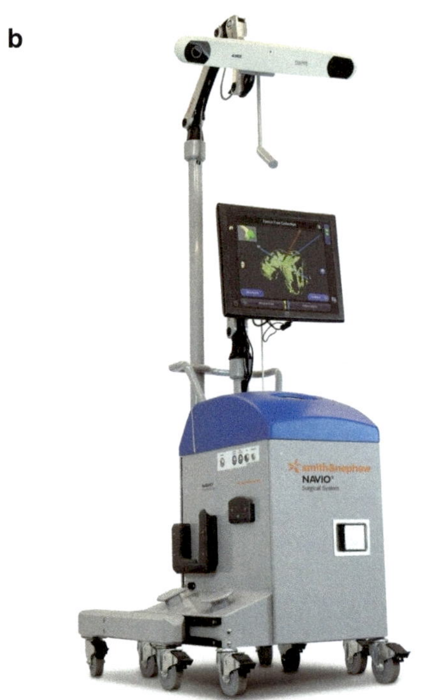

Fig. 9.1 (a, b) Navio handheld robotic sculpting tool (a) and monitor with camera. (Smith & Nephew, Memphis TN)

and safety. The system continuously tracks the position of the patients' lower limb, as well as the handheld burr, so that the limb position and degree of knee flexion can be changed constantly during the surgical procedure to gain exposure to different parts of the knee during registration and bone preparation through a minimally invasive approach.

Indications and Contraindications

The indications and contraindications are identical to those used for conventional approaches to UKA and other robotically assisted methods of UKA. Variations may exist depending on surgeon philosophy, tolerances, or preferences. There are no specific contraindications to the use of the Navio system, although the added duration of surgery early in the learning curve may make it undesirable for some patients until proficiencies with the setup, preparation, and nuances of the surgical procedure are optimized.

Surgical Technique

The patient is positioned supine on the operating table, and the surgical limb is prepped, draped, and positioned in a table-mounted leg holder. Bicortical, partially threaded pins are percutaneously inserted into the metaphysis of the proximal tibia and distal femur. On the tibia, the pins are placed starting approximately 3 cm inferior to the tibial tubercle on the medial side of the tibial crest. On the femur, the pins are placed starting approximately 5 cm superior to the patella with the knee hyperflexed, in order to stretch the quadriceps before pin insertion and to try to avoid inserting the pins through the suprapatellar pouch. Optical tracking arrays are then secured to these transfixion pins, approximately 2 cm above the skin (Fig. 9.2). A tracking system with infrared cameras constantly determines the position of the reflective trackers in space. The knee is taken through a full range of motion, with and without tensioning the collateral ligament on the concavity of the deformity to ensure that the trackers are visible by the camera throughout.

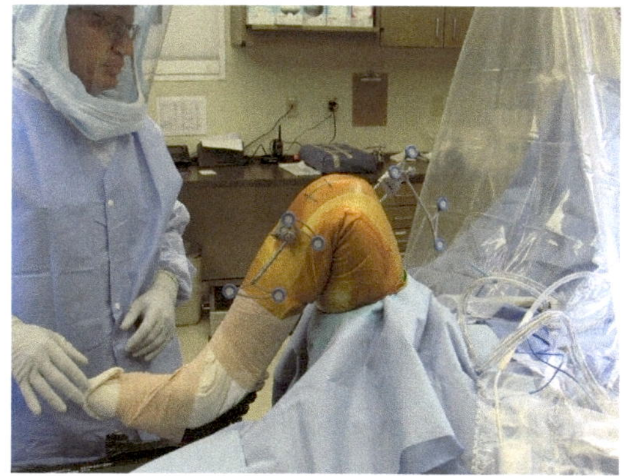

Fig. 9.2 Positioning of bicortical pins and optical trackers in the distal femoral metaphysis, inserted with the knee hyperflexed, approximately 5 cm proximal to the proximal pole of the patella, and proximal tibial metaphysis, approximately 3 cm distal to the tibial tubercle

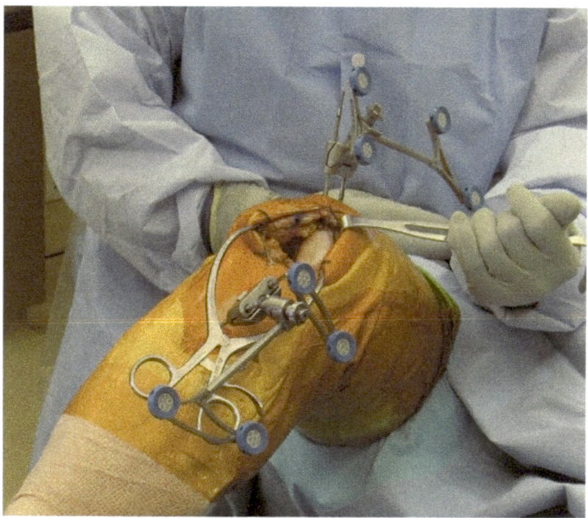

Fig. 9.3 Typical arthrotomy for a medial UKA allows for reasonable joint assessment to confirm appropriate pathology and ample exposure for robotic-assisted surgery

The knee is exposed using a standard arthrotomy, depending on surgeon preference. For medial UKAs an anteromedial skin incision is made from the proximal-medial edge of the patella to a point just proximal and medial to the tibial tubercle (Fig. 9.3); for lateral UKAs a more midline incision is made and carried more proximally, followed by a lateral parapatellar arthrotomy. For purposes of this chapter, we will describe the typical approach and technique used for a medial UKA. A medial parapatellar arthrotomy is made, extending just proximal to the proximal pole of the patella. Care is taken to avoid nicking the trochlear cartilage during arthrotomy; this can be done by making the proximal arthrotomy with the knee either flexed no more than 30° or fully extended (as opposed to making the capsular incision in deep flexion). The joint is inspected to corroborate that the wear pattern is indeed amenable to UKA and osteophytes are removed from the exposed arthritic side of the knee and intercondylar notch.

Limb Registration and Surface Mapping

Since the Navio method is based entirely on intraoperative navigation and registration, the component alignment and sizing, as well as volume and orientation of bone to be removed, are based on the determination of the mechanical and rotational axes of the femur and tibia as well as mapping of the surfaces of the affected condyles. An algorithm is followed that sequentially identifies the hip center (by circumducting the hip), and ankle and knee centers, from which the mechanical axes of the limb, femur, and tibia are determined. The native resting mechanical alignment of the limb is captured in maximal extension, and then the knee is brought through a range of motion to maximum flexion, without tensioning the ligaments, thus establishing the rotational axis of the limb, from which femoral component rotation is ultimately derived (Fig. 9.4). Using the optical probe, multiple points of the distal femur

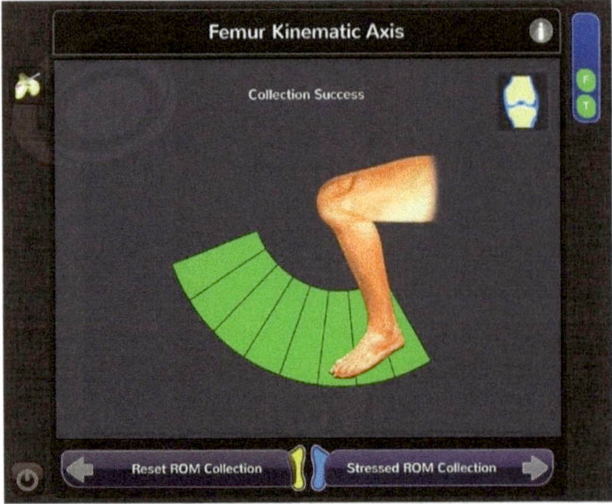

Fig. 9.4 The rotational (kinematic) axis of the limb is established and serves as the reference for rotational alignment of the femoral component

and proximal tibia are registered to determine the boundaries of the surface anatomy and condylar size and shape. The rotational axis of the tibia is based off the orientation of the medial tibial spine (Fig. 9.5a, d). A three-dimensional virtual recreation of the proximal tibia and distal femur is produced by "painting" the condylar surfaces. From this, the component sizes and positions will be determined. In this way, intraoperative mapping supplants the predicate system that required a preoperative CT scan (Fig. 9.6a, b).

Gap Balancing

Another key element of the Navio robotic technique is quantifying dynamically the soft tissue balance of the knee through a full range of motion. An algorithm is followed to establish the tightness or laxity in the hemi-compartment after virtual positioning of the components. After arthrotomy and removal of the medial osteophytes, a valgus stress is applied to the knee (in the case of medial UKA) as it is passively moved from full extension to deep flexion (Fig. 9.7a, b). After the abovementioned surface mapping and three-dimensional planning of implant sizes, their position and orientation are "virtually" established. A graphic representation of gap spacing through an entire range of motion is created. Adjustments can be made in the virtual positioning of the components – including tibial slope and depth of resection or femoral component flexion, anteriorization, and distalization – to achieve the desired soft tissue balance across the entire flexion arc (Fig. 9.7a–d). The goal is to adjust the implant positions and orientations such that the gaps in extension and flexion are balanced according to surgeon preferences, with roughly 2 mm of laxity between the components through a full arc of motion, and avoiding overcorrection of alignment into the opposite compartment (Fig. 9.7c, d). While the positioning and alignment of components is often recognized as the most important element of robotic precision, it may be that the careful quantification of soft tissue balance may be the factor most responsible for improved functional outcomes and equally impactful on implant durability compared to conventional methods. Therefore, the time spent at

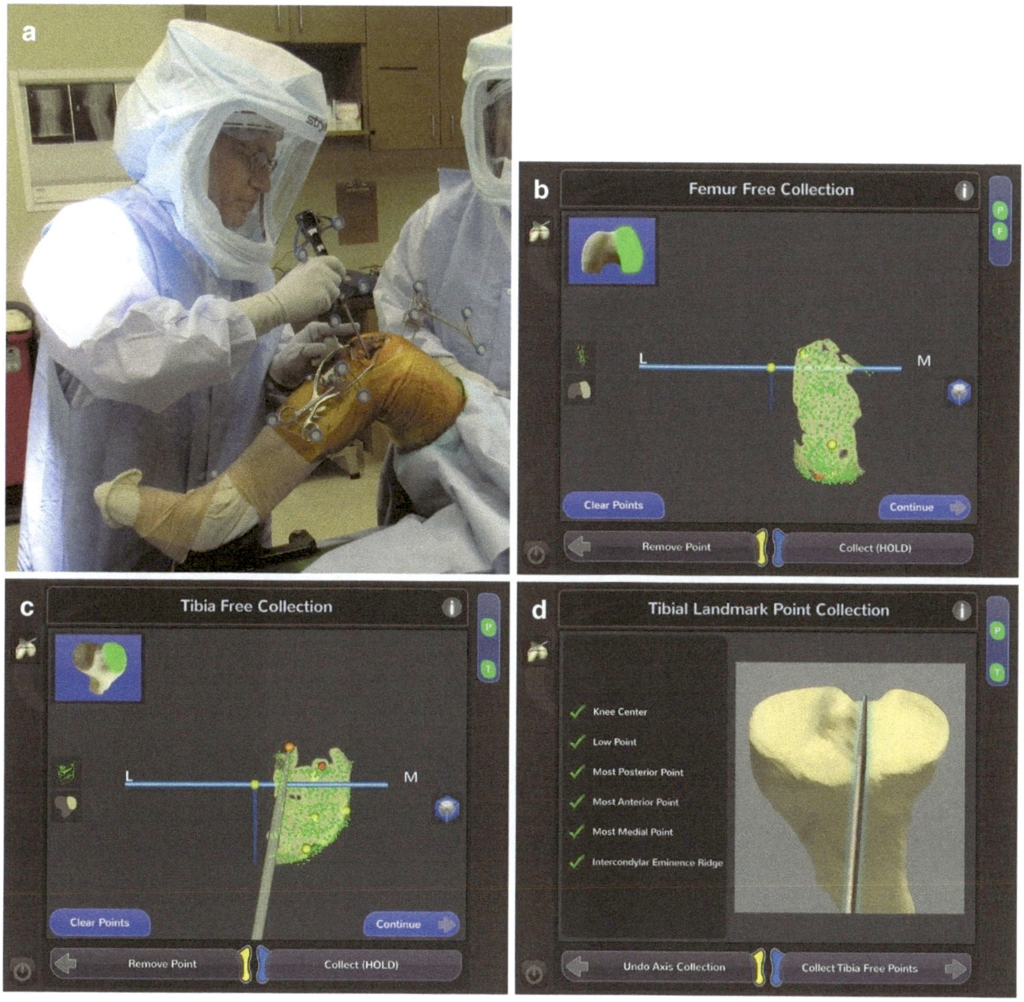

Fig. 9.5 Condylar anatomy is mapped out by "painting" the surfaces of the femoral condyle and tibial hemiplateau with an optical probe (**a**) intraoperative photo, (**b**) mapping of the femoral surface, (**c**) mapping of the tibial surface, and (**d**) rotational alignment of the tibial axis is established along the peak of the medial tibial spine

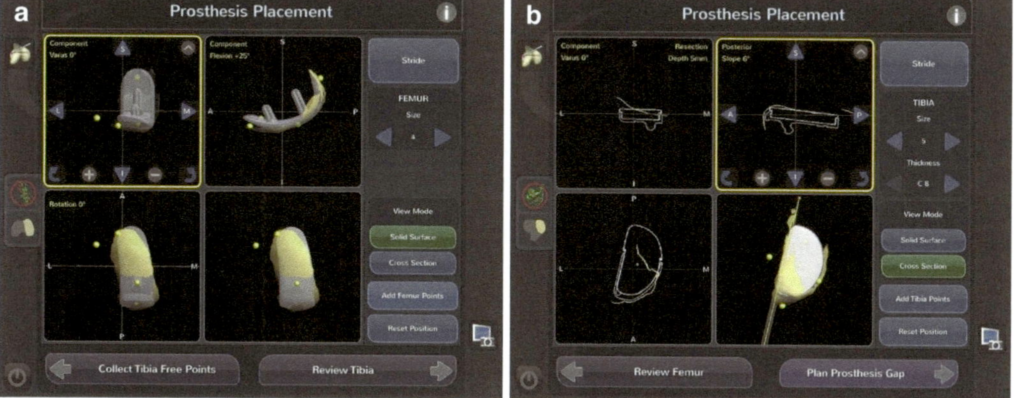

Fig. 9.6 (**a, b**) Provisional sizing and positioning of the femoral and tibial components are planned on the virtual models, based on the mapped condylar surfaces

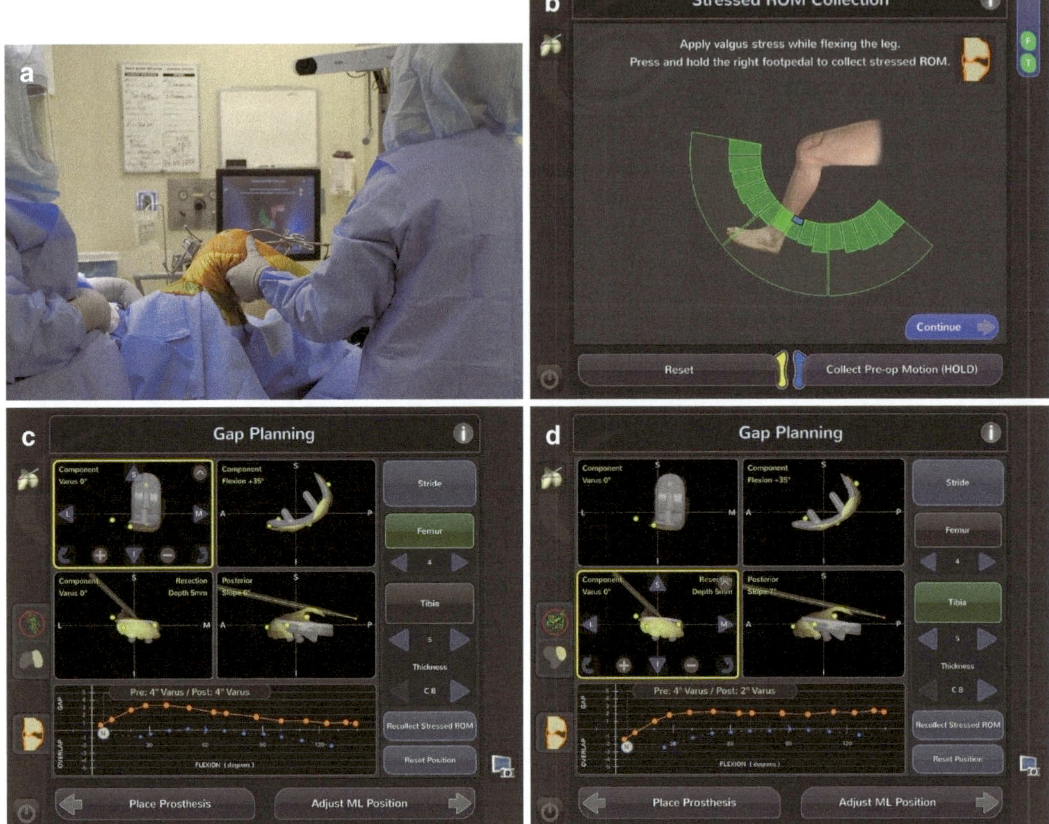

Fig. 9.7 After osteophyte excision, a dynamic soft tissue balancing algorithm is initiated. In the case of a medial UKA, a valgus stress is applied to tension the medial collateral ligament and medial capsule (**a, b**). A virtual graphic representation of gap spacing (relative laxity or tightness) is provided through a full range of motion, and an assessment can be made regarding the planned positions of the femoral and tibial components and anticipated correction of limb alignment. (**c**) In this case, the initial plan showed excessive relative laxity between the components between roughly 20° and 50° and excessive tightness after 90° of flexion. (**d**) Adjustments were made to the tibial slope, and the femoral component was distalized and anteriorized to create a virtual graph that displayed roughly 2 mm of laxity between the components through the entire flexion arc and correction of the limb varus from 4° to 2°

this stage to create a graph depicting the desired soft tissue balance in UKA is critical. Finally, medial and lateral positioning and angular orientation can be planned so that reasonable tracking of the femur on the tibia can be virtually planned and adjustments made as necessary (Fig. 9.8).

Surface Preparation

Once the surfaces have been mapped and the surgical plan and gap balancing have been adjusted, femoral burring is undertaken. Either a 6- or 5-millimeter handheld sculpting burr is used to prepare the bone on the condylar surfaces. The Navio robotic system provides protective control against inadvertent bone removal, through modulating the exposure or speed of a retractable bur. "Exposure-control" mode adjusts the extent to which the bur is exposed beyond a protective sheath. Position data are continuously updated in real time, resulting in the fluid adjustment in the position of the bur tip. When the bur tip is within the field to be removed, it is positioned outside of the cylindrical guard; when it is moved outside of the area, which had been predetermined to be removed, it retracts within the protective sheath. This mode of preparation is ideally suited for the distal condylar surface and portion of the posterior aspect of the femur. In "speed-control"

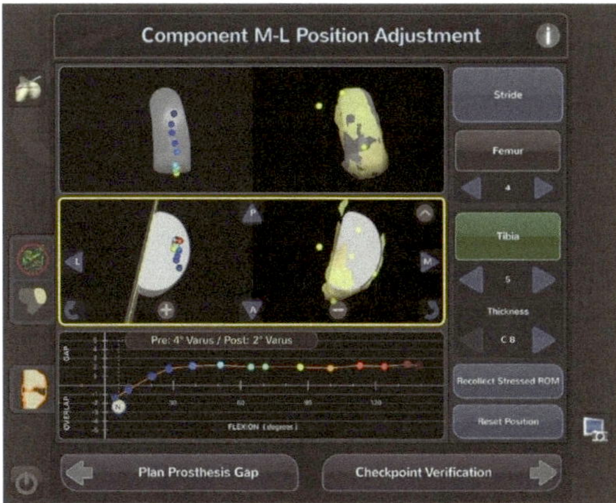

Fig. 9.8 Contact points showing virtually where the femur is anticipated to be tracking on the tibia based on implant position, and soft tissue balance is also shown. Adjustments in position can be made accordingly

mode, a shorter sheath is used that does not cover the bur. Instead, the rotational speed of the bur is modulated based on proximity to the boundaries of the target surface. This allows the bur to spin and remove intended bone, with speed slowing to a stop as the tip reaches the margins of the final preparation position. This mode is ideal for the preparation of the posteriormost portion of the femoral condyle, tibial surface, and femoral and tibial lug holes (Fig. 9.9a–d). Final tibial sizing and lug hole preparation are best done in conjunction with the manual sizer and drill guide, given the difficulty modeling the posterior surface of the tibia earlier in the case, with the femoral condyle intact. This method is most accurate for tibial sizing and ensures accurate anteroposterior translation of the tibial component (Fig. 9.10a, b).

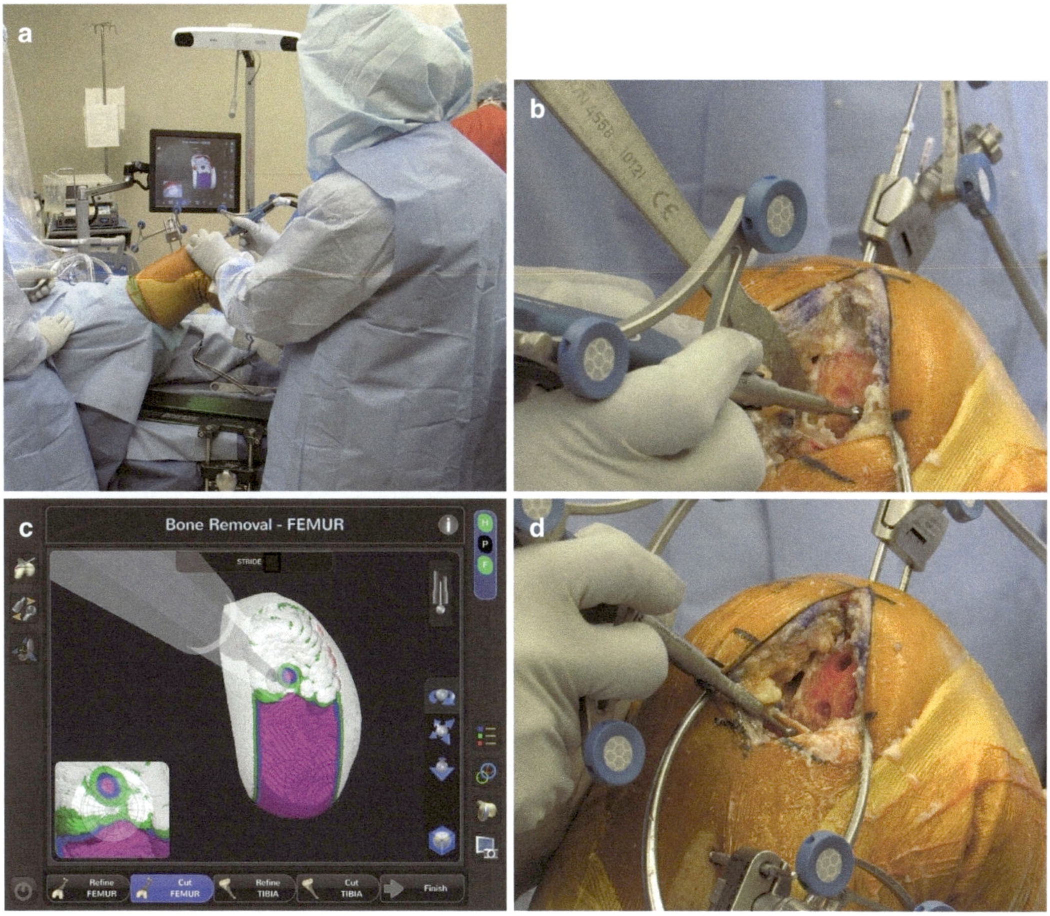

Fig. 9.9 (**a–d**) Real-time and virtual views of femoral and tibial preparation with the 6 mm bur attached to the handheld robotic sculpting tool

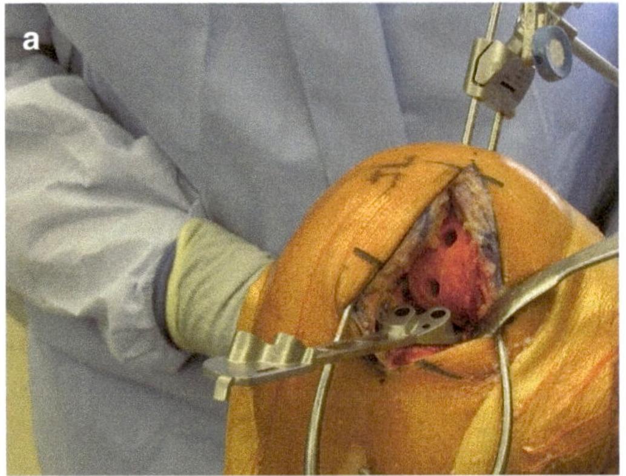

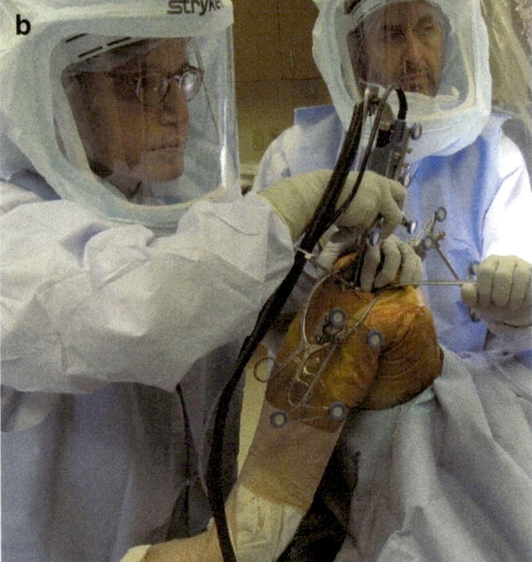

Fig. 9.10 (a, b) Intraoperative view of method of final tibial sizing and tibial lug hole preparation, using the manual guide to optimize component size and AP translation

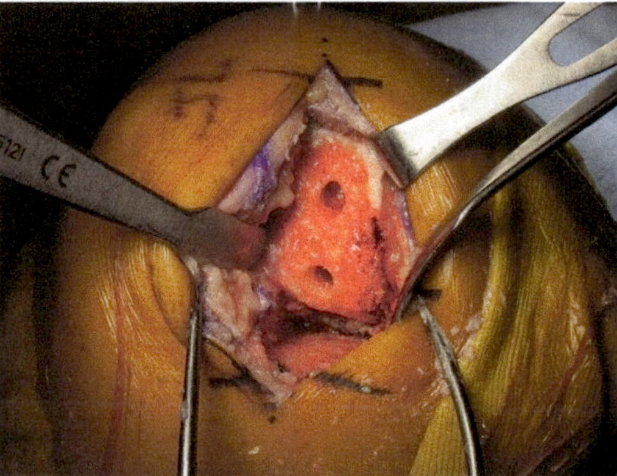

Fig. 9.11 Intraoperative view of the precisely prepared femoral and tibial surfaces

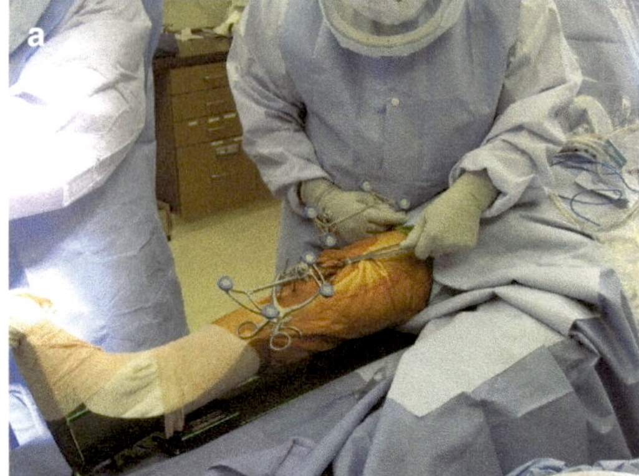

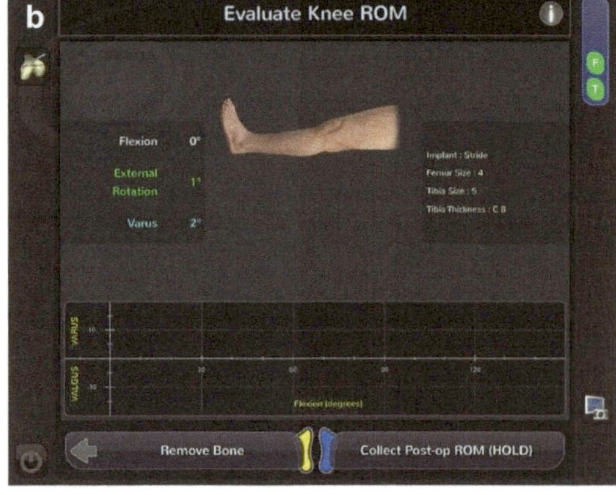

Fig. 9.12 (a, b) With trials in place, limb alignment and soft tissue balance are reconfirmed. In this case, final limb alignment in full extension is 2° varus, consistent with the preoperative plan. A 2 mm shim can be inserted to confirm reasonable balance through a range of motion

Trialing and Implantation

After bone preparation, the surfaces are assessed, and the posterior femoral osteophytes and the remaining peripheral bone that is not covered by the implants are removed (Fig. 9.11). The meniscus is excised and trial components manually impacted into place. Limb alignment, range of motion, implant position, and gap balance can be quantified and compared with the preoperative plan (Fig. 9.12). If necessary, additional bone can be removed by making adjustments to slope or depth of resection in the surgical plan on the computer, depending on where some residual tightness or imbalance may be observed. Once the knee is considered adequately aligned and balanced, the surfaces are irrigated and dried, and final components are manually cemented into place (Fig. 9.13a–e).

Results

In an initial feasibility study of Navio, Smith et al. assessed the accuracy of bone preparation in 20 synthetic lower extremities (10 right and 10 left). Surface preparation and component position were highly accurate, with the root-orientations (flexion-extension, varus-valgus, and rotation) ranging from 1.05° to 1.52° for the femoral implant and 0.66 to 1.32° for the tibial implant; translational errors averaged 0.61 mm, with a maximum of 1.18 mm; and mean surface overcut or undercut was 0.14 mm and 0.21 mm for the femoral and tibial surfaces, respectively

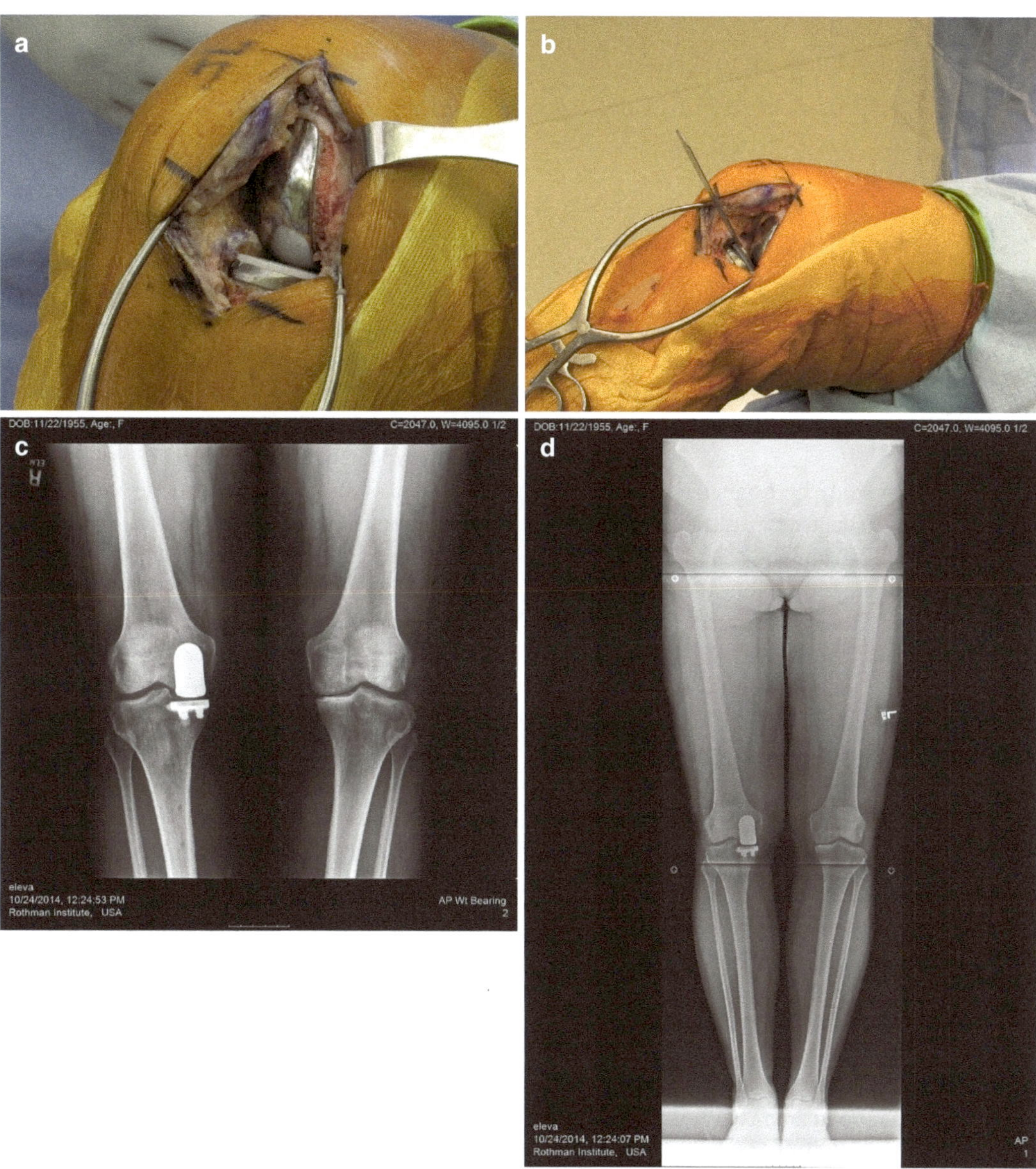

Fig. 9.13 (**a**) Intraoperative appearance of medial UKA cemented into place. (**b**) A 2 mm shim is inserted between the components to pressurize the cement while it cures, with the knee flexed 20–30° to concentrically compress mean-square (RMS) errors across all angular the components. (**c–e**) Standing postoperative anteroposterior (AP) of the limb and knee and lateral radiographs show excellent component position and limb alignment after UKA with Navio robotic tool [38, 39].

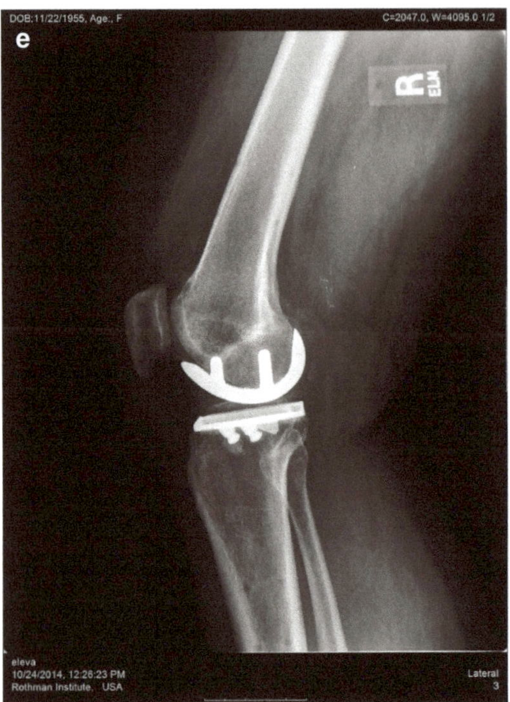

Fig. 9.13 (continued)

Table 9.1 Summary of positioning – robotic techniques vs conventional

RMS error	Mako Rio [19]	Acrobot [13]	Navio PFS [17]	Conventional [19]
Flex-ext (deg)	2.1	2.1	1.8	6.0
Varus-valgus (deg)	2.1	1.7	2.5	4.1
Int-ext (deg)	3.0	3.1	1.7	6.3
Prox-dist (mm)	1.0	1.0	1.3	2.8
Ant-post (mm)	1.6	1.8	1.3	2.4
Med-lat (mm)	1.0	0.6	1.0	1.6

A follow-up study by Lonner et al. evaluated the precision of bone preparation using Navio in 25 cadaveric specimens. The "planned" and "actual" angular, translational, and rotational positions of the components were compared. The RMS angular errors were 1.42–2.34° for the three directions for the femoral implant and 1.95–2.60° for the three directions of the tibial implant. The RMS translational errors were 0.92–1.61 mm for the femoral implant and 0.97–1.67 mm for the tibial implant [25]. The results, further summarized in Table 9.1, highlight comparable precision to image-guided robotic technology and substantially reduced error compared to conventional methods of bone preparation in UKA [21, 25, 28].

A clinical radiographic study by Picard et al. reported on 65 patients undergoing medial UKA using Navio. The planned mechanical axis alignment was compared with the postsurgical alignment using full-length, double-stance, weight-bearing radiographs [40]. The average preoperative alignment was 4.5° mechanical varus (standard deviation = 2.9°, range: 0–12° varus). The average postoperative mechanical axis was corrected to 2.1° (range: 0–7° varus). The postoperative mechanical axis alignment in the coronal plane was within 1° of the intraoperative plan in 91% of the cases. Of the six cases with postoperative alignment greater than 1° from the plan, three resulted from an increase in the thickness of the tibial polyethylene insert implanted. The average difference between the "planned" intraoperative mechanical axis alignment and the postoperative long leg, weight-bearing mechanical axis alignment was 1.8° [40].

In light of the importance of preserving the joint line position in UKA to optimize kinematics and reduce polyethylene stress that is observed with distalizing the joint line, several studies have shown improved femoral joint line position with robotic Navio preparation compared to conventional methods [41]. A retrospective case-control study by Herry et al. compared two matched groups of patients receiving a resurfacing UKA between 2013 and 2016 by either a robotic-assisted ($n = 40$) or conventional ($n = 40$) technique. Restitution of joint line height was significantly improved in the robotic-assisted group compared to the conventional group, which tended to distalize the femoral joint line (+1.4 mm ±2.6 vs +4.7 mm ± 2.4 [$p < 0.05$]) [42]. Likewise, a retrospective case-control study by Fu et al. compared tibial component slope and femoral joint line position in 175 matched medial UKAs performed using a conventional spacer block technique ($n = 52$), image-free robotic system (Navio) ($n = 57$), or CT-based robotic system (Mako) ($n = 66$) by a single surgeon. The mean postoperative posterior slope was highest in the conventional group (8.98°+/−2.83), followed by Mako (7.1°+/−2.5) and then Navio (5.56°+/−2.18). The differences between groups were statistically significant ($p < 0.001$). Importantly, while the senior surgeon attempts to restrict the posterior tibial slope to ≤7°, the percentage of posterior slope outliers >7° were 25%, 5%, and 3.5% for conventional, Mako, and Navio cases, respectively. Furthermore, the joint line was significantly distalized in the conventional group (−1.57 mm+/−1.62) when compared with Navio (−0.3 mm +/− 1.06) ($p < 0.001$) or Mako (−0.26 mm+/−0.98) ($p < 0.001$). There were no differences in joint line between Mako and Navio ($p = 0.65$) in that study [43].

Additionally, robot assistance has been shown to result in a more conservative tibial resection compared to conventional methods [44]. In an analysis of 8421 robotic-assisted UKAs and 27,989 conventional UKAs, Ponzio et al. found that statistically more 8-mm and 9-mm polyethylene inserts – a proxy measure of bone conserving tibial resections – were used in the robotic group (93.6%) than in the conventional group (84.5%) ($P < 0.0001$). Additionally, larger tibial inserts of ≥10 mm – an indication of typically greater tibial resection – were utilized in 6.4% of robotic-assisted cases and 15.5% of conventional cases [44]. This has both physiological and practical implications. First, proximal tibial bone is weaker with more distal resection, and thus it is biomechanically advantageous to minimize bone resection. Second, in the event of a future revision to TKA, reconstruction is more challenging and more likely to require tibial augments and stems when larger tibial resections were made at the time of UKA.

Clinical data is emerging regarding the impact of robotic precision on durability. A recent 2-year clinical study of patients who underwent Navio-assisted UKA (medial 97%; lateral 3%) found the overall implant survivorship (free of failure or revision) to be 99.2%, which was non-inferior when compared to the reference survival rate of 95.7% from the Australian registry. There was one revision encountered during the study, which was due to persistent soft tissue pain, without evidence of loosening, subsidence, malposition, or infection [45]. In a matched case-control study comparing implant position, limb alignment, and revision rate in 160 UKAs performed with either Navio or a conventional technique using the identical implant (HLS Uni Evolution, Tornier®), Batailler et al. found the rate of postoperative limb alignment outliers (±2°) was significantly higher in the control group than in the robotic-assisted group for both lateral UKA (26% in robotic group versus 61% in control group; $p = 0.018$) and medial UKA (16% versus 32%, resp.; $p = 0.038$). Additionally, the coronal and sagittal tibial baseplate position had significantly fewer outliers (±3°) in the robotic-assisted group than in the control group. At a mean follow-up of 19.7 months ±9 for the robotic-assisted group and 24.2 months ±16 for the control group, 5% ($n = 4/80$) of patients in the robotic-assisted UKA group and 9% ($n = 7/80$) in the conventional UKA group required revision to TKA (n.s.d.). In the conventional group, 86% of revisions were due to component malposition or limb malalignment, compared to none in the robotic-assisted group [46]. Current ongoing study is comparing functional outcomes of matched groups of conventional versus Navio-assisted UKA performed by the senior surgeon. Our preliminary unpublished data show accelerated recovery of functional milestones in the robotic group, but analysis at longer follow-up is not yet complete.

Despite the improved precision of robotic UKA, stakeholders – that is, surgeons and administrators of hospitals or surgery centers – have concern that adopting robotic systems may be associated with a lengthy learning period and increased operative time before the surgeon can efficiently and effectively use the technology. In order to address the learning curve for surgical proficiency with Navio, Gregori et al. examined the number of surgeries required to reach "steady-state" surgical time among five experienced arthroplasty surgeons who had no prior surgical experience with this robot [47]. The average surgical time (tracker placement to trial acceptance) among all surgeons across their first 15 cases was 56.8 minutes (range: 27–102 minutes). The average improvement was 46 minutes from the slowest to quickest surgical times, with "cutting" phase decreasing on average by 31 minutes during the initial 15 cases. On average, it took 8 procedures (range: 5–11) to reach a steady-state surgical time, with an average steady-state surgical time of 50 minutes (range: 37–55 minutes).

Unlike its predecessor robotic technology, Navio does not require preoperative mapping utilizing computed tomography (CT) scanning. A study by Ponzio and Lonner found that by switching from a CT scan-based system (Mako, Stryker Mako, Fort Lauderdale, FL) to the Navio system, the avoided per-scan effective dose (ED) of radiation was 4.8 ± 3.0 mSv (approximately equivalent to 48 chest radiographs) [36], thus heeding the US Food and Drug Administration's (FDA) warning that steps be taken to mitigate exposure to avoidable radiation [48].

Conclusion

Navio technology has proven effective in optimizing component alignment, conserving bone resection volumes, restoring joint line, and quantifying soft tissue balance in UKA. Data is only now beginning to emerge that suggests that Navio robotic assistance is improving early functional outcomes and durability in UKA. Further ongoing study will be necessary to better determine whether the added precision of Navio will correlate with better longer-term durability and outcomes than those achieved with conventional methods.

Compared to first-generation image-based robotic systems, without compromising precision or safety, Navio represents considerable savings on multiple levels – including savings of time, inconvenience, and radiation exposure related to the elimination of the preoperative CT scan; savings on space requirements; and savings on capital and per-case costs. These are clear benefits for the key stakeholders – payers, hospitals, surgeons, and patients. Navio dovetails nicely into the transition we are seeing nationwide whereby partial knee arthroplasties are increasingly being performed on an outpatient basis, with greater use in surgery centers rather than hospitals. Its reduced costs, small footprint, and diminished storage needs are perfectly suited for use in these outpatient centers.

References

1. Noticewala M, Geller J, Lee J, et al. Unicompartmental knee arthroplasty relieves pain and improves function more than total knee arthroplasty. J Arthroplast. 2012;27(S8):99–105.
2. Hansen E, Ong K, Kurtz S, Lau E, Lonner JH. Unicondylar knee arthroplasty has fewer complications but higher revision rates than total knee arthroplasty in study of large United States databases. J Arthroplast. [in press].
3. Hansen EN, Ong KL, Lau E, Kurtz SM, Lonner JH. Unicondylar knee arthroplasty in the U.S. Patient population: prevalence and epidemiology. Am J Orthop (Belle Mead NJ). 2018;47(12).
4. Riddle DL, Jiranek WA, McGlynn FJ. Yearly incidence of unicompartmental knee arthroplasty in the United States. J Arthroplast. 2008;23:408–12.
5. Berger RA, Meneghini RM, Jacobs JJ, Sheinkop MB, Della Valle CJ, Rosenberg AG, et al. Results of unicompartmental knee arthroplasty at a minimum of ten years of follow-up. J Bone Joint Surg Am. 2005;87:999–1006.
6. Cartier P, Sanouiller JL, Grelsamer RP. Unicompartmental knee arthroplasty surgery. 10-year minimum follow-up period. J Arthroplast. 1996;11:782–8.
7. Newman J, Pydisetty RV, Ackroyd C. Unicompartmental or total knee replacement: the 15-year results of a prospective randomised controlled trial. J Bone Joint Surg Br. 2009;91:52–7.
8. Pandit H, Jenkins C, Gill HS, Barker K, Dodd CA, Murray DW. Minimally invasive Oxford phase 3 unicompartmental knee replacement: results of 1000 cases. J Bone Joint Surg Br. 2011;93:198–204.
9. Price AJ, Svard U. A second decade lifetable survival analysis of the Oxford unicompartmental knee arthroplasty. Clin Orthop Relat Res. 2011;469:174–9.
10. Australian Orthopaedic Association National Joint Replacement Registry. Available at: https://aoanjrr.dmac.adelaide.edu.au/en.
11. New Zealand Joint Registry. Available at: http://www.nzoa.org.nz/news/new-zealand-joint-registry-thirteen-year-report.
12. Dyrhovden GS, Lygre SHL, Badawy M, Gothesen O, Furnes O. Have the causes of revision for total and unicompartmental knee arthroplasties changed during the past two decades? Clin Orthop Relat Res. 2017;475:1874–86.
13. Epinette JA, Brunschweiler B, Mertl P, Mole D, Cazenave A, French Society for Hip and Knee. Unicompartmental knee arthroplasty modes of failure: wear is not the main reason for failure: a multicentre study of 418 failed knees. Orthop Traumatol Surg Res. 2012;98(6 Suppl):S124–30.
14. Chatellard R, Sauleau V, Colmar M, Robert H, Raynaud G, Brilhault J. Socie te d'Orthope die et de Traumatologie de l'Ouest (SOO). Medial unicompartmental knee arthroplasty: does tibial component position influence clinical outcomes and arthroplasty

survival? Orthop Traumatol Surg Res. 2013;99(4 Suppl):S219–25.

15. Collier MB, Eickmann TH, Sukezaki F, et al. Patient, implant, and alignment factors associated with revision of medial compartment unicondylar arthroplasty. J Arthroplast. 2006;21(6, S2):108–15.

16. Hernigou P, Deschamps G. Alignment influences wear in the knee after medial unicompartmental arthroplasty. Clin Orthop Relat Res. 2004;423:161–5.

17. Hernigou P, Deschamps G. Posterior slope of the tibial implant and the outcome of unicompartmental knee arthroplasty. J Bone Joint Surg Am. 2004;86-A:506–11.

18. Fisher DA, Watts M, Davis KE. Implant position in knee surgery: a comparison of minimally invasive, open unicompartmental, and total knee arthroplasty. J Arthroplast. 2003;18(7, S1):2–8.

19. Hamilton WG, Collier MB, Tarabee E, et al. Incidence and reasons for reoperation after minimally invasive unicompartmental knee arthroplasty. J Arthroplast. 2006;21(6, S2):98–107.

20. Keene G, Simpson D, Kalairajah Y. Limb alignment in computer-assisted minimally-invasive unicompartmental knee replacement. J Bone Joint Surg Br. 2006;88:44–8.

21. Cobb J, Henckel J, Gomes P, et al. Hands-on robotic unicompartmental knee replacement: a prospective, randomised controlled study of the acrobot system. J Bone Joint Surg Br. 2006;88:188–97.

22. Romanowski MR, Repicci JA. Minimally invasive unicondylar arthroplasty: eight-year follow-up. J Knee Surg. 2002;15:17–22.

23. Lonner JH. Indications for unicompartmental knee arthroplasty and rationale for robotic arm-assisted technology. Am J Orthop. 2009;38(S2):3–6.

24. Sinha RK. Outcomes of robotic arm-assisted unicompartmental knee arthroplasty. Am J Orthop. 2009;38(S2):20–2.

25. Lonner JH, Smith JR, Picard F, et al. High degree of accuracy of a novel image-free handheld robot for unicondylar knee arthroplasty in a cadaveric study. Clin Orthop Relat Res. 2015;473:206–12.

26. Lonner JH, Moretti VM. The evolution of image-free robotic assistance in unicompartmental knee arthroplasty. Am J Orthop. 2016;45:249–54.

27. Conditt MA, Bargar WL, Cobb JP, Lonner JH. Current concepts in robotics for the treatment of joint disease. Adv Orthop. 2013;2013:948360.

28. Dunbar NJ, Roche MW, Park BH, et al. Accuracy of dynamic tactile guided unicompartmental knee arthroplasty. J Arthroplast. 2012;27:803–8.

29. Lang JE, Mannava S, Floyd AJ. Specialty update: general orthopaedics: robotic systems in orthopaedic surgery. J Bone Joint Surg Br. 2011;93-B:1296–9.

30. Lonner JH, John TK, Conditt MA. Robotic arm-assisted UKA improves tibial component alignment: a pilot study. Clin Orthop Relat Res. 2010;468:141–6.

31. Conditt MA, Roche MW. Minimally invasive robotic-arm-guided unicompartmental knee arthroplasty. J Bone Joint Surg Am. 2009;91(S1):63–8.

32. Roche M, O'Loughlin PF, Kendoff D, et al. Robotic arm-assisted unicompartmental knee arthroplasty: preoperative planning and surgical technique. Am J Orthop. 2009;38(S2):10–5.

33. Swank ML, Alkire M, Conditt M, et al. Technology and cost effectiveness in knee arthroplasty: computer navigation and robotics. Am J Orthop. 2009;38(S2):32–6.

34. Orthopedic Network News, 2013 Hip and knee implant review. Available at: www.OrthopedicNetworkNews.com. 2013; 24.

35. Medical Device and Diagnostic Industry. 2015. Available at: https://www.mddionline.com.

36. Ponzio DY, Lonner JH. Preoperative mapping in unicompartmental knee arthroplasty using computed tomography scans is associated with radiation exposure and carries high cost. J Arthroplast. 2015;30(6):967.

37. Lonner JH. Robotically assisted unicompartmental knee arthroplasty. In: Austin MS, Klein GR, editors. World clinics: orthopedics: current 112 J.H. Lonner controversies in joint replacement. Philadelphia: Jaypee Brothers Medical Publishers LTD; 2014.

38. Smith JR, Picard F, Rowe PJ. The accuracy of a robotically-controlled freehand sculpting tool for unicondylar knee arthroplasty. J Bone Joint Surg Br. 2013;95(S28):68.

39. Smith JR, Riches PE, Rowe PJ. Accuracy of a freehand sculpting tool for unicondylar knee replacement. Int J Med Robot. 2014;10:162–9.

40. Picard F, Gregori A, Bellemans J, et al. Handheld robot-assisted unicondylar knee arthroplasty: a clinical review. 14th Annual Meeting of the International Society for Computer Assisted Orthopaedic Surgery. Milan, Italy, 2014.

41. Kwon OR, Kang KT, Son J, Suh DS, Baek C, Koh YG. Importance of joint line preservation in unicompartmental knee arthroplasty: finite element analysis. J Orthop Res. 2017;35(2):347–52. https://doi.org/10.1002/jor.23279.

42. Herry Y, Batailler C, Lording T, Servien E, Neyret P, Lustig S. Improved joint-line restitution in unicompartmental knee arthroplasty using a robotic-assisted surgical technique. Int Orthop (SICOT). 2017;41:2265–71. https://doi.org/10.1007/s00264-017-3633-9.

43. Fu H, Manrique J, Yan CH, Chiu KY, Lonner JH. Award paper: joint line restoration and alignment after conventional versus robotic unicompartmental knee arthroplasty. Proceedings of the Hong Kong orthopedic association annual congress, Hong Kong, November 3–4, 2018.

44. Ponzio DY, Lonner JH. Robotic technology produces more conservative tibial resection than conventional techniques in UKA. Am J Orthop. 2016;45(7):E465.

45. Battenberg AK, Netravali NA, Lonner JH. A novel handheld robotic-assisted system for unicompartmental knee arthroplasty: surgical technique and early survivorship. J Robot Surg Springer. 2018; https://doi.org/10.1007/s11701-018-00907-w.

46. Batailler C, White N, Ranaldi FM, Neyret P, Servien E, Lustig S. Improved implant position and lower revision rate with robotic- assisted unicompartmental knee arthroplasty. Knee Surg Sports Traumatol Arthrosc. 2018; https://doi.org/10.1007/s00167-018-5081-5.
47. Gregori A, Picard F, Bellemans J et al. The learning curve of a novel handheld robotic system for unicondylar knee arthroplasty. 14th Annual Meeting of the International Society for computer assisted orthopaedic surgery. Milan, Italy, 2014.
48. Initiative to reduce unnecessary radiation exposure from medical imaging, 2010. Available at: http://www.fda.gov/Radiation-EmittingProducts/RadiationSafety/RadiationDoseReduction/ucm199904.htm. Accessed 20 Feb 2014.

Unicompartmental Knee Arthroplasty Techniques: Mako

10

Martin Roche

The first MAKOplasty was performed in 2006 utilizing an all poly inlay component (Fig. 10.1). The following year, a metal-backed implant was developed and is the standard today (Fig. 10.2). The second-generation RIO Robot was introduced in 2009 and enabled the expansion to medial, lateral, patellofemoral, and bicompartmental knee arthroplasties (Fig. 10.3) [1].

UKAs have shown improved kinematics as related to total knee replacements, less pain from surgery, and a knee that patients prefer [2, 3].

The benefits of "MAKOplasty" still follow the principles of strict patient selection and appropriate planning. Meticulous cementing technique and minimized soft tissue dissection enable consistent results [4].

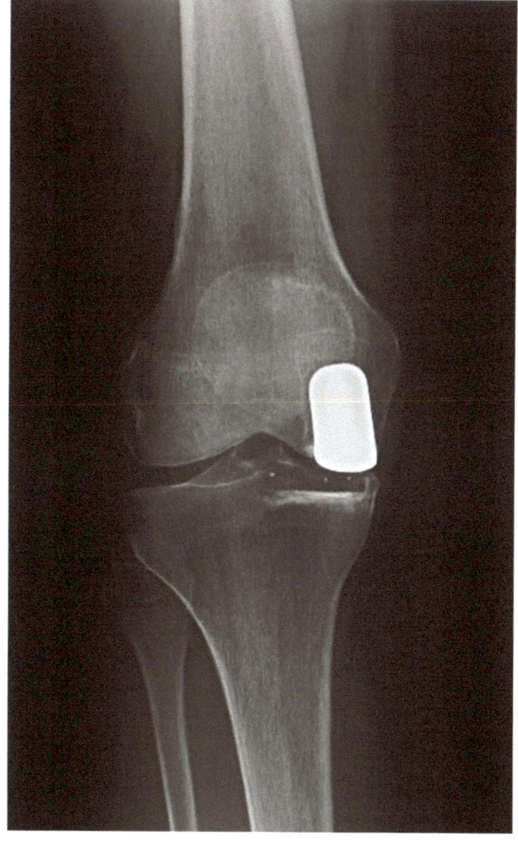

Fig. 10.1 12-year post-op inlay MAKOplasty medial UKR AP view

M. Roche (✉)
Department of Orthopedic Surgery, Holy Cross
Orthopedic Institute, Fort Lauderdale, FL, USA
e-mail: martin@mroche.com

© Springer Nature Switzerland AG 2019
J. H. Lonner (ed.), *Robotics in Knee and Hip Arthroplasty*,
https://doi.org/10.1007/978-3-030-16593-2_10

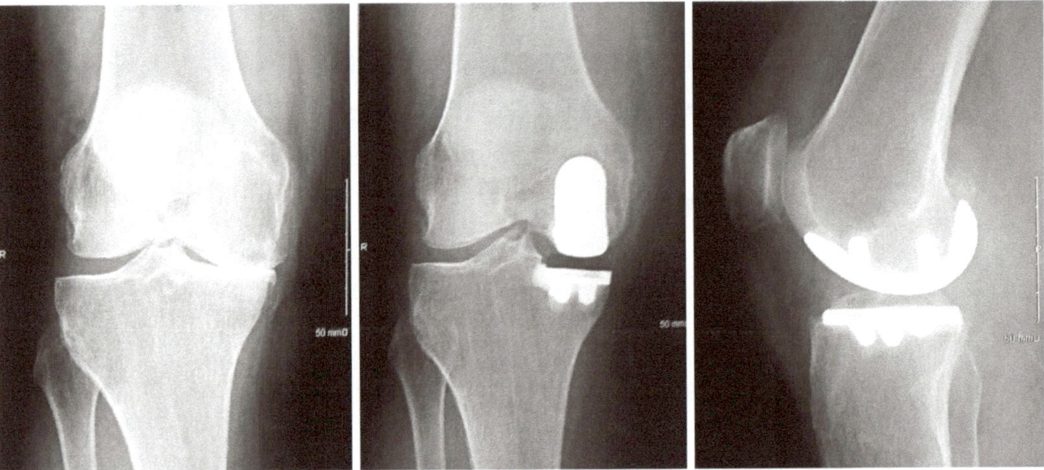

Fig. 10.2 10-year post-op medial onlay MAKOplasty AP- pre-op; AP- post-op – Lat- postop– Lat view

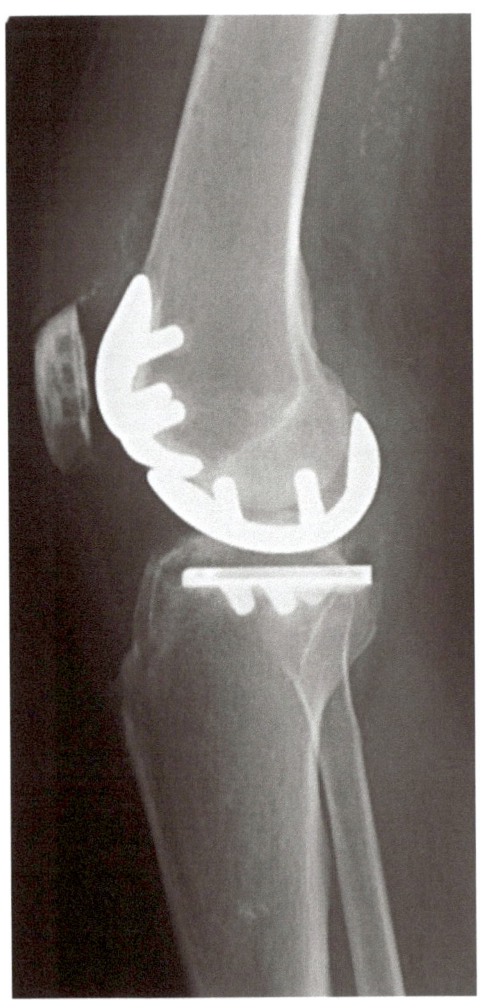

Fig. 10.3 Lateral view onlay bicompartmental MAKOplasty 8 years post-op

The Robotic System

(a) Software

The application software begins with a CT scan of the patient's affected lower limb. This CT scan includes the hip, knee, and ankle joint. This enables anatomic implant matching and positioning, with evaluation of the joint pathology including intra- and extra joint deformities.

The CT scan is 3D reconstructed and then preoperative outlined to enable accurate verification and validation of the patient's anatomy during the procedure. The software is depicted on a graphic user interface in the operating room and is the focus of the surgeon during surgery.

(b) Hardware

The Robotic base houses the motors and extends out an arm that has 6 degrees of freedom. The motorized burr or saw blade is attached to the end of the arm to allow surgeon control of the instrument.

Multiple sensors are utilized to control safety and feedback during utilization of the burr or saw.

The navigation system is an infrared optical tracking system that requires stabile reflective sensors that are attached to the patient's femur and tibia through bone pins. The robotic arm is tracked as well and validated with an independent sensor array [5, 6].

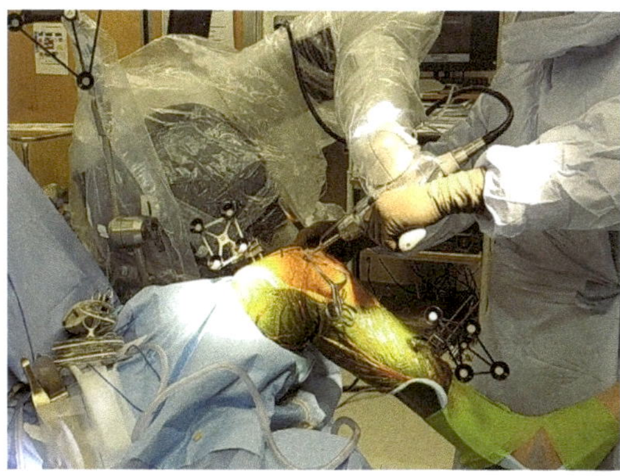

Fig. 10.4 Robotic arm and burr entering operative knee with tracking sensors

Checkpoints in the femur and tibia are utilized to confirm that no unintended loss of registration prior to cutting has occurred. The Robotic system is sterilely draped and positioned for full access to the surgical field (Fig. 10.4) [7]

(c) Implants

The Femoral and Tibial components are specific to the system, with a range of compatible sizes. The femur is CoCr and the tibial baseplate is titanium. The tibial polyethylene sizes extend from 6 mm to 9 mm and are gamma sterilized. The implants are cemented.

Surgical Planning Phase

The surgeon evaluates the patient's preoperative CT scan and can adjust the implants for an anatomic fit. This enables the appropriate slope, rotation, cortical rim fit to be obtained. The joint line and depth of resection are initially set. Other pathologies can be defined such as the extent of avascular necrosis and any subchondral cysts. This imaging-based approach allows preoperative implant selection and accurate registration to minimize error and improve intra-op efficiencies.

Patient Positioning and Surgical Exposure

The patient is positioned in a standard supine fashion. The operative knee is examined. The knee is tested for range of motion, ligamentous stability and correctability of the deformity. The operative leg is prepped, draped and placed in a dynamic and articulating leg holder, making sure full range of motion can be achieved. A tourniquet is usually applied and used.

Medial UKA

A medial arthrotomy is performed to enter the diseased compartment. The incision can be minimized as the surgeon can place the knee in various positions to allow the burr or saw to safely prepare the bone without direct visualization and preventing soft tissue trauma (Fig. 10.5). Minimally invasive approach was popularized by Dr. Repicci and has become a "standard" approach [8]. He cited the potential advantages of decreased blood loss, less tissue trauma and morbidity, as well as earlier recovery and easier rehabilitation. With minimally invasive procedures using conventional cutting guides, visualization is reduced leading to potential errors in implant placement, limb alignment, cement technique, and bone preparation (Fig. 10.5) [9–11].

Most advocates of minimally invasive knee surgery champion an arthrotomy that does not invade the quadriceps femoris tendon. Also, eversion of the patella is avoided. In the case of robotic-assisted surgery, the loss of direct visualization is offset by the haptic boundaries and tracking of the joint spatially through a range of motion that is created by the system as a safeguard. The knee is stabilized and positioned in angles for maximal access, the MCL and patellar tendon protected, and robotic arm brought into field of surgery. This approach can be made more extensile in the occasional case requiring concomitant patellofemoral resurfacing [10].

Lateral UKAs

Lateral UKRs are commonly approached with a lateral longitudinal incision, although this also varies by surgeon preference. Most of the work and exposure are done in extension and midflexion to relax the lateral pull of the patella. The tibia must be internally rotated anteriorly to conform to the femur in extension based on the "screw home "mechanism. The femur must be

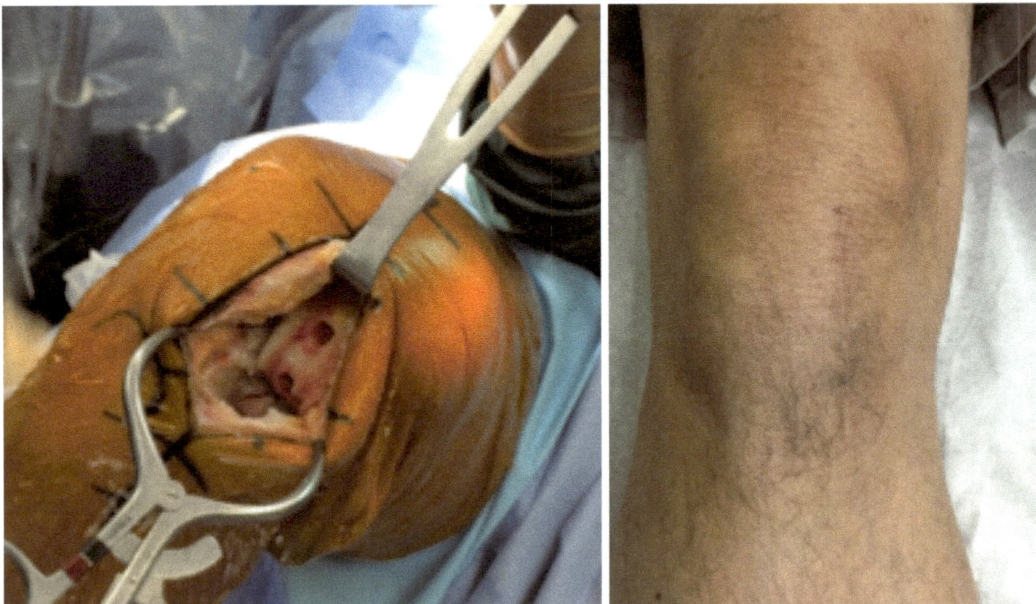

Fig. 10.5 Minimally invasive approach after bone prep of medial robotic UKR and post-op scar

lateralized and verticalized as well. The positioning of the femoral component should accommodate the femoral divergence of the lateral condyle when the knee is flexed; in that way, impingement with the tibial spines will be avoided when the knee is brought into extension. The flexion gap can be difficult to balance, with its inherent laxity, and a worn or dysplastic posterior femur. Care must be taken not to overstuff the flexion gap, which will drive the extension gap into varus mal-alignment [9].

Occasionally, the popliteus has to be recessed due to impingement. During insertion of the femur, placing the knee in extension, and then flexing the knee aides in placement, as the lateral patellar pull is neutralized.

Benefits of Robotic Technology

A robotic-assisted platform enables the surgeon to utilize a pre-op computer-assisted planning system and a tactile guidance system intraoperatively.

Achieving accurate alignment of the tibial component in unicompartmental knee arthroplasty with use of conventional instrumentation is inconsistent, with outliers beyond 2° of the preoperatively planned alignment occurring in as many as 40–60% of knees, particularly when minimally invasive surgical approaches are used. One study found a large range in tibia component alignment, with a mean of 6° (standard deviation, 4°) and a range from 18° varus to 6° valgus in 221 consecutive knees that underwent unicompartmental knee arthroplasty performed through a minimally invasive approach [11].

These errors are compounding, as an inaccurate tibial resection in the coronal, sagittal, and rotational planes leads to gap imbalance, malalignment, malrotation, impingement, and edge loading (Fig. 10.6) [12, 13].

Roche and Coon have reported the accuracy of the RIO system in accurate implant placement [14, 15]. Coon et al. radiographically compared 44 manually implanted UKAs to 33 robotically implanted. The accuracy of implant positioning with robotic arm assistance was improved by a factor of 2.8 in the sagittal plane and an average RMS error of 3.2° in the coronal plane as compared with the accuracy of manual, jig-based instrumented UKAs. Roche et al. radiographically measured postoperative implant placement accuracy on a series of 43 UKA patients. Average RMS errors were 1.9° in the coronal plane and 1.7° in the sagittal plane.

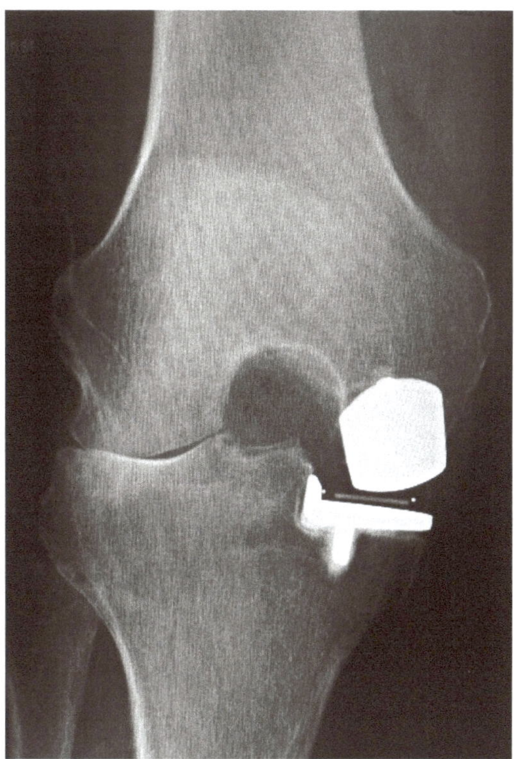

Fig. 10.6 Accelerated lateral joint degeneration due to overcorrection of limb and coronal implant impingement

While the robotic arm ensures accurate implant placement, many additional factors are required for a surgeon to achieve a successful surgical outcome. The ability to perform the predicted surgical plan consistently and precisely is related to proper implant sizing and positioning specific to the patients' anatomy. Optimizing the tension/balance of the collateral and cruciate ligaments through entire range of motion [16], actualizing smooth implant-cartilage transitions through cartilage mapping software, and the ability to minimize bone resection and tissue injury during surgery with haptic boundaries are the benefits of haptically controlled robotic assistance in UKA.

Through a minimal incision, optimized implant placement and soft tissue balancing enables a rapid rehabilitation program that enables patients to return to activities of daily living or resume work with shortened recovery times.

Consistent Execution of Surgical Plan

The system reduces variability, improves safety, while maintaining surgical efficiencies. The learning curve is consistent and independent of surgeon experience and volume. Accuracy is a key differentiator. Robotic UKA is 2 to 3 times more accurate and 3 times more reproducible than manual UKA [11, 13, 14]. This is critical as most common technical errors lead to early implant failure. The ability to recreate the joint line, slope, and implant position allows the knee to achieve early motion and potentially improve outcomes. Knowing the implant size preoperatively minimizes trays, and the surgical execution and leg positioner minimizes the need for surgical retraction affecting line of sight.

Pre-resection Plan Customization

Registration Phase

Femoral and Tibial tracking pins are placed and stabilized, and the sensors are positioned for the infrared tracking system to follow the positions of the leg and navigated robotic arm through a full range of motion. During pin placement, care is taken not to impinge on the quadriceps tendon, and care is needed in the osteopenic bone. Check points are placed in a stable area while avoiding any stress holes around the final implant. The robotic arm is tracked through a series of cubic maneuvers and registered. The Limb is registered to obtain the mechanical axis and the bones are registered utilizing sharp probes that contact the bone and are validated to the patients CT scan.

Customization of Plan

The knee is inspected to ensure a stable ACL and that the patellofemoral and lateral cartilage is healthy. If other compartments are felt to be arthritic and require resurfacing, the plan can now be adjusted to include other compartments, and cartilage can be mapped to ensure a smooth transition of components.

The osteophytes are removed, and the knee can now be evaluated. The surgeon now can correct the limb deformity based on the ligament tension and confirm that overcorrection has not occurred throughout a full range of motion.

(A) Four poses are commonly utilized to evaluate alignment and gap distances (Fig. 10.7)
- 0°: This pose defines any flexion contractures and enables the surgeon to adjust the femoral component size to ensure the tibia will not impinge on the femoral cartilage in full extension
- 10°: uncouples the screw home mechanism and relaxes the posterior capsule. The surgeon can determine the initial alignment and add a valgus force until the mcl is tensioned while ensuring the limb alignment has not been overcorrected.
- 45°: maintains the same angular force and establishes the mid-flexion laxity.
- 90°: maintains the same tension with the femur stabilized to define flexion gap.
- The knee is now taken through a full range of motion to evaluate kinematic rollback and implant-to-implant articulation (Fig. 10.8).

(B) Based on these corrected angles, the plan can now be modified. The graph will depict the gap distances between the bone models, and with a goal of obtaining a 2 mm gap between components, the implant positions can be adjusted accordingly. The joint line is respected and over-resection of the tibia is avoided.

(C) The third step is to now confirm central tracking of the femur on the tibia to avoid implant edge loading that could lead to early loosening. Cartilage mapping can be utilized to ensure a smooth transition especially with an associated trochlear implant.

The final plan is now loaded on the graphic computer screen and the surgeon prepares to

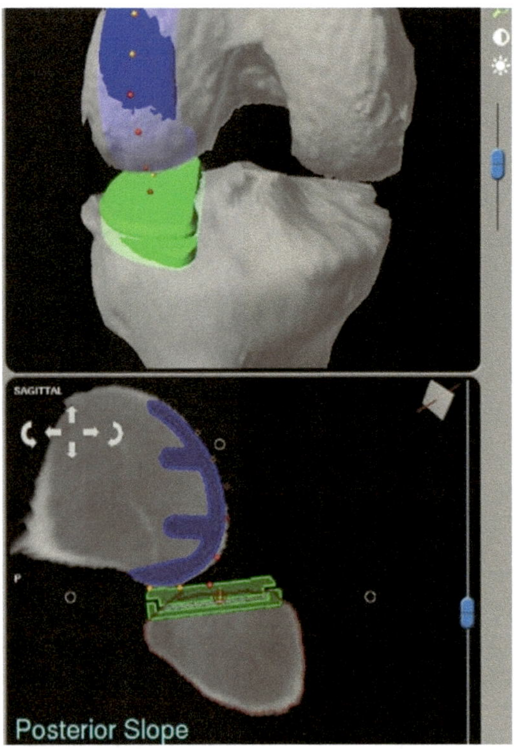

Fig. 10.8 Dynamic kinematic knee assessment – dots depict central implant tracking

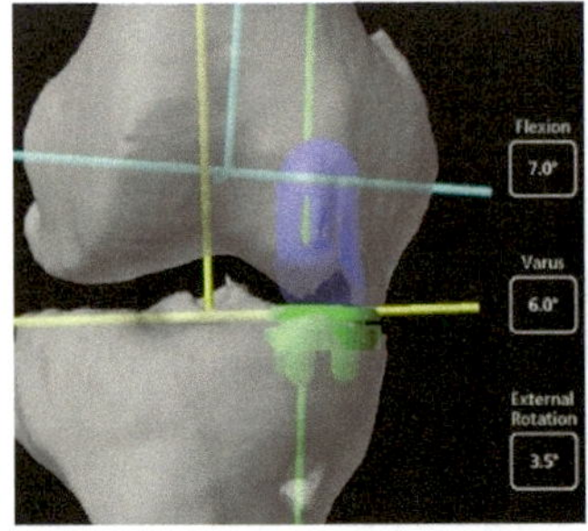

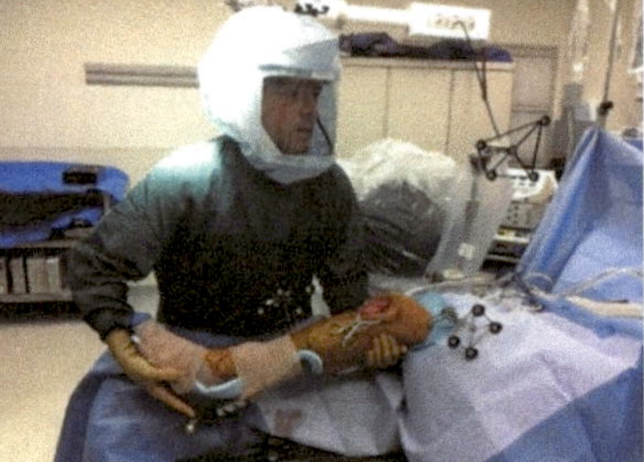

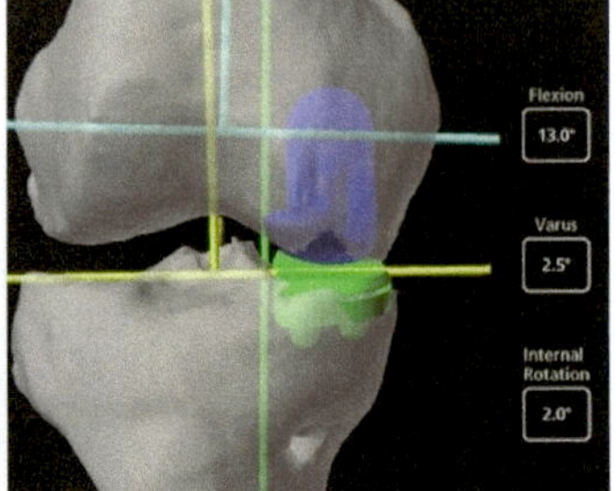

Fig. 10.7 Surgeon defines corrective alignment and gaps prior to bone resections

resect the appropriate thickness and angular implant positions. This approach allows a truly customized plan by achieving kinematic balance without disrupting the soft tissue envelope.

This integrated planning with accurate execution helps prevent common errors that lead to pain and early revision [4, 17, 18]:

- Overcorrection
- Flexion-extension Instability
- Patellar impingement
- Implant edge loading
- Implant overhang/underhang
- Implant malrotation-malalignment (coronal/sagittal/rotational)
- Tibial over-resection, joint line error
- ACL/MCL injury

Surgical Execution

The leg is stabilized with a mobile leg holder to avoid any velocity traps when the knee suddenly moves that would cause the robot to shut down the burr or saw function while allowing the incisional mobile window to be minimized.

The volume of the implant is depicted in green, and the surgeon is instructed to remove this defined bone volume. The surgeon can utilize the burr/saw combination for efficiency.

Haptic borders are defined and presented during surgical bone preparation. "Haptics" is the art of giving tactile, visual and auditory feedback during bone preparation. This allows the surgeon to work efficiently and commonly interact with the user screen, rather than solely trying to visualize inside the knee joint (Fig. 10.9). If the surgeon tries to violate the haptic boundaries, an auditory and visual red area is produced to enable the surgeon to refine his or her approach. If the haptic wall is violated, the system will shut the robotic arm down for safety [1, 5, 19].

A retractor on the mcl can be used. The medial meniscus is not initially resected, in order to help protect the MCL and medial capsule. The femur or tibia can be approached first.

The burr or saw is placed in the entry plane "approach mode" and the trigger is compressed. While the trigger is pressed, the robotic arm performs surgeon-controlled motorized alignment to align the cutting tool to the stereotactic boundary and to position the cutting tool at the Engage Line.

Once motorized alignment is completed, the system mode changes from "Approach Mode" to "Cutting Mode," in which the cutting tool is constrained to the stereotactic boundary and is ready to cut the bone. This change from "Approach Mode" to "Cutting Mode" is visualized on the user screen. The surgeon can visualize the cutting action in 3 different planes. The stereotactic

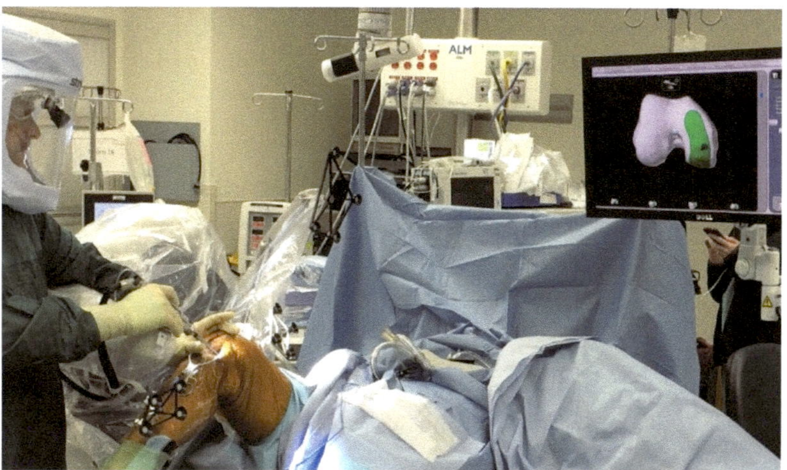

Fig. 10.9 Surgeon interacting with computer screen during burring utilizing haptics

interface constrains the surgeon to the field of bone preparation.

Once the bone prep is completed, the robotic arm is holstered moving the cutting tool away from the knee joint. When the cutting tool passes the Exit Line, stereotactic control is disabled. The cutting tool will once again be in "Approach Mode." Following the planar cuts, the femoral keel and postholes for the femur and tibia are prepared with the haptically controlled motorized burr. Meniscal remnants and residual osteophytes are now removed.

The cut surfaces can be checked for accuracy, and the trial implants are impacted. The leg is now evaluated to confirm appropriate alignment, stability and range of motion. If any refinements are required, the plan can be adjusted and the robotic arm re-engaged. If thicker poly trials are required, they can be inserted and the limb re-evaluated.

Once the trialing is accepted, the bone is dried and the implants are cemented. Commonly the tibia is cemented first and any excess cement is now removed from the rim. The femur is cemented and the trial poly is inserted to allow the implant to cure in compression. The knee should be held in mid-flexion to allow a concentric compression and avoid rocking the tibial implant.

Once the cement has hardened, the tourniquet is let down and the knee irrigated. The final poly is inserted and impacted. The bones pins and check points are removed and sites are irrigated and closed.

The standard fascia and skin closure is performed. No drains are used. The operative dressing is applied and a cryo pad applied.

Pain Control and Discharge

Regional adductor canal sensory blocks can supplement the postoperative pain. General or spinal anesthetic is used with peri-capsular blocks. The patient is ambulated within 2 hours and discharged home.

Home exercises are given, with minimal formal physical therapy. The Patient advances their activity as tolerated over the first 4–6 weeks.

Complications

Patient selection is still critical for any UKA system and implant selection. The Robotic system does not improve outcomes for poor patient selection. Utilizing a CT scan requires overall limb cortical and joint anatomy accuracy when defining the surgical plan. The surgeon should visualize the plan preoperatively.

Navigation allows accurate tracking of the robotic arm and limb. Care to confirm reflective sensors are stable and no OR lights are interfering with the IR tracking is essential. If validation is lost during surgery, specific steps are utilized to re-register and confirm accuracy prior to bone resection. Education of the surgical team to respect the tracking arrays is required. Bone pins should be placed in a uni-cortical fashion, with care not to spear the quadriceps tendon. The check points are placed in stable areas, but not directly under the implant surface as they can lead to stress risers and fracture.

Potential issues with the robotic system breakdown during surgery are infrequent, and the system is tested prior to patient induction. The burr and saw blade need to be attached and stability confirmed and then cleared with specific registration accuracy.

The defined resection levels and limb alignment have to respect the joint line and minimize tibial bone resection that can lead to post-op complications. Cementing technique is critical as retained cement can break off and require post-op arthroscopy to remove the loose body. Early recovery can lead to issues of tibial bone stress edema due to excessive activity, and stress risers secondary to navigation pins are well documented.

Outcomes

With any new adopted technology; evaluation of outcomes, patient satisfaction, and economic metrics [20] are required to enable widespread adoption.

The 2017 Australian Registry published the 1-year revision data for all UKAs at 2.2%, while

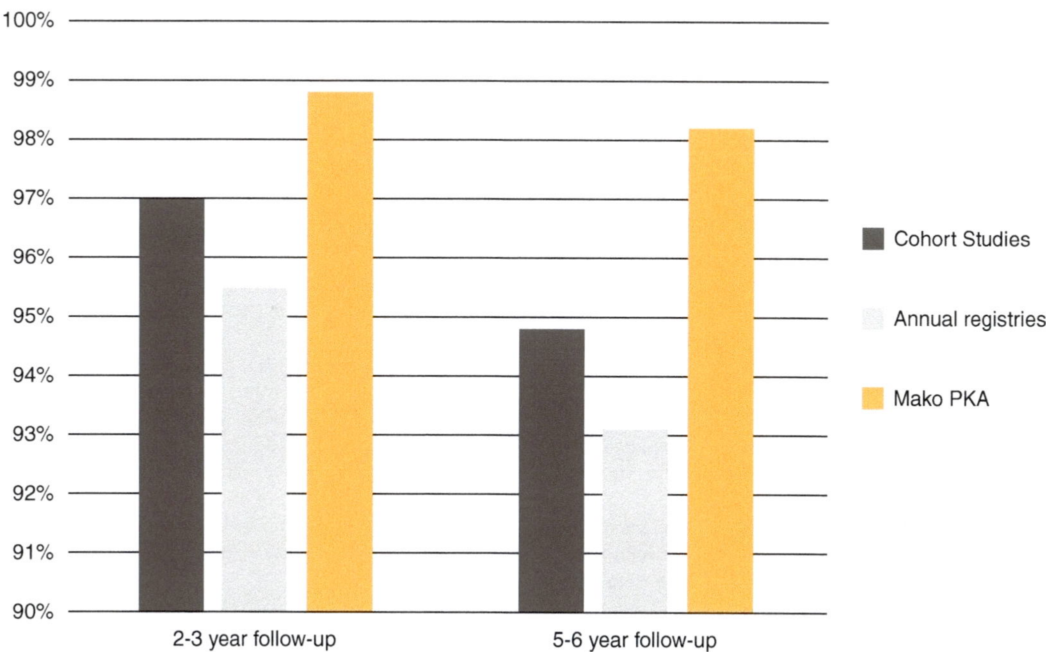

Fig. 10.10 MAKOplasty medial UKR implant survival outcomes

the Mako-robotic-enabled UKA had a cumulative revision rate of 0.8% at 1 year [21]. A multicenter study of over 900 medial MAKOplastys at 2 years reported a 1.2% cumulative revision rate with a Kaplan-Meier survivorship rate at 2 years: 99.1% [22].

An RCT reported on 139 patients that were manually instrumented mobile bearing UKAs vs. a robotic-assisted UKA. They reported greater accuracy, lower post-op pain scores, and 2× more excellent results with the robotic-assisted surgery [12].

A multicenter study reported a 5 year 1.8 revision rate and a 90% patient satisfaction rate [23].

UKA is cost-effective compared to TKA if annual conversion rate is <4% in 78-year-old patients [24]. The data supports the overall value in the adoption of robotic-assisted unicompartmental surgery [20–22] (Fig. 10.10).

Summary

With any advanced technology integration, the benefits to the surgeon must be focused on improving patient outcomes. Patients are requesting new technology, and hospitals are looking to grow their market share and developing profitable service lines. Surgeons need to validate the overall "value" of the technology. Variables include efficiencies, safety, consistency, and cost [23, 24].

The benefits of Robotics center on a consistent execution of the surgical plan. The ability to customize the surgery to an individual's knee pathology is due to the flexibility of the system. Anatomically fitting the implants; adjusting the plan to optimize alignment, implant position, and gaps; and then consistently executing the plan lead to improved post-op outcomes and patient satisfaction.

To date, over 100,000 robotic-assisted MAKOplasty procedures have been successfully performed worldwide. This enhanced technology has been shown to have a consistent learning curve and can provide similar outcomes for surgeons of various expertise and case volumes [25].

The ability to customize each procedure to the patient's disease progression and soft tissue envelope has been shown to provide excellent patient satisfaction and early recovery.

Mid-term results are excellent, with long-term data required to enable continued adoption and capital investment.

Future applications and implant designs will be enabled by the ability to attach various instruments to the robotic arm, and explore the continued operative efficiencies with a larger ambulatory presence.

References

1. Roche M, et al. Robotic arm-assisted unicompartmental knee arthroplasty: preoperative planning and surgical technique. Am J Orthop (Belle Mead NJ). 2009;38(2 Suppl):10–5.
2. Zuiderbaan HA, et al. Unicompartmental knee arthroplasty versus total knee arthroplasty: which type of artificial joint do patients forget? Knee Surg Sports Traumatol Arthrosc. 2017;25(3):681–6.
3. Borus T, Roberts D, Fairchild P, Christopher J, Branch S, Conditt MA, Matthews J, Pirtle K, Baer M. UKA patients return to function earlier than TKA patients. ISTA 27th Annual Congress; September 24–27, 2014, Kyoto, Japan.
4. Hamilton WG, Collier MB, Tarabee E, McAuley JP, Engh CA Jr, Engh GA. Incidence and reasons for reoperation after minimally invasive unicompartmental knee arthroplasty. J Arthroplasty. 2006;21(6 Suppl 2):98–107.2198 2006.
5. Van der List, Jelle P, Chawla H, Pearle AD. Robotic-assisted knee arthroplasty: an overview. Am J Orthop. 2016;45(4):202.
6. Gomes P. Surgical robotics: reviewing the past, analysing the present, imagining the future. Robot Comput Integr Manuf. 2011;27(2):261–6.
7. Roche M. Robotic-assisted unicompartmental knee arthroplasty. Clin Sports Med. 2014;33(1):123–32.
8. Repicci JA, Eberle RW. Minimally invasive surgical technique for unicondylar knee arthroplasty. J South Orthop Assoc. 1999;8(1):20–7. discussion 27.
9. Conditt MA, Franceschi G, Bertolini D, Khabbaze C, Rovini A, Nardaccione R. Unicompartmental lateral knee arthroplasty using the robotic arm system. ISTA 27th Annual Congress; September 24–27, 2014, Kyoto, Japan.
10. Borus T, Brilhault J, Confalonieri N, Johnson D, Thienpont E. Patellofemoral joint replacement, an evolving concept. Knee. 2014;21:S47–50.
11. Citak M, Suero EM, Citak M, Dunbar NJ, Branch SH, Conditt MA, Banks SA, Pearle AD. Unicompartmental knee arthroplasty: is robotic technology more accurate than conventional technique? Knee. 2013;20(4):268–71.
12. Bell S, Anthony I, Jones B, et al. Improved accuracy of component positioning with robotic-assisted Unicompartmental knee arthroplasty: data from a prospective, randomized controlled study. Bone Joint Surg Am. 2016;98(8):627–35. https://doi.org/10.2106/JBJS.15.00664.
13. Lonner JH, John TK, Conditt MA. Robotic-arm assisted UKA improved Tibial component alignment: a pilot study. Clin Orthop Relat Res. 2009;468(1):141–6.
14. Roche MW, Augustin D, Conditt MA. Accuracy of robotically assisted UKA. J Bone Joint Surg Br. 2010;92-B(SUPP_I):127.
15. Coon TM, Driscoll MD, Conditt MA. Robotically assisted UKA is more accurate than manually instrumented UKA. J Bone Joint Surg Br. 2010;92-B(SUPP_I):157.
16. Roche MW, Branch S, Lightcap C, Conditt MA. Intra-operative assessment of the soft tissue envelope is integral to the planning of UKA components. World Arthroplasty Congress, April 15–18, 2015, Paris, France.
17. Ridgeway SR, et al. The effect of alignment of the knee on the outcome of unicompartmental knee replacement. J Bone Joint Surg Br. 2002;84(3):351–5.
18. Aleto TJ, et al. Early failure of unicompartmental knee arthroplasty leading to revision. J Arthroplast. 2008;23(2):159–63.
19. Lonner JH. Robotic-arm assisted unicompartmental knee arthroplasty. Semin Arthroplast. 2009;20(1):15–22.
20. Moschetti WE, Konopka JF, Rubash HE, Genuario JW. Can robot-assisted unicompartmental knee arthroplasty be cost-effective? A Markov decision analysis. J Arthroplast. 2016;31(4):759–65.
21. National Australian Joint Replacement Registry 2017 Annual Report.
22. Pearle AD, van der List JP, Lee L, Coon TM, Borus TA, Roche MW. Survivorship and patient satisfaction of robotic-assisted medial unicompartmental knee arthroplasty at a minimum two-year follow-up. Knee. 2017;24(2):419–28.
23. Kleeblad LJ, Coon TM, Borus TD, Pearle AD. Survivorship and patient satisfaction of robotic-assisted medial unicompartmental knee arthroplasty at a minimum five-year follow-up. European Knee Society 2017 annual meeting. London, England. Poster No. P54. April 19–21, 2017.
24. Slover J, et al. Cost-effectiveness of unicompartmental and total knee arthroplasty in elderly low-demand patients: a Markov decision analysis. JBJS. 2006;88(11):2348–55.
25. Branch SH, Erdos T, Conditt MA, Jinnah RH, Christopher J. The learning curve of robotically assisted UKA. 13th EFORT Congress, May 23–25, 2012, Berlin, Germany.

Patellofemoral Arthroplasty: NAVIO

Brian Hamlin

Patellofemoral arthroplasty (PFA) is a well-recognized procedure for the treatment of isolated patellofemoral arthrosis of the knee [1, 2]. Indications/Contraindications for the procedure are well documented in the literature [3]. Despite the successful outcomes that many patients experience with this procedure, there remains a significant complication, reoperation, and revision rate, particularly with inlay style implants [4]. Progression of tibiofemoral disease is the most common reason for late failures; early patellar instability occurs more frequently with inlay than onlay style trochlear implants. Controlling trochlear component rotational alignment relative to the anteroposterior axis of the femur has reduced problems related to patellar tracking [4]. The precision necessary to place the trochlea implant can be challenging, and surgeon error in component positioning may lead to patellar maltracking as well as mechanical symptoms, such catching and clunk. Although surgical techniques and patellofemoral implants have improved, a robotically assisted technique for placement of the trochlea implant should allow the surgeon to achieve more predictable results.

NAVIO: Imageless Robotic Assistance

The NAVIO robotic sculpting tool is a hand-held semi-active robotic technology for accurate bone shaping [5] (Fig. 11.1). The instrumentation for the system is simplified with minimal equipment/trays being required, and the operative footprint is small (Figs. 11.2 and 11.3). Preoperative imaging such as MRI or CT is not required. Instead the system allows for a registration of the patient's anatomy within the surgical workflow using an optical probe. The NAVIO system provides control of bone removal by either modulating the speed or the exposure of the motorized bur. In exposure control, the technology tracks the position of the handpiece and bur relative to the intended cut plan and adjusts the exposure of the bur beyond a static guard to modulate cutting. In speed control, the system modulates the rotational speed of the bur based on proximity to the target surface. The system has been shown to be extremely accurate and more precise than what can be achieved with standard instrumentation [6, 7].

B. Hamlin (✉)
Department of Orthopaedics, Magee Womens Hospital of UPMC, Pittsburgh, PA, USA

© Springer Nature Switzerland AG 2019
J. H. Lonner (ed.), *Robotics in Knee and Hip Arthroplasty*,
https://doi.org/10.1007/978-3-030-16593-2_11

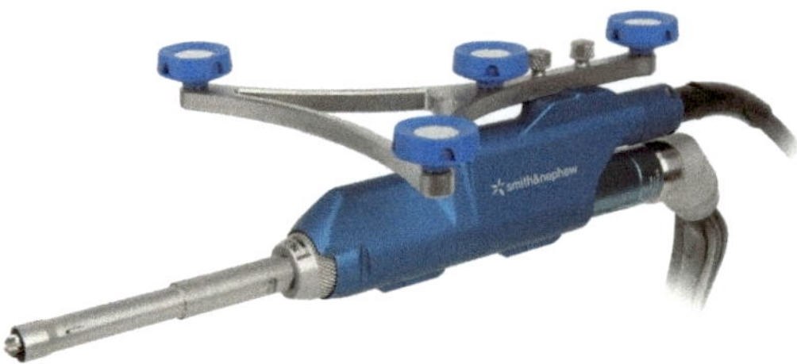

Fig. 11.1 NAVIO Precision Freehand Sculpting tool in exposure control mode. (Courtesy of Smith & Nephew, Memphis, TN, USA)

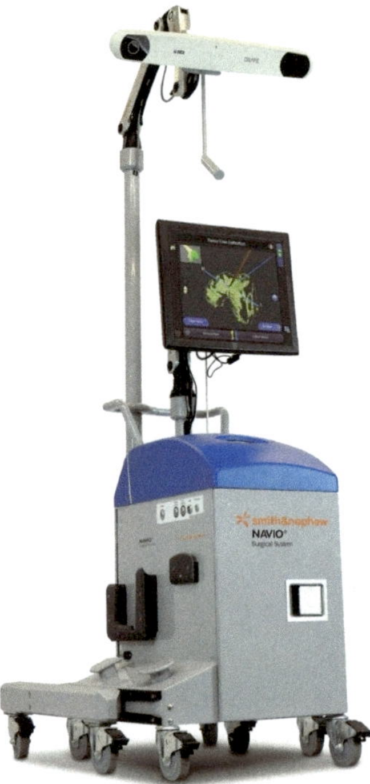

Fig. 11.2 NAVIO Optical Camera and Base unit which houses the computer, bur power supply, and interactive computer screen. (Courtesy of Smith and Nephew, Memphis, TN, USA)

Surgical Technique: NAVIO

The majority of procedures are performed under a spinal anesthetic. All patients receive appropriate preoperative intravenous antibiotics prior to incision. At the surgeon's discretion, patients may also receive 1 gram of intravenous tranexamic acid unless contraindicated. A standard medial parapatellar approach is made to the knee under tourniquet control. Care should be taken to protect the normal meniscal and articular cartilage surfaces that are not being replaced. The isolated disease of the PF joint is confirmed, and then peripheral osteophytes are removed. The patella is prepared in standard fashion. With the knee in full extension, the patella is everted and held with a tenaculum. A transverse cut is performed so to give a uniform thickness across the patella, parallel to the anterior surface. Medialization of the patellar button will assist with patellar tracking. In general, the amount of articular surface resected should be replaced with an equally thick polyethylene button. Ideally the remaining patellar thickness after resection should be at least 15 mm, leaving a composite thickness of 23–24 mm. However, many patients with advanced disease of the patellofemoral joint will have decreased patellar bone stock, patellar wear, and dysplasia (especially of the lateral facet), and care should be taken to avoid over-resecting and leaving an overly thin patella of less than 12 mm. While overstuffing of the patella should be avoided, in these circumstances, slight overstuffing may be necessary.

Optical tracking pins are placed in the femur, and the femoral landmarks/anatomy are registered with an optical probe (Fig. 11.4). A bone morph/virtual model is then created within the software (Fig. 11.5). The surgeon uses the graphic user interface to optimize component size and position (Fig. 11.6). The system allows for either an inlay or onlay component. The surgeon has complete freedom in implant position and can control rotation, depth, flexion, and extension of the implant. Therefore one can plan a perfect transition from the implant to the patients' native surrounding condylar cartilage and determine the femoral rotation deemed most appropriate given the patient's trochlear and condylar anatomy (Fig. 11.7). While some surgeons prefer to position the prosthesis perpendicular to the anteroposterior axis of the femur for all patients, others opt for slight inset (and thus internal rotation) relative to the trochlear peaks.

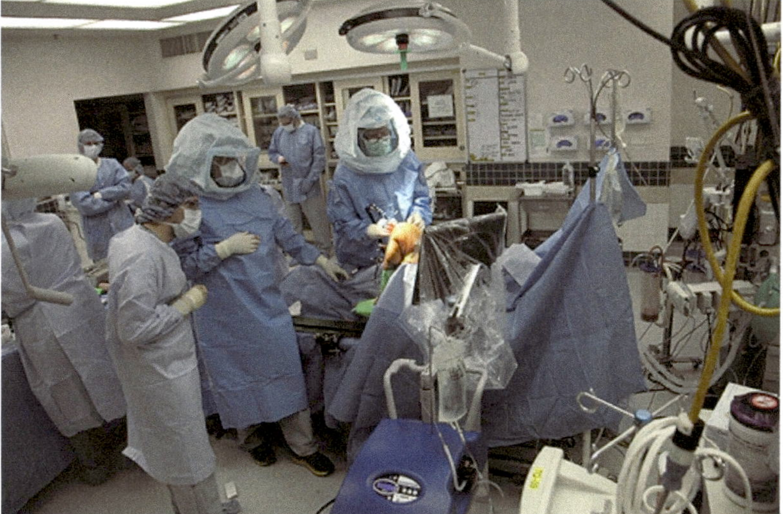

Fig. 11.3 A relatively small operative room footprint is needed to accommodate the NAVIO unit

With robotic planning, this can be quantified before precise surface preparation. Additionally, the trochlear implant should be optimally positioned so that it is flush with the anterior femoral cortex proximally and the condylar surfaces distally to limit chance of mechanical symptoms and patellar catching.

After sizing and positioning the implant, the NAVIO handheld burr is used for bone removal (Fig. 11.8). The surgeon is guided with an active user interface to complete the bone preparation. Exposure control mode is used initially for the bulk of the planned bony removal. Speed control can then be used for fine details as well as preparation of lugholes. Upon completion of the bone removal, trialing of the implants occur. If a tourniquet is being used, it can be released to judge patellar tracking. If component position has been optimized but poor tracking persists, consideration should be given to other measures such as releasing the lateral retinaculum and/or medialization of the tibial tubercle.

In addition to patellar stability, the transition of the patella tracking from trochlea implant to native cartilage should be carefully assessed to assure there is no sudden change that could cause mechanical symptoms. If trialing shows issues with the position of the trochlea, the plan within the software can be easily changed.

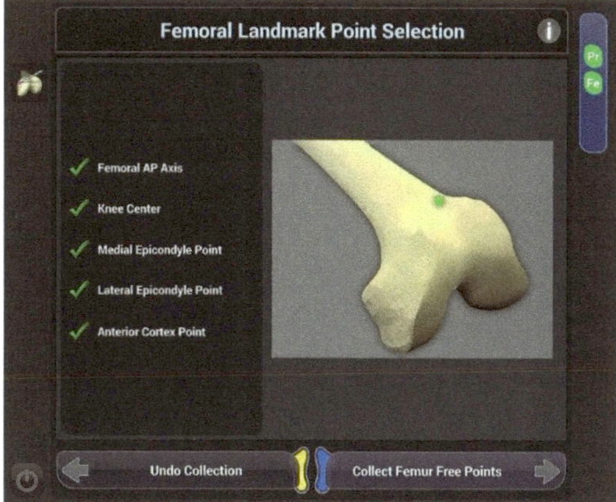

Fig. 11.4 Optical probe registers femoral landmarks

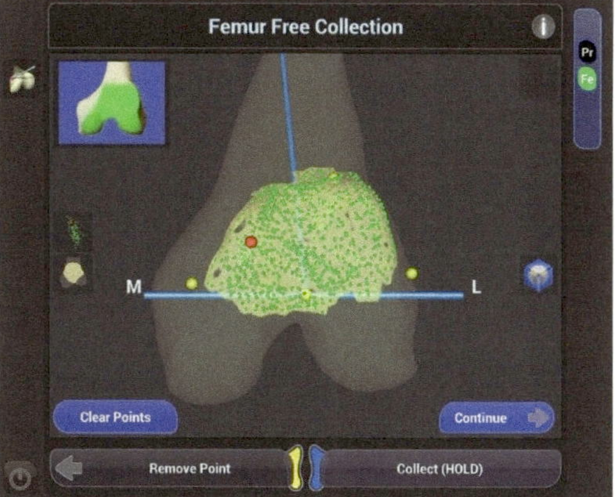

Fig. 11.5 Femoral surface is painted to build the virtual model using the optical probe

Further bone shaping can be performed to match the new plan before cementation of the final implants.

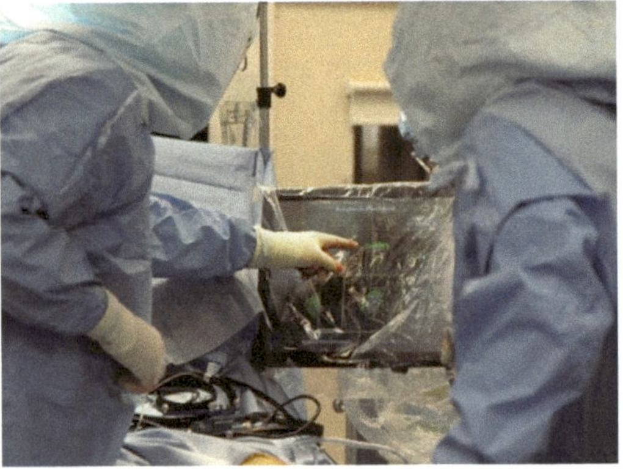

Fig. 11.6 Surgeon can easily manipulate the implant using the GUI to plan for an ideal implant size and position

Postoperative Care

The majority of patients receive a multimodal approach to pain management including acetaminophen, selective Cox-2 inhibitor, gabapentin, and judicious use of opioids. A periarticular injection is also performed to assist with postoperative pain control. All patients are mobilized on the day of surgery. Patients are typically discharged on postoperative day 1. PFA can be performed in the outpatient setting if one wishes.

Patients are enrolled in an outpatient physical therapy regimen concentrating on range of motion and safe ambulation initially. A walking aid is encouraged until patients demonstrate good control of their quadriceps. Physical therapy introduces strengthening and functional exercises

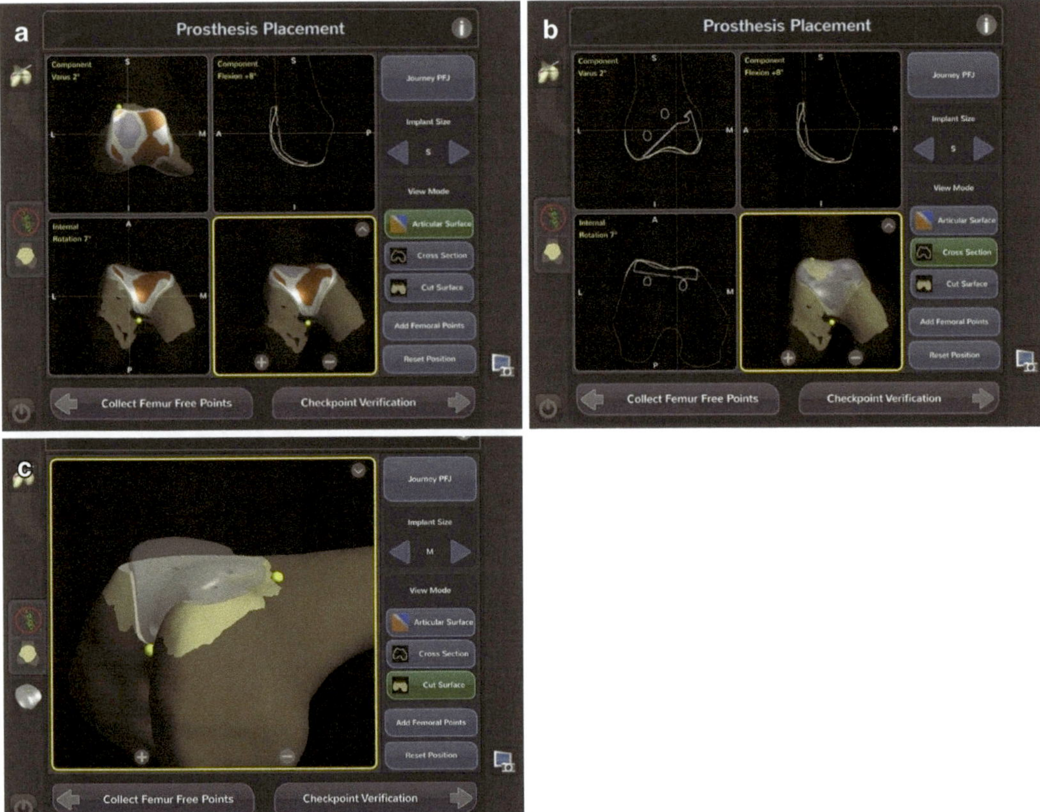

Fig. 11.7 (**a–c**) Prosthesis placement is idealized for depth, flexion, extension, and rotation. If necessary err on the side of a slightly recessed implant in relation to the patient's native cartilage

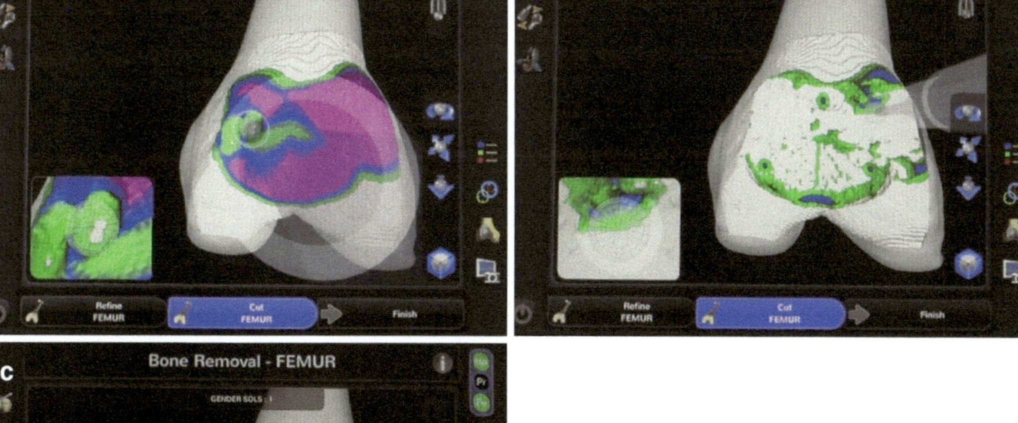
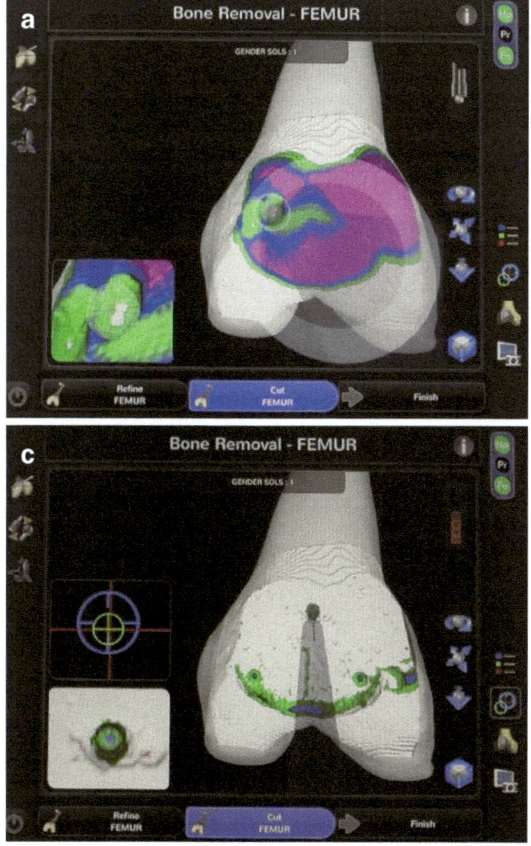

Fig. 11.8 (**a–c**) Exposure control mode is used for bulk of the bone removal. Speed control can be used for fine-tuning as well as placement of lug holes

over several weeks before transitioning to a home exercise program.

The majority of patients can return to most activities by 3 months postoperatively with the understanding it can take 6 months to a year to be fully recovered. No restrictions are placed with regard to activity.

Conclusion

Robotic preparation is an effective way to prepare the trochlear surface in PFA. The NAVIO robotic sculpting tool provides a vehicle for quantifiable preoperative virtual templating and planning and precise surface preparation. Following sound principles of patient selection, precise robotic

surgical technique and postoperative care can facilitate successful recovery and outcomes of surgery.

References

1. Osarumwense D, et al. Patellofemoral joint arthroplasty: early results and functional outcome of the Zimmer Gender solutions Patello-Femoral joint system. Clin Orthop Surg. 2017;9(3):295–302.
2. Akhbari P, et al. The Avon Patellofemoral joint replacement: mid-term prospective results from an independent centre. Clin Orthop Surg. 2015;7(2):171–6.
3. Pisanu G, et al. Patellofemoral arthroplasty: current concepts and review of the literature. Joints. 2017;5(4):237–45.
4. Dy CJ, Franco N, Ma Y, Mazumdar M, McCarthy MM, Gonzalez Della Valle A. Complications after

patello-femoral versus total knee replacement in the treatment of isolated patello-femoral osteoarthritis. A meta-analysis. Knee Surg Sports Traumatol Arthrosc. 2012;20(11):2174–90.

5. Lonner JH. Robotically assisted unicompartmental knee arthroplasty with a handheld image-free sculpting tool. Orthop Clin North Am. 2016;47(1):29–40.

6. Smith JR, Riches PE, Rowe PJ. Accuracy of a freehand sculpting tool for unicondylar knee replacement. Int J Med Robot. 2014;10(2):162–9.

7. Lonner JH, et al. High degree of accuracy of a novel image-free handheld robot for unicondylar knee arthroplasty in a cadaveric study. Clin Orthop Relat Res. 2015;473(1):206–12.

Patellofemoral Arthroplasty Technique: Mako

12

Jesua Law, Aaron Hofmann, Bradley Stevens, and Alexandria Myers

Isolated patellofemoral arthritis is not uncommon and a well-recognized variant of the osteoarthritic (OA) knee with no clear consensus in treatment. McAlindon et al. [1] demonstrated isolated patellofemoral arthritis in as many as; 11% of men and 24% of women, older than 55 years old. Davies et al. [2] demonstrated isolated patellofemoral OA in 9.2% of patients with symptomatic osteoarthritis of the knee. Nonoperative and many forms of operative treatments have failed to demonstrate long-term effective results in the setting of advanced patellofemoral OA. Total knee arthroplasty has demonstrated long-term and excellent results; however, many surgeons are hesitant to perform a TKA in younger patients with isolated patellofemoral arthritis. Mont et al. [3] have demonstrated that as many as 19% of patients experience residual anterior knee pain when TKA is performed for isolated patellofemoral OA. Patellofemoral arthroplasty is an effective procedure in the properly selected patient which can theoretically preserve the natural tibiofemoral biomechanics and kinematics.

Patellofemoral arthroplasty was first described by McKeever [4] in 1955, using a design that resurfaced either the trochlea or the patella. Blazina et al. [5] and Lubinus [6] both described newer PFA designs with reasonable short-term results in 1979; however, up to 30% of cases had complications due to excessive polyethylene wear or maltracking related to malalignment [7–9]. Contemporary PFA prostheses utilize ultrahigh molecular weight polyethylene (UHMWPE) and have reduced patellar maltracking problems associated with older designs. Appropriately positioned trochlear inlay designs and onlay designs have reduced component malposition, whereas the previous inlay designs placed the trochlear component in excessive internal rotation, thereby causing patellar instability and maltracking.

Outcomes and longevity of patellofemoral arthroplasty are directly related to component position and precise surgical technique. Due to the narrow window of error with trochlear component positioning, some authors have advocated the use of robotic-assisted patellofemoral arthroplasty (RA-PFA). RA-PFA with the Mako system uses a preoperative CT scan to allow accurate templating and placement

J. Law (✉)
Department of Orthopedics, Valley Orthopedic Surgery, Modesto, CA, USA

A. Hofmann
Department of Orthopaedic Surgery, Center for Precision Joint Replacement, Salt Lake Regional Medical Center/Hofmann Arthritis Institute, Salt Lake City, UT, USA

B. Stevens · A. Myers
Hofmann Arthritis Institute, Salt Lake City, UT, USA

© Springer Nature Switzerland AG 2019
J. H. Lonner (ed.), *Robotics in Knee and Hip Arthroplasty*,
https://doi.org/10.1007/978-3-030-16593-2_12

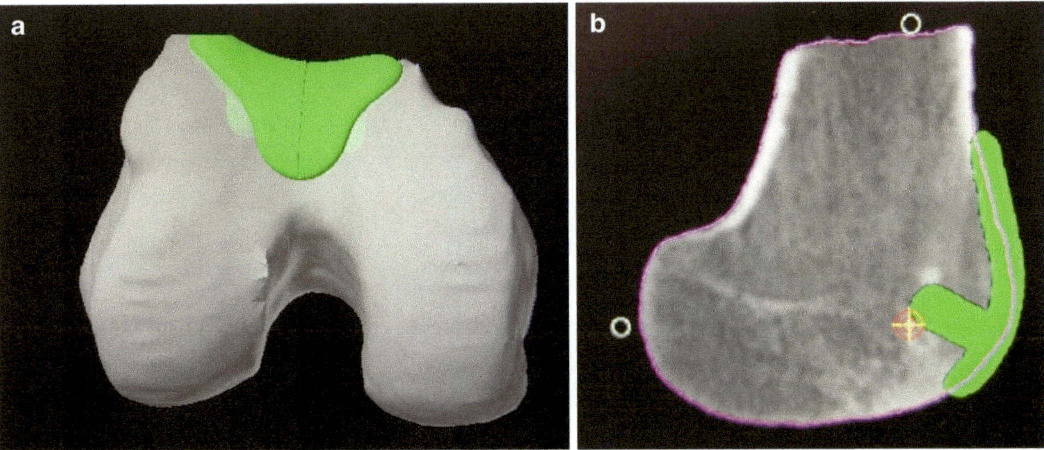

Fig. 12.1 (**a**) A three-dimensional reconstruction model utilizing a patient's preoperative CT scan to overlay the intended trochlear component. Notice the component does not enter the femoral notch or overhang medial or laterally. (**b**) Sagittal image of the planned trochlear component overlay onto patients preoperative CT scan

of the trochlear prosthesis, with consideration given to the rotational alignment of the component relative to the patient's native anatomy (Fig. 12.1).

Imaging

Weight-bearing AP and midflexion PA radiographs are needed to ensure that there is no tibiofemoral osteoarthritis; however, weight-bearing AP radiographs often underestimate the amount of tibiofemoral arthritis. The midflexion PA radiograph is needed to rule out posterior condylar wear, and axial radiographs should be evaluated to identify trochlear dysplasia or patellar tilt/subluxation [10] (Fig. 12.2). MRI images and previous arthroscopic photographs should be reviewed if available [11]. Prior to the use of RA-PFA surgery, the patient is required to obtain a preoperative CT scan for evaluation of the patient's anatomy, and this will be uploaded to the robotic software for 3D modeling and preoperative and intraoperative planning.

Clinical Evaluation

The clinical evaluation should start by ruling out other causes for anterior knee pain including

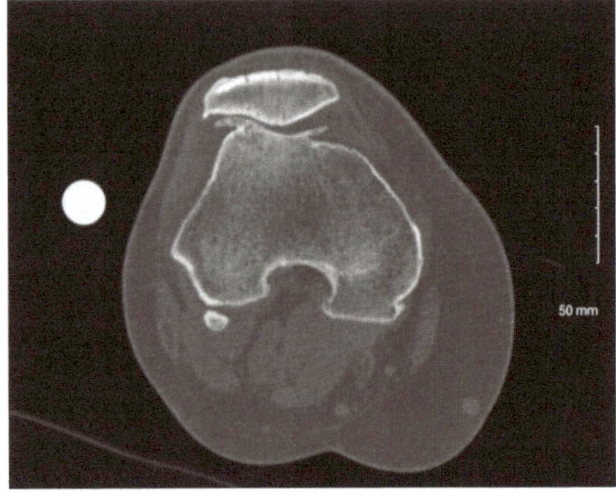

Fig. 12.2 Preoperative CT image demonstrating lateral patellar subluxation

quadriceps/patellar tendonitis, pes anserine bursitis, or meniscal tears prior to considering PFA. Key elements of the patient's history need to be evaluated to elucidate a history of trauma, patellar subluxation or·dislocations, as well as previous treatments (both surgical and nonsurgical). Patients with patellofemoral degeneration will complain of anterior knee pain that worsens when going upstairs, squatting, or sitting for a prolonged time. Physical exam should demonstrate tenderness to palpation to the medial/lateral facets of the patella and a positive patellar

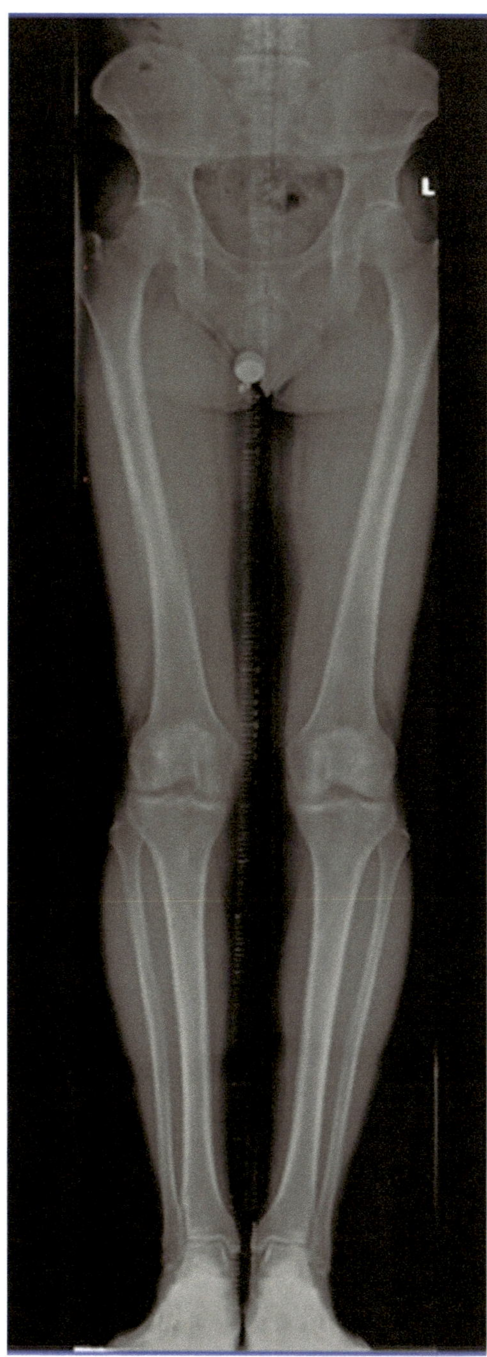

Fig. 12.3 Preoperative long-cassette standing X-ray assessing patient's leg alignment and Q angle

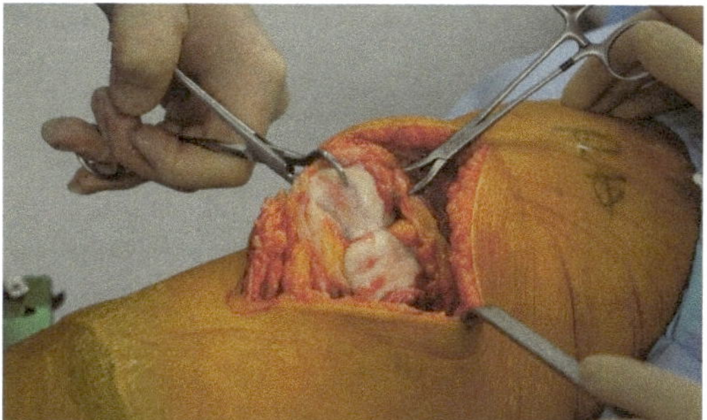

Fig. 12.4 Intraoperative evaluation demonstrates extensive degenerative changes isolated to the patellofemoral articulation

Indications

Potential candidates for isolated patellofemoral arthroplasty are patients with osteoarthritis or posttraumatic patellofemoral joint degeneration affecting daily activities. Radiographs and physical exam findings noted earlier should confirm the diagnosis of extensive patellofemoral joint degeneration (Fig. 12.4). If previous arthroscopy pictures or reports are available, these should be evaluated for extensive grade 3 or above chondromalacia limited to the patellofemoral joint, as these patients may also be surgical candidates if symptomatic [12]. Patellofemoral malalignment or dysplasia-induced degeneration is a common indication for PFA. Patients with excessive Q angles should have a tibial tubercle realignment before or during the PFA [12].

Contraindications

Patients with systemic or inflammatory arthropathy, patella baja, chondrocalcinosis, Outerbridge grade 3 or 4 in the tibiofemoral articulation, or those patients with less than grade 3 chondromalacia of the patellofemoral articulation are not candidates for isolated patellofemoral arthroplasty. It is important that the clinician spend time to evaluate the tibiofemoral articulation because with the current prosthesis designs, the most common cause of failed PFA is progression of tibiofemoral osteoarthritis. Tauro et al. [9] demonstrated 8% medial or lateral compartment osteoarthritic

grind test. Patellofemoral crepitance is common, and the physician should also assess for patellar tracking, and take note of the patient's Q angle (Fig. 12.3).

progression at 8 years, and Kooijman et al. [13] demonstrated a 23% progression at 15 years. Active infection is an absolute contraindication to knee arthroplasty, which includes PFA, and uncorrected patellofemoral instability/malalignment is a relative contraindication and should be addressed prior to or during the patellofemoral arthroplasty as discussed earlier. Typically, the physical exam should demonstrate no evidence of knee flexion contractures, with a minimum of 100° degree knee range of motion, as knee contractures are suggestive of knee pathology that extends past the patellofemoral compartment of the knee [12]. Medial and lateral joint line tenderness may be a sign of underlying tibiofemoral chondral damage or meniscal damage and may be a contraindication for isolated PFA unless the suspicion is that the pain is referred from the patellofemoral compartment (as confirmed with MRI). Patients should be counseled on expectations and outcomes; those with chronic narcotic use, chronic regional pain syndromes, or psychogenic pain are not suitable candidates.

Surgical Technique Using the Mako Robotic System

The primary purpose of preoperative templating, in robotic-assisted patellofemoral arthroplasty with the Mako system, is for accurate implant sizing and alignment relative to the patient's bony anatomy. It should be noted that with this system, a preoperative CT scan is needed for the robotic recognition of the patient's anatomy, and any adjacent metallic artifact in the operative or non-operative leg may reduce its accuracy. It is important for the surgeon to remember that surgical outcomes are maximized by proper patellar and trochlear implant sizing and positioning, as well as meticulous surgical dissection. During templating of the trochlear component, it is important to sufficiently externally rotate the trochlear component so that it is aligned perpendicular to the AP axis of the femur and parallel to the epicondylar axis (Fig. 12.5).

When selecting the trochlear implant size, it is important to choose a trochlear prosthesis that

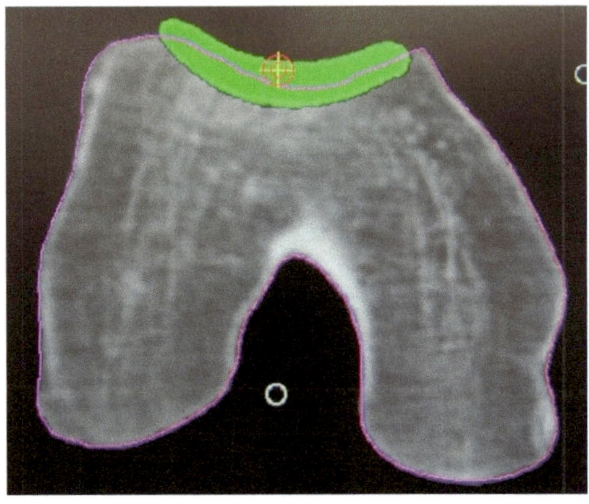

Fig. 12.5 Preoperative templating demonstrating the trochlear component perpendicular to the AP axis of the femur (Whiteside's Line) and parallel to the epicondylar axis

gives broad anterior coverage, but does not overhang medially/laterally and does not extend into the intercondylar notch, which would cause ACL impingement. The trochlear prosthesis should be templated to rest level with the adjacent condylar cartilage, or countersunk by 1 millimeter, and should have a smooth transition between the anterior femoral cortex and the trochlear implant.

In our technique, an anterior skin incision is made with the knee flexed at a 45° degree angle, and the arthrotomy is performed medial to the skin incision. While performing the arthrotomy, the surgeon must be mindful to avoid damaging the underlying articular cartilage of the tibiofemoral compartments while also avoiding damage to the intermeniscal ligament. A muscle sparing approach, such as the subvastus approach, is used while ensuring sufficient mobility of the patella to allow for trochlear prosthesis insertion (Fig. 12.6). Once the arthrotomy has been performed, it is important to take note of all the intraarticular structures in the knee including the ACL, PCL, and medial and lateral tibiofemoral compartments of the knee and ensure that no extensive chondromalacia is present. During intraoperative inspection, if there is more diffuse chondromalacia or ACL/PCL deficiency is noted, we would advise considering performing a total knee arthroplasty instead of an isolated RA-PFA.

Next, "education" of the robotic system is performed to calibrate the robotic recognition software. This is performed by fixating three-dimensional probes into the patient's femur for spatial recognition as well as selecting several predetermined areas to the patient's native anatomy for computer recognition and confirmation (Fig. 12.7). After this has been performed, the robotic burring device will assist the surgeon with the templated resection of the trochlea (Fig. 12.8). It is important that intercondylar osteophytes be removed after calibra-

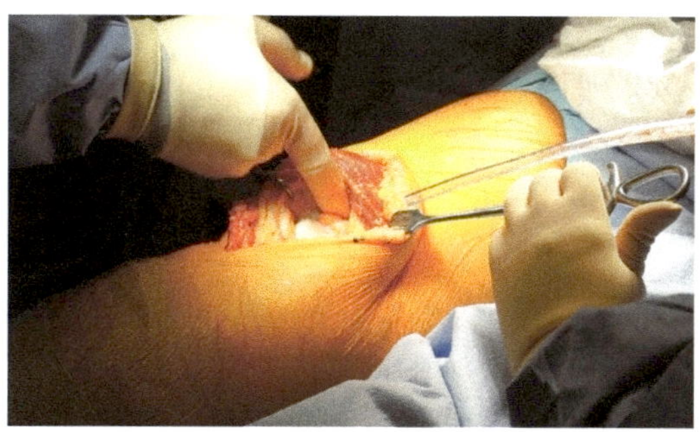

Fig. 12.6 Muscle sparing subvastus approach demonstrated. All components of the knee are evaluated (extensive patella wear noted to the left of the surgeon's finger), and care is taken not to damage the anterior horn of the meniscus or intermeniscal ligament

tion but prior to termination of the case to ensure no ACL impingement will occur. As stated earlier, preparation of the trochlear bed should be either flush or within 1 mm of surrounding femoral articular cartilage. The patella is resurfaced using standard TKA principles, including medialization of the patellar component, and a measured resection technique should be utilized to avoid overstuffing the patellofemoral joint. Resection of the lateral patellar facet should be performed to improve patellar tracking and avoid lateral patellar impingement.

Once all bony preparation has been performed, trial implants should be placed, and the patellar alignment and tracking should be assessed. Lateral retinacular balancing is performed using an inside out "peeling" technique, recessing the retinaculum from the lateral patellar facet without formally releasing the capsule. Patellar tilt, subluxation, and catching should be scrutinized at this point, and adjustments should be made if necessary. Once satisfied with placement, size, and patellar tracking of the trial implants, the final implants should be inserted using standard cement techniques. Soft tissue balancing is performed by closing the capsule in 20–30° of knee flexion [14] (Fig. 12.9).

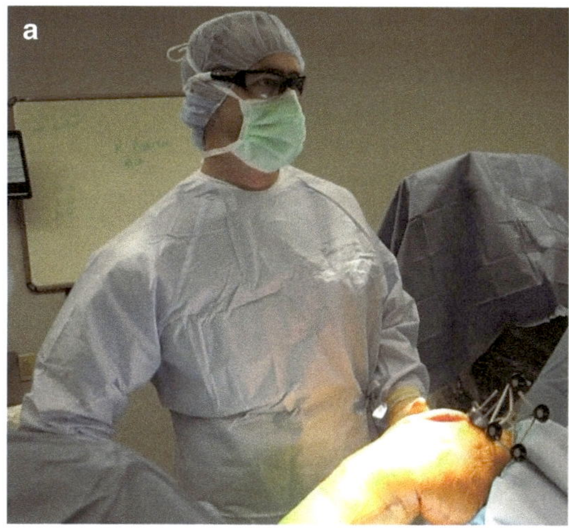
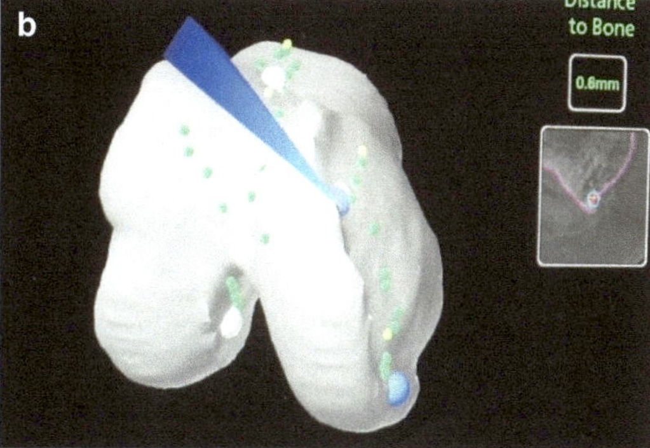

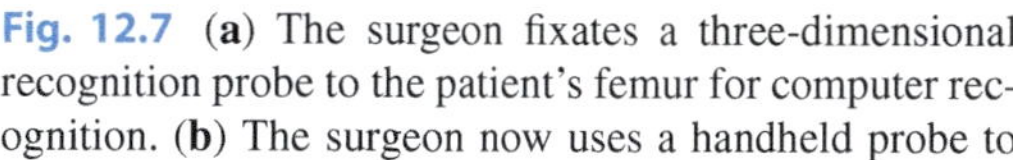

Fig. 12.7 (a) The surgeon fixates a three-dimensional recognition probe to the patient's femur for computer recognition. (b) The surgeon now uses a handheld probe to pinpoint several key features of the patient's anatomy for further computer recognition and calibration

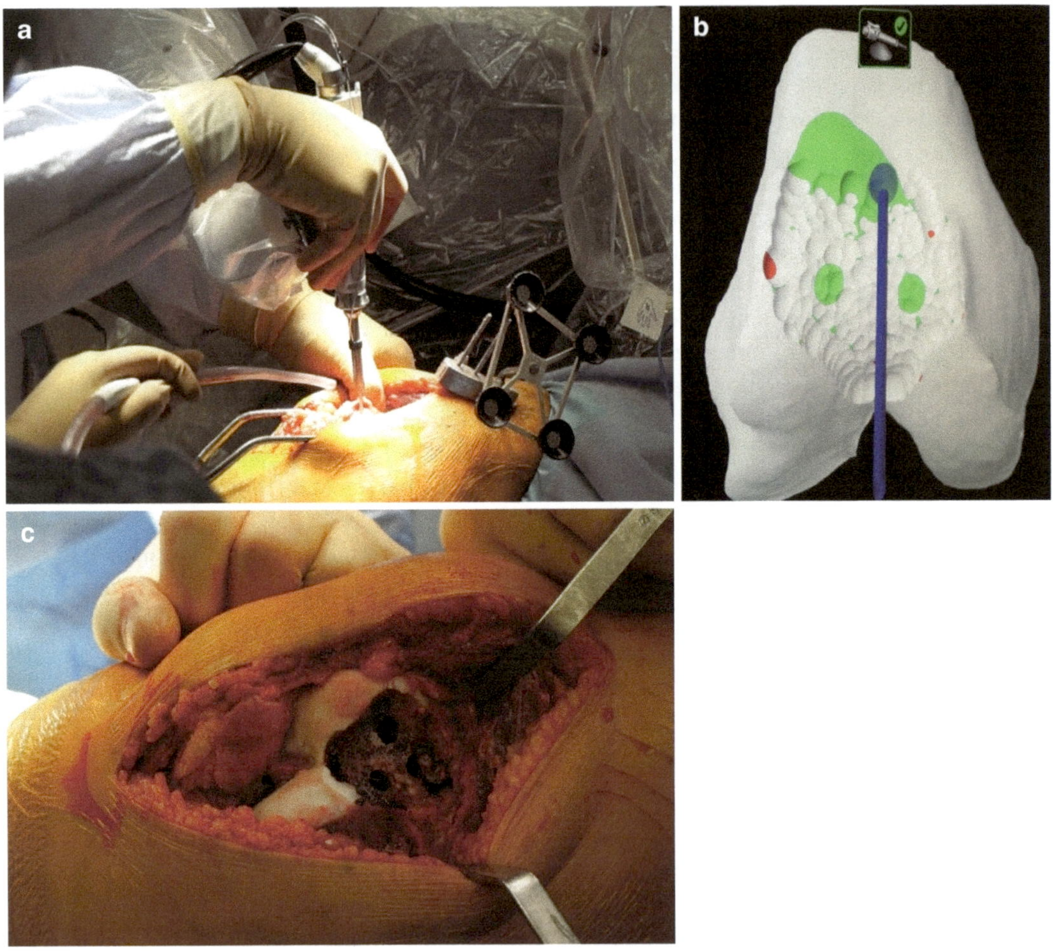

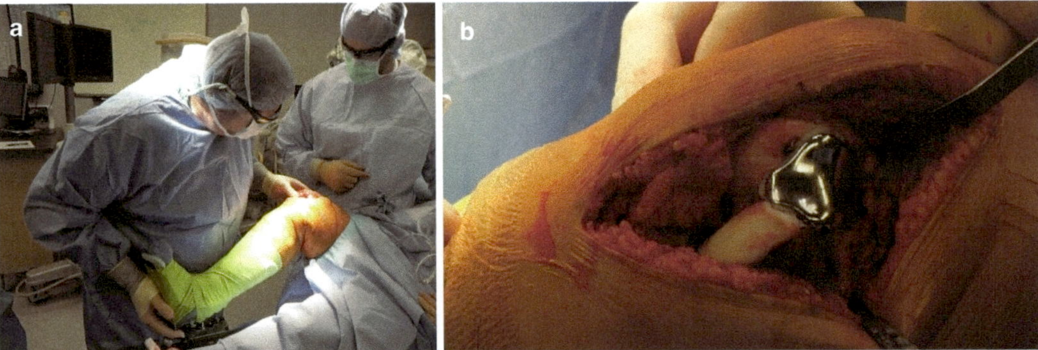

Fig. 12.8 (**a**) Intraoperative photo demonstrating robotic-assisted osteotomy of the trochlea. (**b**) Real-time robotic-aided feedback giving the surgeon cues as to the depth of his resection (green color on screen signifies more resection is needed; white is the appropriate depth of resection, and red signifies too deep of a resection). (**c**) Final trochlear resection performed utilizing robotic assistance

Fig. 12.9 (**a**) Trial implants are temporarily placed, and patellar tracking is assessed. (**b**) Final trochlear and patellar component fixed in place using standard cement techniques. (**c**) Intraoperative photo demonstrating both patellar and trochlear components

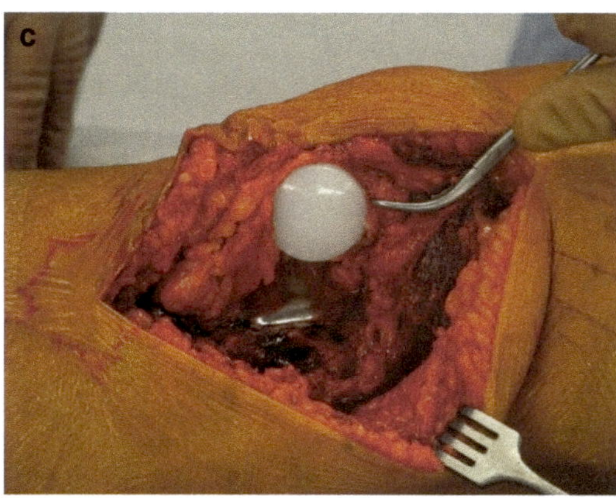

Fig. 12.9 (continued)

Results

There are currently no publications analyzing the results of RA-PFA, although reports of conventionally performed PFA using sound techniques and designs may serve as surrogate measures of outcomes of PFA until further data is collected [14–17]. Hofmann et al. in 2009 [18] retrospectively reviewed 40 conventional PFAs in 34 patients, with a mean 30-month follow-up. Ninety-five percent of the patients were satisfied with their procedures and had significant improvements in Tegner scores. There were two revisions for traumatic injuries; otherwise there were no failures. In our current unpublished study, we evaluated 37 robotic-assisted PFAs in 31 patients performed by 4 fellowship-trained arthroplasty surgeons. At a mean 4-year follow-up, this study demonstrated an average final KOOS score of 96.43 points and a Tegner score of 93.95 points. Pain scores were markedly improved from an average preoperative VAS score of 7.8 to 1.01 postoperatively. Five knees were converted to TKA at final follow-up due to tibiofemoral osteoarthritis progression. There were no cases of aseptic loosening in this patient population.

Discussion

Robotic patellofemoral arthroplasty is a new and innovative way to treat isolated patellofemoral arthritis. Careful patient selection, selection of components of sound design, and meticulous surgical technique are important considerations to obtaining acceptable outcomes [19]. The surgeon should adhere to key surgical principles, including the use of proper muscle sparing exposures, avoidance of femoral notching, avoidance of internal rotation of the trochlear component, utilizing a measured patella resection technique to avoid over-tensioning the patellofemoral joint, and proper soft tissue balancing upon closure. Patients should be counseled about the potential for patellar instability (particularly with internally rotated inlay-style designs) as a short-term complication and later progression of tibiofemoral osteoarthritis as the most common long-term complication. Further study will be necessary to determine whether there is a benefit to performing PFA with robotic assistance compared to conventional techniques in terms of patellar tracking, functional outcomes, and durability.

References

1. McAlindon TE, Snow S, Cooper C, Dieppe PA. Radiographic patterns of osteoarthritis of the knee joint in the community: the importance of the patellofemoral joint. Ann Rheum Dis. 1992;51:844–9.
2. Davies AP, Vince AS, Shepstone L, Donell ST, Glasgow MM. The radiographic prevalence of patellofemoral osteoarthritis. Clin Orthop Relat Res. 2002;402:206–12.
3. Mont MA, HAAS S, Mullick T, Hungerford DS. Total knee arthroplasty for patellofemoral arthritis. J Bone Joint Surg Am. 2002;84:1977–81.
4. McKeever DC. Patella prosthesis. J Bone Joint Surg Am. 1955;37-A:1074–84.
5. Blazina ME, Fox JM, Del Pizzo W, Broukin B, Ivey FM. Patellofemoral replacement. Clin Orthop. 1979;144:98–102.
6. Lubinus HH. Patella glide bearing total replacement. Orthopedics. 1979;2:119–27.
7. Arcierio RA, Major MC, Toomy HE. Patellofemoral arthroplasty: a three to nine year follow up study. Clin Orthop. 1988;330:60–71.
8. Argenson JN, Guillaume JM, Aubaniac JM. Is there a place for patellofemoral arthroplasty? Clin Orthop. 1988;236:60–71.
9. Tauro B, Ackroyd CE, Newman JH, Shah NA. The Luminus patellofemoral arthroplasty. J Bone Joint Surg (Br). 2001;83-B:696–701.
10. Lonner JHJ. Patellofemoral arthroplasty. J Am Acad Orthop Surg. 2007;15(8):495–506.

11. Wheaton AJ, Casey FL, Gougoutas AJ, et al. Correlation of T1rho with fixed charge density in cartilage. J Magn Reson Imaging. 2005;20:519–25.
12. Leadbetter WB, Ragland PS, Mont MA. The appropriate use of patellofemoral arthroplasty: an analysis of reported indications, contraindications and failures. Clin Orthop Relat Res. 2005;436:92.
13. Kooijman HJ, Driessen APPM, van Horn JR. Long-term results of patellofemoral arthroplasty: a report of 56 arthroplasties with 17 years of follow up. J Bone Joint Surg (Br). 2003;85-B:836–40.
14. Leadbetter WB, Kolisek FR, Levitt RL, Brooker AF. Patellofemoral arthroplasty: a multi-centre study with minimum 2-year follow-up. Int Orthop. 2008;33:1597–601.
15. Ackroyd CE, Newman JH, Evans R, Eldridge JD, Joslin CC. The Avon patellofemoral arthroplasty: five year survivorship and functional results. J Bone Joint Surg Br. 2007;89:310–5.
16. Mont MA, Johnson AJ, Naziri Q, Kolisek FR, Leadbetter WB. Patellofemoral arthroplasty 7-year mean follow-up. J Arthroplast. 2012;27(3): 358–61.
17. Konan S, Haddad FS. Midterm Outcome of Avon Patellofemoral Arthroplasty for Posttraumatic Unicompartmental Osteoarthritis. J Arthroplast. 2016;31:2657–9.
18. Hofmann AA, Clark CD, Ponder C, Hoffman M. Patellofemoral replacement: the third compartment. Semin Arthro. 2009;20:29–34.
19. Glassman AH, Lachiewicz PF, Tanzer M, editors. Orthopedic knowledge update: hip and knee reconstruction. 4th ed. Rosemont: American Academy of Orthopaedic Surgeons; 2011.

Cécile Batailler, Nathan White, E. Servien,
P. Neyret, and Sébastien Lustig

Treatment of limited osteoarthritis of the knee remains a challenging problem. Non-operative treatments often provide only limited pain relief and functional improvement. Joint preserving surgery, such as realignment osteotomy or tibial tubercle osteotomy, has an established yet limited role. Furthermore, patient selection and indications for joint preservation surgery have important points of difference from those for arthroplasty. For isolated but advanced osteoarthritis, unsuitable for joint preserving surgery, unicompartmental knee arthroplasty (UKA) can be a good treatment option, offering several potential advantages including better function and easier postoperative recovery.

Bicompartmental osteoarthritis is not rare, comprising almost 58% of the population which consult for knee osteoarthritis [1]. Many patients who undergo total knee arthroplasty (TKA) have bicompartmental arthritis, involving either the medial or lateral tibiofemoral compartment plus the patellofemoral compartment, and have no significant deformity, excellent motion, and intact cruciate ligaments. For these patients, some sur-

geons perform a bicompartmental knee arthroplasty (BiKA) to bridge the gap between UKA and TKA. In the same manner, a high percentage of patients who undergo patellofemoral arthroplasty (PFA) or medial/lateral UKA later develop progressive osteoarthritis in another compartment and are often converted to TKA. These patients could potentially benefit from a modular approach to resurfacing the degenerating compartment.

Although generally considered a more complicated procedure than TKA, BiKA provides the same theoretical advantages as UKA, when compared to TKA. Preservation of the intercondylar eminence with both of the cruciate ligaments, restoration of normal kinematics and gait, preservation of bone stock, maintenance of the rotational axis, maintenance of normal leg morphology, normal patella level, and tracking and conservation of proprioception are the fundamental characteristics supporting partial arthroplasties.

BiKA can refer to arthroplasty of the patellofemoral compartment plus the medial or lateral compartment, or both medial and lateral femorotibial compartments. This surgery is very demanding and rarely performed. Recently developed robotic-assisted systems aim to improve the clinical efficacy of knee arthroplasty, by providing optimized component positioning and dynamic ligament balancing. These robotic-assisted systems improve accuracy, thereby reducing the number of outliers, and would seem ideally suited to demanding surgery such as bicompartmental knee arthroplasty. Despite the assistance

C. Batailler (✉) · S. Lustig
Department of Orthopedic Surgery, Hôpital de la
Croix Rousse, Lyon, France
e-mail: cecile.batailler@chu-lyon.fr

N. White
Park Clinic Orthopaedics, Melbourne, VIC, Australia

E. Servien · P. Neyret
Albert Trillat Center, Orthopedic Surgery, Lyon North
University Hospital, Lyon, France

© Springer Nature Switzerland AG 2019
J. H. Lonner (ed.), *Robotics in Knee and Hip Arthroplasty*,
https://doi.org/10.1007/978-3-030-16593-2_13

provided by advanced robotics, many surgical steps must be undertaken unaided, and a large degree of technical skill is required on the part of the surgeon. This chapter describes the surgical technique, along with helpful tips, and reports some outcomes of robotic-assisted BiKA.

Indications

The indications for BiKA should be based on both clinical and radiological criteria, and are in general the same as for UKA, with the difference of bicompartmental arthritis. The primary indication for BiKA is thus painful osteoarthritis affecting two compartments (Figs. 13.1 and 13.2). The second major indication is the patient with a medial/lateral UKA or a PFA, who develops progressive osteoarthritis in another compartment, while satisfying other criteria for deformity and stability.

The anterior cruciate ligament (ACL) should be healthy or reconstructed. Laxity is evaluated clinically as well as on lateral X-rays with ante-

rior stress. On stress views, an anterior translation greater than 10 mm or a posterior saucer-shaped indentation can reflect ACL deficiency.

Preoperative deformity in the frontal plane should be limited to a tibiofemoral angle of 194° for lateral UKA (i.e., overall valgus less than 14°) or 170° for medial UKA (i.e., overall varus less than 10°). Reducibility must also be judged on an anteroposterior X-ray with a varus or valgus stress. Full correction is not required, as the aim is to demonstrate correction of the part of the deformity caused by intra-articular wear rather than the entire deformity.

Finally, preoperative range of motion must be normal or nearly normal, with flexion greater than 100° and flexion contracture of no more than 10°. No limitations of weight and age are recommended, although BiKA is especially suitable for young and active patients with body mass index (BMI) <32 and high functional expectations.

We consider any form of inflammatory arthritis an absolute contraindication to BiKA due to the potential for rapid degeneration in the remaining compartment.

Preoperative Exams

Radiographic analysis includes anteroposterior and lateral views of the knee, full length bilateral standing radiographs, varus and valgus stress radiographs, and a skyline view at 30° of knee flexion.

On X-ray the surgeon should assess the preoperative valgus/varus deformity, its reducibility, signs of ACL insufficiency (anterior tibial translation greater than 10 mm, posterior tibial erosion), and narrowing of the patellofemoral joint space. Tibiofemoral subluxation in the AP view also indicates ACL insufficiency and is therefore a contraindication for BiKA.

Robotic-assisted BiKA using the Navio system doesn't require supplementary imaging, such as CT scan or MRI. All planning is performed at the beginning of the surgery, after knee mapping.

Occasionally, MRI is undertaken when there is a clinical question regarding the competence of the ACL, or the integrity of the compartment which is considered to be unaffected. A CT scan can be performed to assess risk factors for patellar instability before PFA.

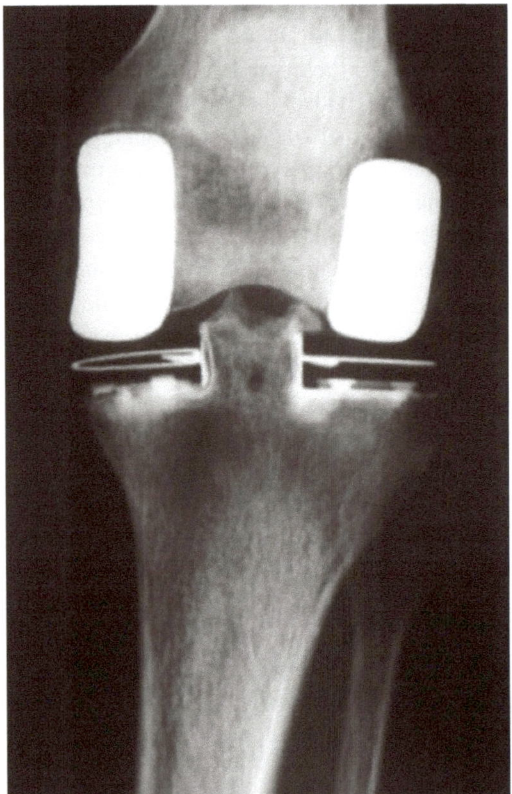

Fig. 13.1 A 63-year-old lady, 2-year follow-up after bicompartmental UKA

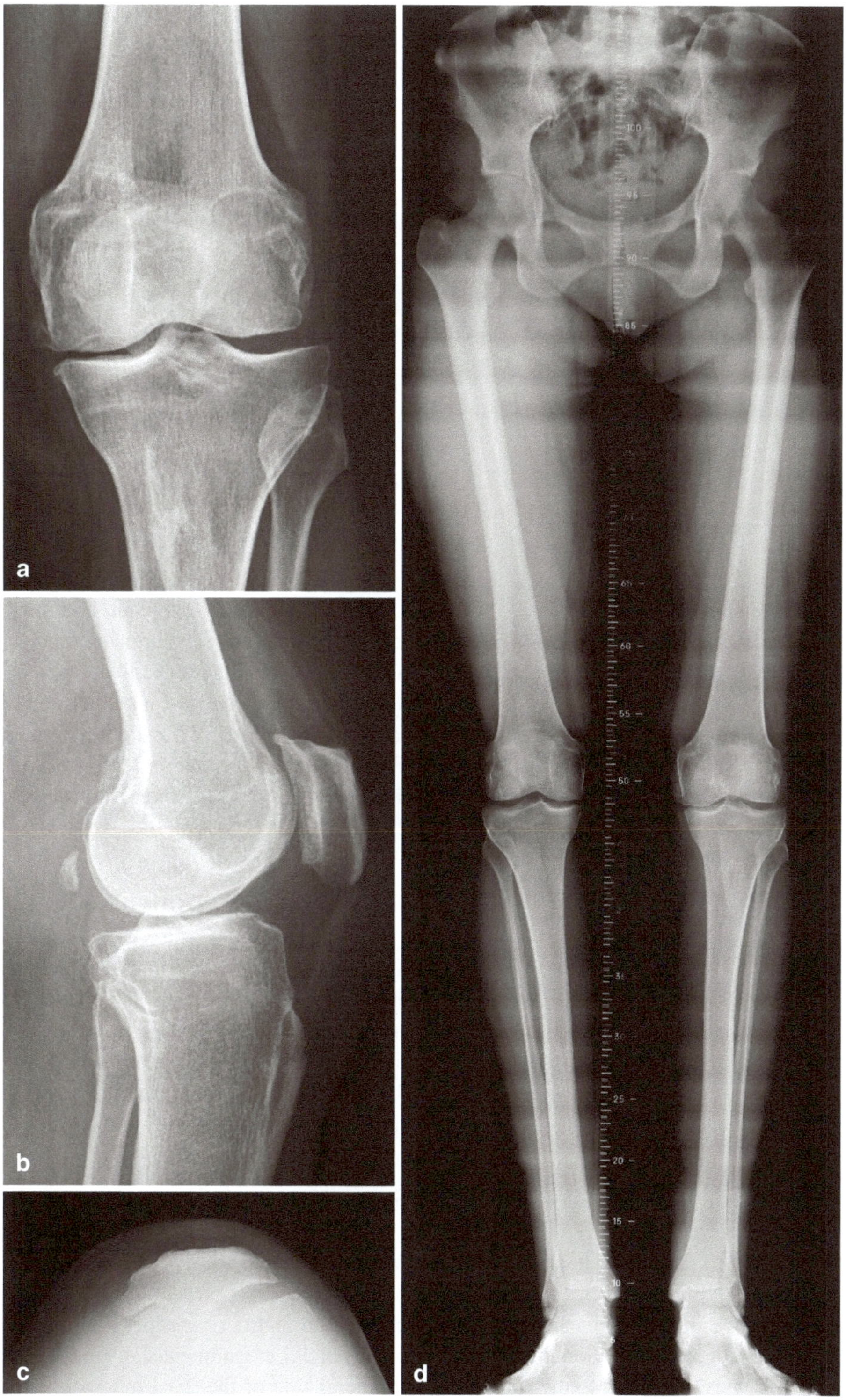

Fig. 13.2 (**a–g**) Young and active patient (53 yo) with symptomatic medial tibiofemoral osteoarthritis associated with patellofemoral osteoarthritis. The lateral compartment and the cruciate ligaments are safe. The varus defor-mity (HKA: 176°) is reducible on the X-ray with valgus stress. The patella is subluxed with an osteoarthritis stade IV of Iwano. A bicompartmental knee arthroplasty has been performed with a medial UKA and a PFP

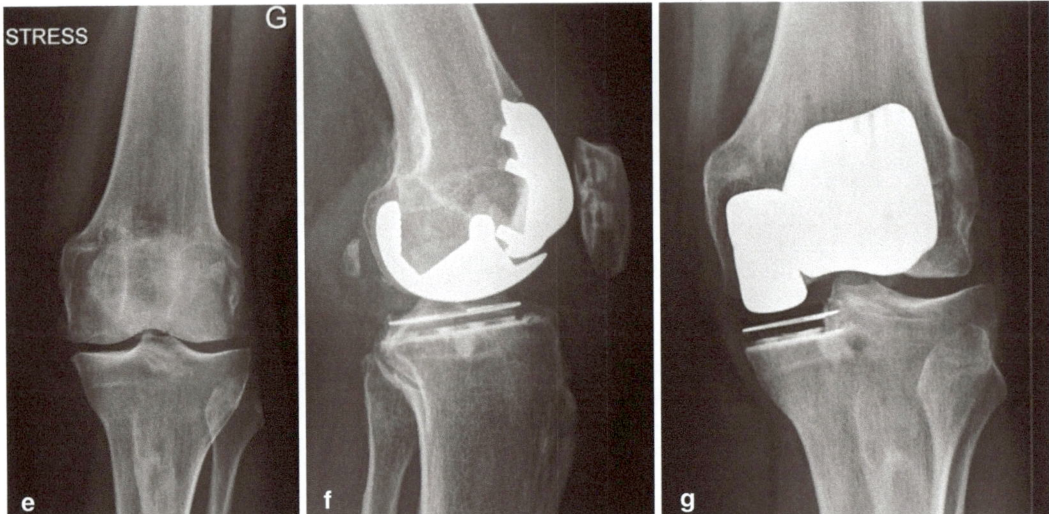

Fig. 13.2 (continued)

Surgical Technique

Which Implant Type?

Two types of BiKA can be used: a single, monolithic implant and non-linked independent implants. We have a preference for the non-linked independent implants, and we described the technique with these. Performing both arthroplasties separately allows optimal positioning of each implant. In this way, the trochlea of the PFA can be placed in the correct rotation, with the optimal depth to allow both good patella tracking and avoidance of overstuffing the patellofemoral joint. For medial and lateral UKA, coronal, sagittal, and rotational alignment can be independently determined while avoiding edge loading and overcorrection. Non-linked implants also allow size interchangeability between compartments, to accommodate potential variability in femoral geometry and aspect ratios between patients and compartments of the knee. In modular bicompartmental resurfacing, the size of the gap between the transitional edge of the trochlear component and the proximal edge of the femoral component of the UKA may vary according to the patients.

Implanting a modular bicompartmental resurfacing device, with or without robotics, is technically easier than implanting a monolithic device

[2]. With a monolithic implant, both implant sizing and alignment are significant challenges due to variability in alignment and morphology of the distal femur [3]. Morrison et al. had a revision rate of 14% of their 21 Journey-Deuce BiKA to TKA for persistent pain after 1 year postoperatively, with a trend for increased revision rate at 2 years of follow-up [4].

Anesthesia and Positioning

The procedure can be performed either under general or regional anesthesia. The patient is placed supine on a standard operating table, with a positioner allowing the knee to be flexed and held at 90° and with or without tourniquet, according to surgeon preference.

Surgical Approaches

Medial/Lateral UKA and PFA

The skin incision measures 12–16 cm, with its upper limit 3–4 cm superior to the proximal pole of the patella, extending distally toward the medial or lateral side of the tibial tuberosity and ending 2 cm under the joint line. First, the medial/lateral UKA is undertaken using trans-quadricipital approach (via the quadriceps tendon) or subvastus

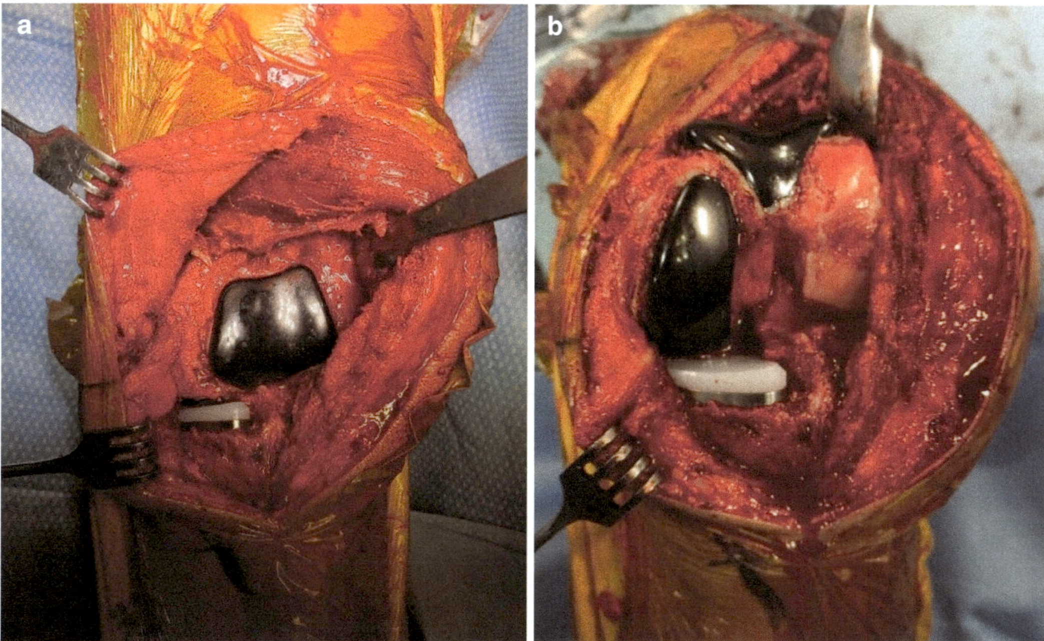

Fig. 13.3 (**a** and **b**) A subvastus approach can be used for medial UKA associated with PFP and allows a good exposure

approach for medial UKA and PFA (Fig. 13.3). Then the PFA is performed, with the trial implants of the UKA in place. The definitive implants are positioned after all trials.

Medial and Lateral UKA

The skin incision measures 10 to 14 cm, and its upper limit is 1–2 cm over the proximal pole of the patella, extending distally toward the medial or lateral side of the tibial tuberosity and ending 2 cm under the joint line. The scar is on the side of the concavity of deformity. Each UKA is performed by a subvastus arthrotomy (medial and lateral). Firstly, the UKA of the side which is most worn (usually in the concavity) is performed, prior to the other tibiofemoral UKA.

Steps with the Robotic-Assisted System (Navio)

For each compartment, the anatomic landmarks, the acquisition phases, and the planning must be performed independently before each arthroplasty. However, the navigation pins are not changed.

After percutaneous insertion of bicortical pins into the proximal tibia and distal femur and attachment of optical tracking arrays, mechanical and rotational axes of the limb are determined intraoperatively by establishing the hip and knee centers (and the center of ankle for UKA). Either the kinematic, anteroposterior (Whiteside), or transepicondylar axes of the knee are identified and selected to determine the rotational position of the femoral component. The condylar anatomy and tibial plateau anatomy, or the trochlea anatomy, are mapped out by "painting" the surfaces with the optical probes (Fig. 13.4). A virtual model of the knee is created.

For medial or lateral UKA, a dynamic soft tissue balancing algorithm is initiated. With an applied valgus stress to tension the medial collateral ligament (for medial UKA) or a varus stress to tension the lateral structures (for lateral UKA), the three-dimensional positions of the femur and the tibia are captured throughout a passive range of knee motion. Implant sizes, position, and orientation are "virtually" established. A graphic representation of gap spacing through an entire range of flexion is created, and determination is made regarding whether

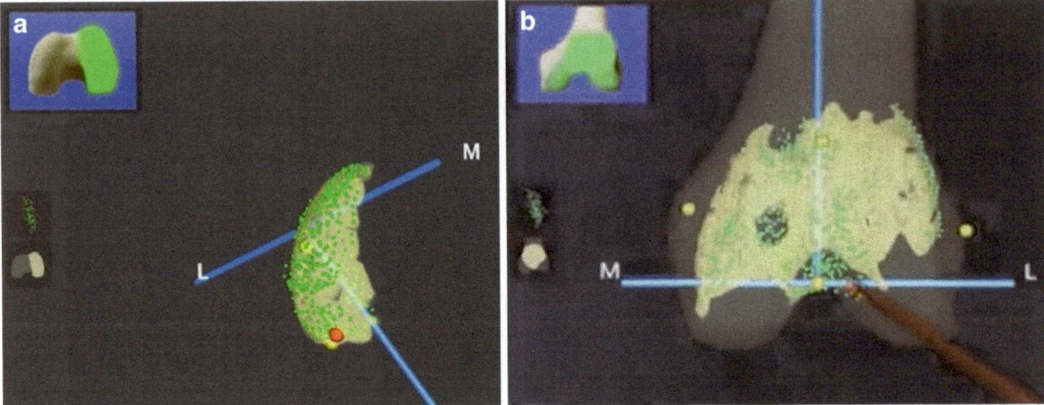

Fig. 13.4 (**a** and **b**) The condylar anatomy for UKA or the trochlea anatomy for PFP are mapped out by "painting" the surfaces with the optical probes to create a virtual model of the knee

the planned position of the femoral and tibial components is adequate or adjustments can be made to achieve the desired soft tissue balance (Fig. 13.5). By adjusting the implant positions, including tibial slope, depth of resection, and anteriorization or distalization of the femoral component, virtual dynamic soft tissue balance can be achieved.

For PFA, a virtual model of the knee is created after the trochlear mapping. There is no dynamic acquisition. The trochlear implant is planned with the three-dimensional representation in all spatial plans (Fig. 13.6).

When planning is complete, a handheld sculpting burr is used to prepare the bone on the condylar, tibial, or trochlear surfaces (Fig. 13.7). The Navio PFS system modulates the exposure of the burr tip beyond the protective sheath. These position data are continuously updated in real time. After bone preparation, the surfaces are assessed and trial components impacted into place for assessment of range of motion and stability. For medial or lateral UKA, limb alignment, range of motion, implant position, and gap balance can be quantified and compared with the preoperative plan.

Features of Each Compartment

Knowledge of the surgical principles, and relevant tips, unique to each compartment, is essen-tial. These features remain the same with or without a robotic-assisted system.

Following BiKA, mechanical alignment must be close to 180° with 1–2° of persistent deformity in the concavity.

Medial UKA

The tibial cut should be performed perpendicularly to the tibial axis. The tibial resection should be minimal (4–5 mm), just below medial osteophytes. The slope of the tibial cut should reproduce the natural slope in the medial compartment, or a little less, to protect the ACL.

The size of the femoral component is the largest size that will not overhang the junction between the remaining articular cartilage and the cut end of the distal femur, to avoid patellar conflict. Usually the femoral component is as close as possible to the intercondylar notch, without conflict with tibial eminences. The rotation of the femoral component follows the native rotation of the medial condyle. The femoral alignment should be checked in flexion and extension.

During the trials, with the knee in extension or in flexion, a 2-mm spacer should be able to be inserted into the space between tibial and femoral components.

Lateral UKA

The tibial cut should be at 90° to the tibial axis. It is very important to perform a minimal tibial

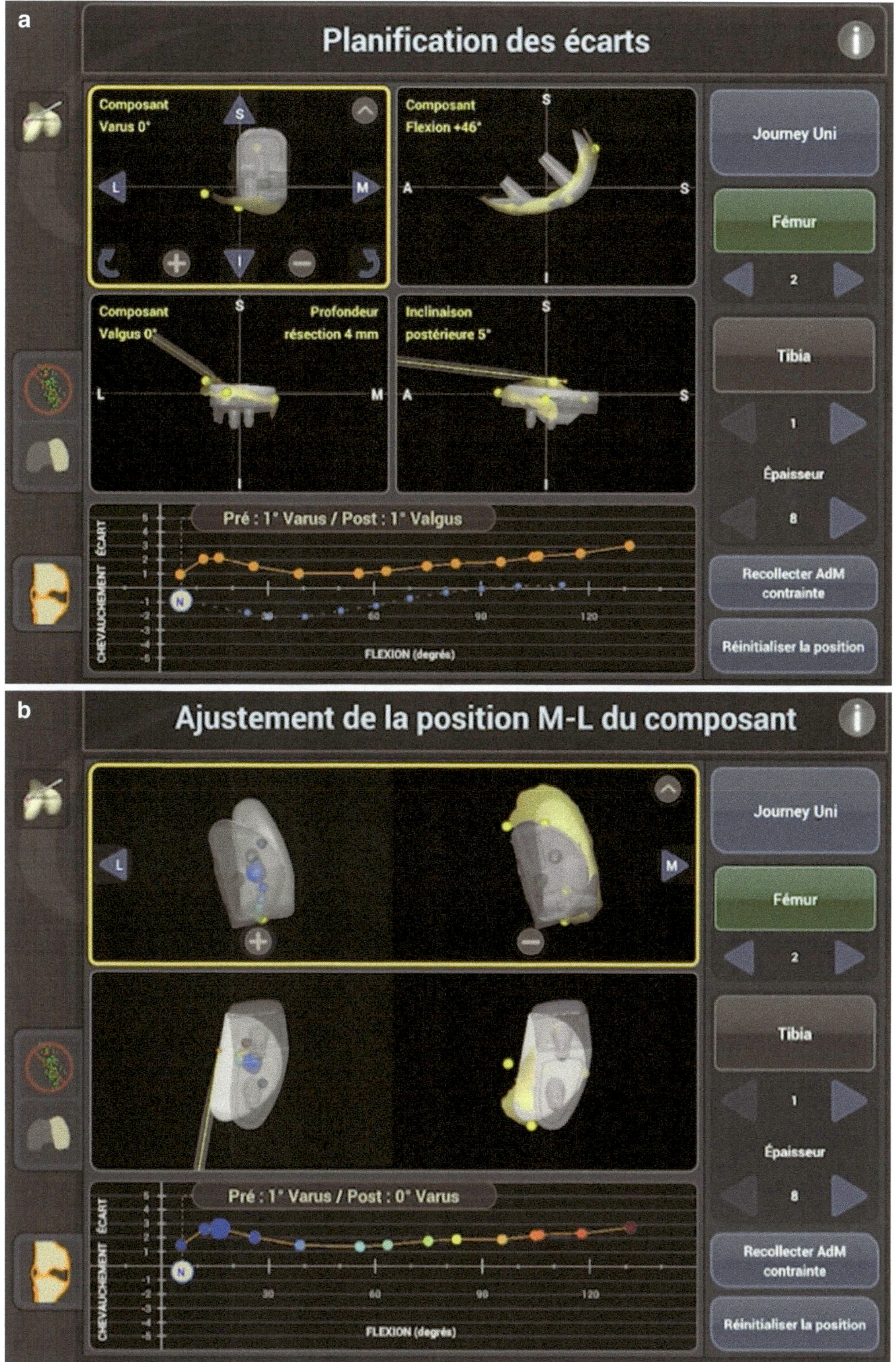

Fig. 13.5 (**a** and **b**) Implant position and orientation of UKA are "virtually" established to obtain a satisfying alignment and a good dynamic soft tissue balance. A graphic representation of gap spacing and the implants alignment through an entire range of flexion is created to appreciate this planning

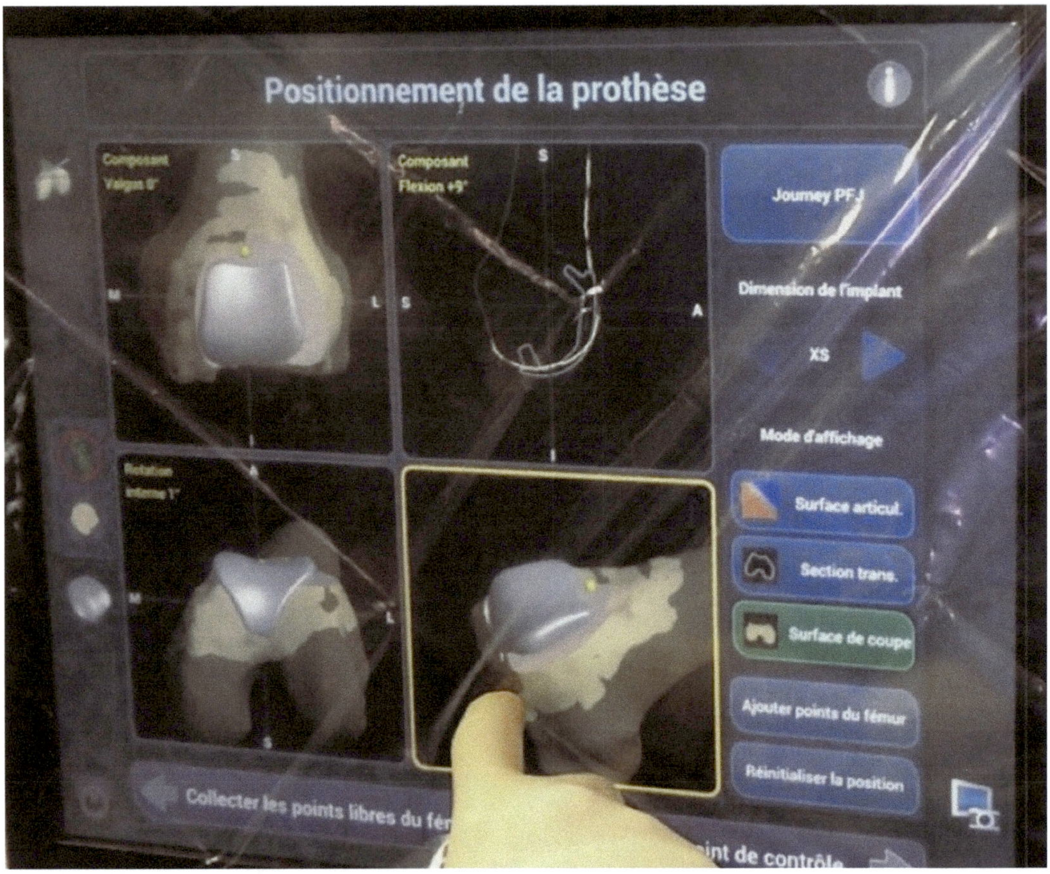

Fig. 13.6 For patellofemoral arthroplasty, a virtual model of the knee is created after the trochlear mapping to plan the trochlear implant position in all spatial plans

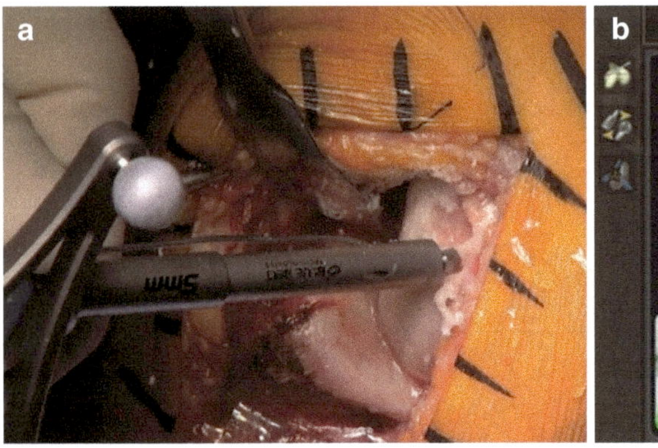
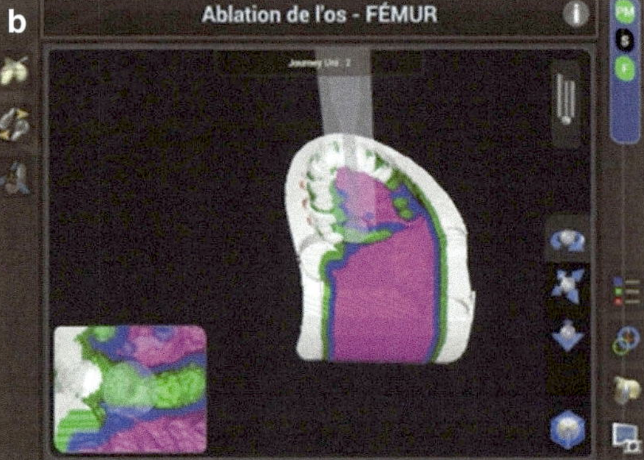

Fig. 13.7 (**a** and **b**) A handheld sculpting burr is used to prepare the bone on the condylar, with an automatic feedback system, to remove only the necessary bone according to the plan. The Navio PFS system modulates the exposure of the burr tip beyond the protective sheath

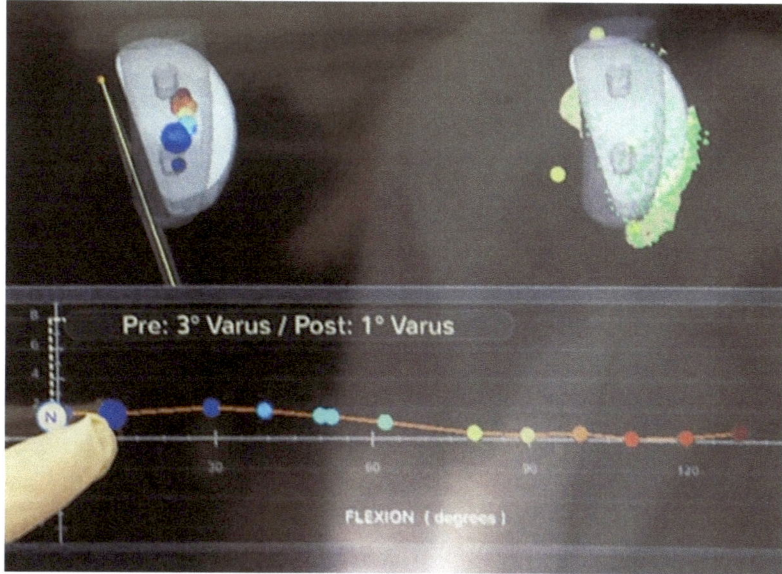

Fig. 13.8 During robotically assisted UKA, the "screw home" mechanism is easily identified. This picture of the planning during robotically assisted UKA shows the position of both implants in extension, with the difference in rotation

resection (4 mm maximum) because it is the femoral side that is most often affected by lateral compartment osteoarthritis. The slope of the tibial cut should reproduce the natural slope in the lateral compartment to avoid being tight in flexion (anterior slope) and to protect the ACL (high posterior slope). Because the lateral tibial plateau undergoes an external rotation due to the "screw home" mechanism, the line of the sagittal cut will have some internal rotation, thus crossing the patellar tendon.

The distal femoral cut should be minimal to allow for a distalized femoral implant that compensates for the wear of the femur. With condylar hypoplasia, the femoral component should not reproduce the femoral anatomy, but should augment the dysplastic condyle both distally and posteriorly.

Positioning must take into account the "screw home" mechanism as the knee comes into extension. Thus the tibial implant should be as close as possible to the tibial eminences and should have 10–15° of internal rotation (Fig. 13.8). Furthermore, the femoral positioning in flexion should exaggerate the lateral rotation and be positioned laterally, sometimes on the lateral osteophytes.

Patellofemoral Arthroplasty

The design of the patellofemoral prosthesis is essential to good patellar tracking and satisfying outcomes. The trochlear geometry of the Journey PFJ (anterior cut onlay-style implant) is asymmetric, implanted in neutral rotation relative to the anteroposterior axis of the femur, with a lateralized trochlear groove in extension to obtain good patellar tracking through a range of motion.

The femoral component must reproduce the trochlear size to avoid anterior "overstuffing" and persistent pain. The transition between the trochlea and condyles should be smooth. The orientation of the femoral component is essential and is affected by the presence of preoperative patellar maltracking. Sometimes, the femoral component should be translated laterally, with some external rotation relative to the plane of the patellar, to centralize the patella and optimize tracking (Fig. 13.9).

Complications

Specific complications related to robot-assisted UKA/PFA include issues with pin placement, longer initial operative times, and case conversion owing to mechanical or hardware issues. The pin tracts for the optical tracking arrays create a stress riser in the cortical bone, which poses a risk for fracture; therefore, it is highly advised that the tracking pins be inserted in the metaphyseal regions of the femur and tibia rather than the diaphyses, to

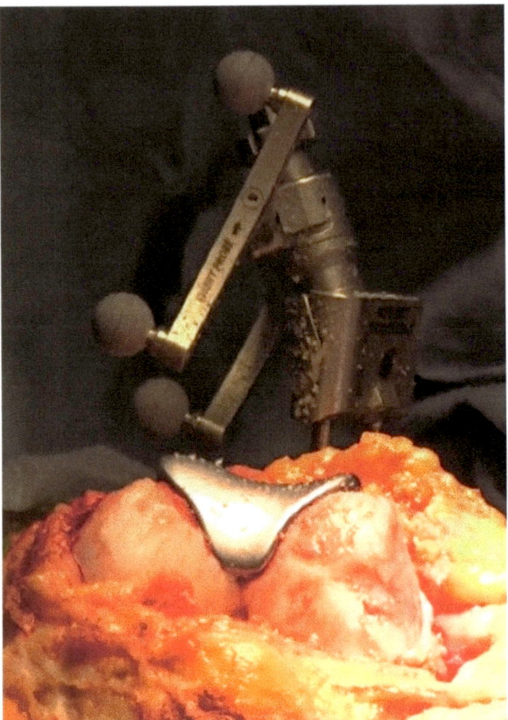

Fig. 13.9 The femoral component must reproduce the trochlear size to avoid anterior "overstuffing." This femoral component is a little translated laterally with some degrees of external rotation relative to the patellar plane to recenter the patella and optimize the patellar tracking

minimize fracture risk. Incorrect pin placement could also theoretically cause neurovascular injury. There is also a risk of inadvertent soft tissue trauma during bone preparation with the robotic tool [5].

Medial and Lateral UKA

Typical complications observed after UKA with conventional techniques may also occur with robotic control, including prosthetic loosening, polyethylene wear, progressive osteoarthritis of the unresurfaced compartments of the knee, infection, stiffness, instability, and thromboembolic complication.

During a BiKA combining medial and lateral UKA, the main risk is tibial spine fracture or avulsion. Parratte et al. described 4 cases in 100 BiKAs [6]. These cases were all immediately treated by

internal fixation, with a combination of cancellous screws and suture anchors. In the described cases, the outcomes after this complication were the same as for other patients. Misalignment after BiKA, particularly overcorrection, can cause excessive stress on the contralateral compartment, and either a wear or a loosening of the implants, or wear of an unresurfaced tibiofemoral compartment.

Patellofemoral Arthroplasty

Early postoperative complications of PFA include persistent anterior knee pain, patellar catching or snapping, patellar maltracking or instability, and extensor mechanism disruption. Increased peripatellar pain may be an early consequence of "overstuffing" of the patellofemoral joint through the placement of an implant that is thicker than the amount of bone and cartilage that is resected. These complications are essentially linked to the position of the PFA [7]. The robotic-assisted system is helpful to try to reduce the malposition of the PFA [8]. There is no specific complication of PFA in BiKA with non-linked independent implants.

Outcomes

In the literature, very few studies have described robotic-assisted BiKA. Some authors describe outcomes after BiKA without robotic assistance, while others report outcomes after robotic-assisted UKA.

One study reports outcomes of bicompartmental arthroplasty (PFA associated with medial or lateral UKA) with the Mako system [9]. This paper found that BiKA, without distinction whether lateral or medial, reliably alleviated pain and improved the Oxford Knee Scores, from 18 ± 6 (range 10–28) to 36.43 ± 8.56 (range 8–48) ($p < 0.0001$). There was one patient with poor functional outcome. Twenty-four out of 29 patients (83%) had good to excellent outcome, at a mean follow-up of 27 months.

A second paper, by Lonner et al., examined a series of 12 consecutive modular BiKAs implanted with robotic arm assistance [2]. The mean knee ROM significantly improved from 100° of flexion preoperatively to a mean of 126° of flexion. Improvements in WOMAC scores and KS scores were also statistically significant with a minimum follow-up of 6 months.

The outcomes of BiKA are related to a variety of factors, including patient-related factors, implant design, alignment, and fixation. Patient selection significantly influences outcomes following BiKA.

Parratte et al. found that after at greater than 2 years, contemporary unlinked BiKA (bi-UKA and medial UKA with PFA) was associated with greater comfort during everyday activities (forgotten knee) and better functional outcomes, compared to TKA [6]. On a series of 100 bicompartmental arthroplasties (medial and lateral UKA), Parratte et al. described 91% of satisfied or very satisfied patients at a mean follow-up of 11.7 years. The remaining 9% were non-satisfied patients, who underwent revision before 4 years for aseptic loosening [10]. The few studies describing range of movement after BiKA generally report satisfactory range of motion, with most achieving flexion greater than 120° without pain, and complete extension [11–13].

BiKA has demonstrated mixed results in regard to durability, with one study showing a 17-year survival to revision, radiographic loosening, or disease progression of 78% in the bi-UKA group and 54% in the med-UKA/PFA group. The main cause of revision was aseptic loosening of the tibial implant (medial and/or lateral). Revision for symptomatic patellofemoral osteoarthritis is not frequent [6].

Revision, if required, is often carried out without difficulty, using a primary implant TKA. Occasionally the employment of augments and stems is required. The use of revision TKA implants is generally not necessary after combined PFA and medial/lateral UKA. The use of revision type prostheses, including hinge prostheses, may be a little more common after a BiKA combining medial and lateral UKA [6, 13].

Conclusion

Bicompartmental knee arthroplasty is a demanding surgery, which provides good functional results and a high rate of satisfaction. In the available literature, excellent long-term clinical and radiological outcomes have been achieved, with a survivorship similar to that of classic UKA. The ideal candidate for BiKA is a young patient affected by medial or lateral tibiofemoral osteoarthritis, with patellofemoral compartment involvement. Robotic assistance can be very helpful to position the implants and to allow a less invasive approach during this demanding surgery. However, very few studies report functional outcomes after robotic-assisted BiKA. Another scenario is the development of patellofemoral osteoarthritis after UKA or medial/lateral tibiofemoral osteoarthritis after PFA. For these cases, the suitability of robotic-assisted systems is less certain, because intraoperative registration and mapping are affected by the presence of prior PFA and UKA. Perhaps this indication will be further assessed in the future with robotic-assisted systems.

References

1. Ledingham J, Regan M, Jones A, Doherty M. Radiographic patterns and associations of osteoarthritis of the knee in patients referred to hospital. Ann Rheum Dis. 1993;52:520–6.
2. Lonner JH. Modular bicompartmental knee arthroplasty with robotic arm assistance. Am J Orthop (Belle Mead NJ). 2009;38:28–31.
3. Palumbo BT, Henderson ER, Edwards PK, Burris RB, Gutierrez S, Raterman SJ. Initial experience of the Journey-Deuce bicompartmental knee prosthesis: a review of 36 cases. J Arthroplast. 2011;26:40–5.
4. Morrison TA, Nyce JD, Macaulay WB, Geller JA. Early adverse results with bicompartmental knee arthroplasty: a prospective cohort comparison to total knee arthroplasty. J Arthroplast. 2011;26:35–9.
5. Lonner JH. Robotically assisted unicompartmental knee arthroplasty with a handheld image-free sculpting tool. Orthop Clin North Am. 2016;47:29–40.
6. Parratte S, Pauly V, Aubaniac JM, Argenson JN. Survival of bicompartmental knee arthroplasty at 5 to 23 years. Clin Orthop Relat Res. 2010;468:64–72.
7. Lustig S, Magnussen RA, Dahm DL, Parker D. Patellofemoral arthroplasty, where are we

today? Knee Surg Sports Traumatol Arthrosc. 2012;20:1216–26.

8. Cossey AJ, Spriggins AJ. Computer-assisted patellofemoral arthroplasty: a mechanism for optimizing rotation. J Arthroplast. 2006;21:420–7.

9. Tamam C, Plate JF, Augart M, Poehling GG, Jinnah RH. Retrospective clinical and radiological outcomes after robotic assisted Bicompartmental knee Arthroplasty. Adv Orthop. 2015;2015:747309.

10. Parratte S, Ollivier M, Opsomer G, Lunebourg A, Argenson JN, Thienpont E. Is knee function better with contemporary modular bicompartmental arthroplasty compared to total knee arthroplasty? Short-term outcomes of a prospective matched study including 68 cases. Orthop Traumatol Surg Res. 2015;101:547–52.

11. Argenson JN, Parratte S, Bertani A, Aubaniac JM, Lombardi AV Jr, Berend KR, et al. The new arthritic patient and arthroplasty treatment options. J Bone Joint Surg Am. 2009;91(Suppl 5):43–8.

12. Isaac SM, Barker KL, Danial IN, Beard DJ, Dodd CA, Murray DW. Does arthroplasty type influence knee joint proprioception? A longitudinal prospective study comparing total and unicompartmental arthroplasty. Knee. 2007;14:212–7.

13. Shah SM, Dutton AQ, Liang S, Dasde S. Bicompartmental versus total knee arthroplasty for medio-patellofemoral osteoarthritis: a comparison of early clinical and functional outcomes. J Knee Surg. 2013;26:411–6.

Stefan W. Kreuzer, Stefany J. K. Malanka, and Marius Dettmer

Patients suffering from osteoarthritis (OA) of the knee who have failed conservative management have a number of surgical treatment options. For cases where OA has affected more than one compartment of the knee but has not yet progressed to all three, bicompartmental knee arthroplasty (BiKA) is an option. With the rise of navigated surgery and robotic assistance in arthroplasty, MAKOplasty, the technology set by Stryker MAKO, has become an established surgical option for individuals suffering from early to mid-stage osteoarthritis (OA). In this chapter, we describe the indications for MAKO bicompartmental knee arthroplasty, the potential benefits, and the general and specific techniques associated with each subtype of bicompartmental knee arthroplasty that can be performed using the MAKO system.

MAKO Bicompartmental Configurations

There are three possible configurations for MAKO bicompartmental knee arthroplasty. The medial bicompartmental (medial BiKA) configuration combines medial unicondylar arthroplasty (medial UKA) with patellofemoral joint arthroplasty (PFA) (Fig. 14.1). This is the most common multi-compartment configuration, as due to anatomical and biomechanical characteristics of the knee, in most cases, osteoarthritis is usually more prominent in the medial compartment. The lateral bicompartmental (lateral BiKA) configuration combines lateral unicondylar arthroplasty (lateral UKA) with patellofemoral joint arthroplasty (PFA) and is less common. The third configuration, which is more commonly referred to as bi-unicompartmental knee arthroplasty (Bi-UKA), involves both medial and lateral UKAs (Fig. 14.2). There is the possibility of replacing all three compartments separately (medial UKA, lateral UKA, and PFA), which has been performed by the author. However, in such cases it may be more prudent to opt for a conventional TKA as the complexity of replacing three individual compartments is very high and the indications are very narrow; therefore, this procedure will not be included in this chapter.

Officially, MAKO only recognizes the medial bicompartmental configuration as it is currently the only FDA-approved MAKO bicompartmental

S. W. Kreuzer (✉)
INOV8 Orthopedics/Memorial Bone and Joint Research Foundation, Houston, TX, USA
e-mail: skreuzer@inov8hc.com

S. J. K. Malanka · M. Dettmer
Memorial Bone and Joint Research Foundation, Houston, TX, USA

© Springer Nature Switzerland AG 2019
J. H. Lonner (ed.), *Robotics in Knee and Hip Arthroplasty*,
https://doi.org/10.1007/978-3-030-16593-2_14

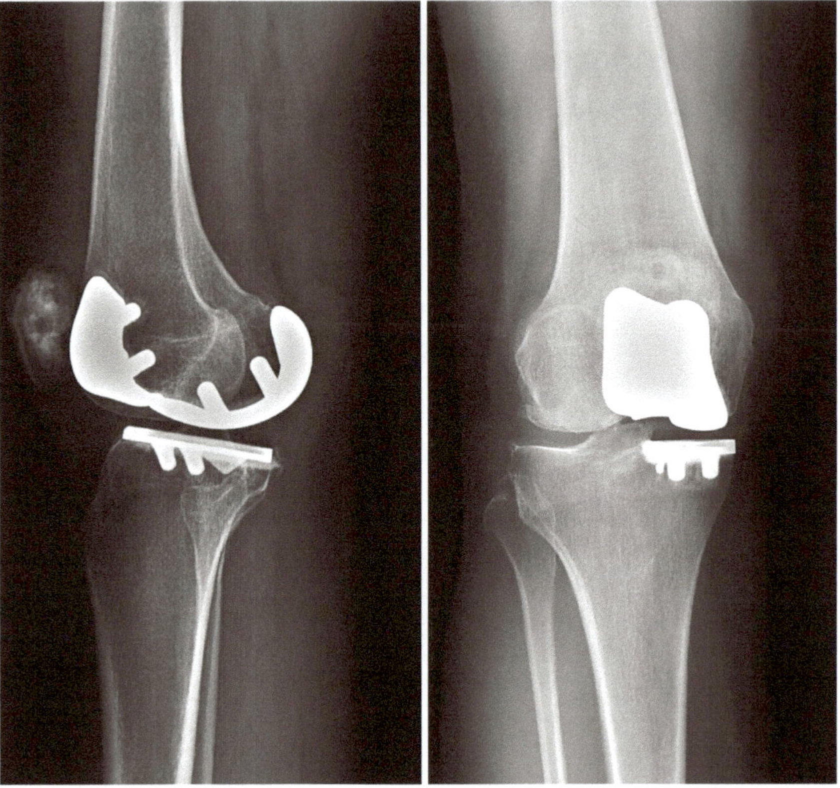

Fig. 14.1 Lateral and AP views of medial and patellofemoral implants after MAKO medial bicompartmental knee arthroplasty

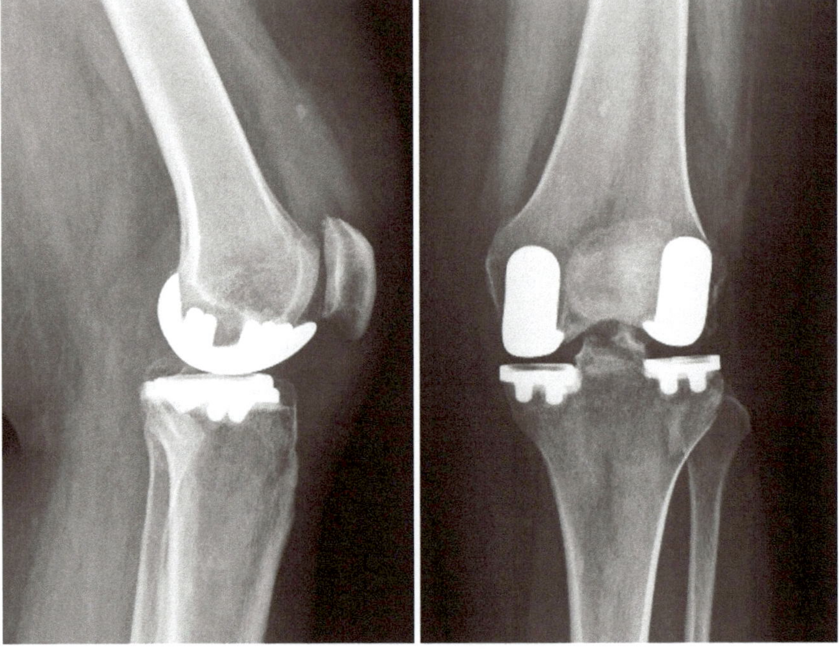

Fig. 14.2 Lateral and AP views of medial and lateral implants after MAKO bi-unicompartmental knee arthroplasty

application. Furthermore, the manufacturer refers to this configuration as the MAKO MCK, or "multicompartmental knee," in line with the Restoris MCK line of partial knee implants. The remaining bicompartmental configurations are considered off-label uses of the MAKO Restoris MCK implant system. While beyond the scope of this chapter, it is worth noting that as mentioned above it is possible to perform a tricompartmental knee arthroplasty using a combination of medial UKA, lateral UKA, and PFA; however, this too remains an off-label use of the Restoris MCK implants and is rarely performed.

Indications for MAKO Bicompartmental and Bi-unicompartmental Knee Arthroplasty

The ideal candidate for MAKO BiKA and Bi-UKA is a young and relatively healthy patient with high activity levels (i.e., those presenting with high activity levels, as indicated by rating scales such as the UCLA Activity score [1]) and who participates in high-impact sports (including cycling, downhill skiing, hiking, tennis, etc.), with a BMI below 30. This contradicts early indications that suggested that only older patients with low activity levels are good candidates for partial knee arthroplasty; however, more recent studies have demonstrated that younger patients with higher functional demands can benefit greatly from bicompartmental knee arthroplasty and have comparable, if not better, outcomes [2–4]. Further indications for this treatment type include severe pain and previous failure of conservative treatment.

On physical exam, candidates should demonstrate a range of motion of a minimum of 110° in the affected knee, with any flexion contracture limited to less than 5°. Patients undergoing medial BiKA should have angular deformity no greater than 8° of varus, while patients undergoing lateral BiKA should have angular deformity no greater than 4° of valgus. For patients undergoing Bi-UKA, the affected knee should be very close to neutral alignment, with angular deformity no greater than 4° of varus or valgus.

Contraindications for MAKO BiKA and Bi-UKA include septic osteoarthritis (OA), rheumatoid arthritis, post-traumatic OA with severe deformity, or any other severe deformity exceeding the aforementioned criteria. Although debatable, it is now our thought that patients ≥65 years of age should not be considered for BiKA or Bi-UKA unless they are extremely active, as described above.

Rationale for Use and Potential Drawbacks

Bicompartmental knee arthroplasty offers greater bone and tissue preservation over conventional TKA, as both BiKA and Bi-UKA preserve the intercondylar eminence and therefore the ACL and PCL ligaments. This in turn preserves the natural kinematics of the knee, providing rotational stability, along with restraint against anterior and posterior translation of the tibia relative to the femur during extension and flexion, respectively. Furthermore, the bone and tissue preservation offered with MAKO BiKA and Bi-UKA facilitates any future revisions by allowing relatively easier conversion to TKA, in the event that it becomes necessary in the future. The surgical approach is less invasive and thus leads to decreased blood loss and damage to surrounding healthy tissue. Consequently, this can mean decreased post-operative pain and a shorter recovery time for patients, and is thought to lead to better functional outcomes. This assumption was confirmed in a recent study aimed at investigating the potential benefits of Bi-UKA in comparison to total knee replacements for younger patients. The authors found that there were significant benefits regarding patient-reported outcomes such as the perceived ability to perform activities of daily living and the subjective rating of symptoms after surgery [5]. Moreover, the use of a robotic system has been shown to decrease the learning curve usually associated with tradiional instrumentation-based UKAs, whereas there is no evidence for additional risk to patients during the learning phase [6].

It should be noted that in modular BiKA and Bi-UKA, where multiple implants are involved, a high level of accuracy is required for implant alignment to optimize implant longevity and functional outcomes. Indeed, studies have shown that robotic assistance in these surgeries offers a high level of precision that contributes to higher reproducibility and improved outcomes [5]. The MAKO BiKA and Bi-UKA also use a proprietary implant system, the Restoris MCK system, which is designed specifically for use with the MAKO robotic arm and software system. This tight integration of hardware and software promotes precision and accuracy, with the drawback that there are no other options available for implant design and composition available. The procedure can also possibly lead to reliance on robotic haptic feedback and computer templating if performed with high frequency in comparison to manual surgery. Another drawback to the use of robotic assistance with MAKO BiKA and Bi-UKA is that there is an increased cost, not only for the robot but also for the two sets of implants. Lastly, the high complexity of this procedure makes this more technically difficult and also increases operative time. Still, with these considerations, MAKO BiKA and Bi-UKA remain a highly beneficial option for certain patients.

General Surgical Methods for MAKO Medial BiKA, Lateral BiKA, and Bi-UKA

All patients undergoing MAKO BiKA or Bi-UKA require CT scans of the operative limb to be obtained prior to surgery to allow for 3D visualization of the patient's unique anatomy [5]. This is conducted under the same protocol as for MAKO UKA. CT scans are obtained through the hip and ankle in 5-mm-thick slices, in addition to 1-mm-thick slices through the knee, and are then converted to DICOM format and uploaded to the MAKO Tactile Guidance System (TGS) [7, 8]. Software is then used to template the implant sizes, positioning, and alignment and to provide initial guidelines for bone resection [7]. All templated data is reviewed for feasibility preoperatively and is confirmed using intraoperative bony landmark registration to confirm optimal component placement.

Following patient positioning, sterile draping, and tourniquet inflation, an anteromedial parapatellar incision from the superior aspect of the patella to approximately 2 cm below the tibial plateau is performed. A medial parapatellar arthrotomy is then used to dissect through soft tissue layers through the medial capsule. Once the medial compartment is exposed, fat tissue and damaged or visible meniscus tissue can be trimmed, and the patella is retracted laterally off the femoral trochlea.

Tracker arrays are placed for kinematic tracking of soft tissue balancing; a tibial tracker array is fixed percutaneously in the proximal tibia, while the femoral tracker array is fixed in the distal femur through the arthrotomy. Patient landmarks in the proximal femur and distal tibia are then verified by circumducting the hip, then registering points on the medial malleolus and then the lateral malleolus. Checkpoint screws are placed in cortical bone at the distal femur and the proximal tibia to detect any position changes of the tracker array. Bone registration points on the tibial and femoral surfaces are then collected and compared with the preoperative model prepared from the CT scans to confirm the actual three-dimensional geometry of the structures [5, 8]. As such, osteophytes should not be removed prior to this registration. Kinematic tracking allows for assessment of mechanical alignment, ligament laxity, and flexion extension gaps in order to recreate a balanced joint. For accurate balancing, it is critical that all osteophytes and adhesions are removed after the registration is completed. The methods used for bone registration and soft tissue balancing vary depending on the selected bicompartmental approach and the varus/valgus alignment of the knee, and as such these methods will be described in greater detail when discussing each specific bicompartmental approach.

Based on the measurements obtained during kinematic tracking, which are compared against the 3D model of the native joint, the MAKO TGS defines parameters for bone resection. The checkpoint screws must be re-registered prior to bone resection to confirm and accept these parameters. The RIO arm, which uses a burr for cutting, is moved into the surgical field. Haptic feedback guides the surgeon, as the operator can only move the burr within the defined parameters; if the surgeon attempts to move the burr outside this area, the arm will exert increased resistive force in combination with provision of tactile feedback, preventing bone resection beyond the spatial limits determined by the TGS.

Once the predetermined portion of bone has been resected, the trial implants are placed in an order specific to the bicompartmental approach. Polyethylene insert thickness and additional bone resection needed are determined by the desired final varus/valgus alignment angle, the surgeon's feel, and the data obtained through kinematic tracking. Any overhanging bone or cartilage will be removed using a rongeur. After soft tissue balancing has been performed to confirm proper balancing and fit between components, the trial implants are removed. It is critical that the bone is irrigated extensively to remove any debris from the cancellous bone that could lead to post-operative irritation, and is dried using a CO2 Lavage System (such as CarboJet, Kinamed Inc., Camarillo, CA) to allow for optimal cement fixation. Two cement batches are used to ensure uniform application, and the components are seated in the cement mantle using special impactors, again in an order specific to the bicompartmental approach.

Surgical Methods and Considerations for MAKO Medial BiKA

Registration for MAKO medial BiKA is based on the protocol for MAKO medial UKA, with some additional registration points on the anterior cortex and the trochlear groove. A digitizer wand (Fig. 14.3) is used to trace over the articular and surrounding non-articular surfaces of the medial condyle, the femoral trochlea groove, and the anterior cortex, along with the medial tibial pla-

teau, medial tibial condyle, anterolateral (Gerdy's) tubercle, anterior intercondylar area, and tibial tuberosity (Fig. 14.4a, b). Following bone registration, it is critical that all osteophytes are removed and the medial gutter is re-established for accurate balancing. Any adhesions in the posterior capsule of the posterior medial condyle and contracted tissue along the medial tibial plateau must be released prior to soft tissue balancing.

Soft tissue balancing for a varus knee is performed by applying a physiologic (gentle) valgus stress over a range of joint positions (a minimum of four poses, although the author usually captures around ten poses), including full extension (approx. 10°), mid-flexion (30°–60°),

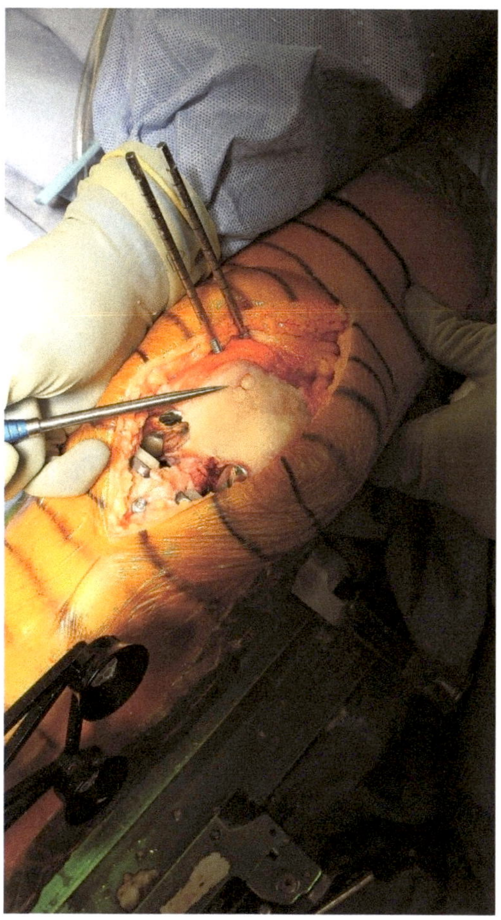

Fig. 14.3 A digitizer wand is used to register bony landmarks for confirmation of the 3D model of the knee

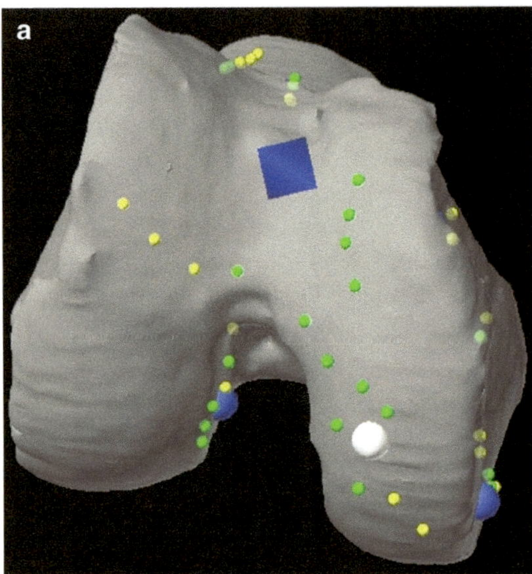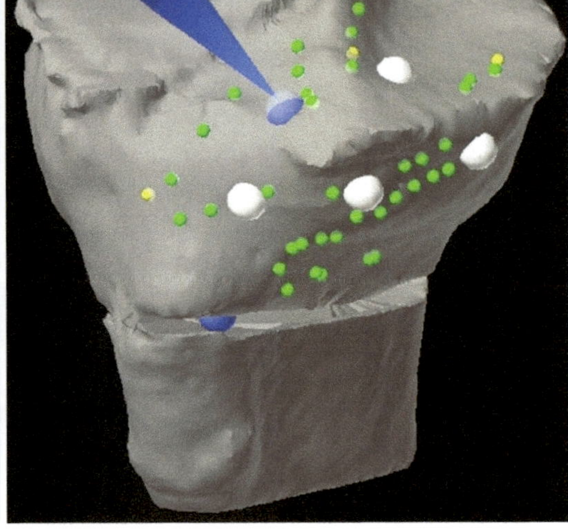

Fig. 14.4 Registration points on the (**a**) medial femoral condyle, cortex, and trochlear groove and (**b**) medial tibial plateau, medial tibial condyle, anterolateral (Gerdy's) tubercle, anterior intercondylar area, and tibial tuberosity in MAKO medial bicompartmental knee arthroplasty

flexion (approx. 90°), and full flexion (110°–120°), and captured via kinematic tracking [9]. The valgus stress tests open the arthritic medial compartment joint space to restore tibiofemoral alignment along the mechanical axis to a relative pre-arthritic state by creating moderate tension to the MCL [10]. Adequate tension on the MCL is necessary to maintain proper joint space throughout the full range of motion [7]. Additional cartilage points are obtained in the area of transition between the implant and remaining cartilage to further fine-tune implant position to avoid a step-off between the implant and the remaining cartilage.

Once soft tissue balancing has been completed and the implant sizes have been determined, the calculated area of bone is resected—starting with the medial femoral condyle and then the medial tibial plateau and finally the femoral trochlea. Trial implants are placed and the operative knee is passively flexed and extended over a full range of motion to further confirm soft tissue balancing via kinematic tracking. Further adjustments can be made to the surgical plan if necessary, as the MAKO TGS software will calculate new parameters for bone resection if needed. Finally, for the PFA, the patellar implant thickness is determined using calipers to measure the preoperative patellar thickness with the leg in full extension. Saw and drill guides are used to allow for manual resection of the articulating surface. Once the desired joint alignment has been achieved, the bone is irrigated and prepared as described earlier, and the final implants are cemented in the following order if only one batch of cement is utilized: the tibial implant followed by the femoral implant and the patellofemoral implant. The patella button is placed and cementing is achieved using a clamp assembly. Alternatively, if two batches are utilized, the sequence is as follows: the patellofemoral and tibial implants with the first batch and the femoral implant and patella button with the second batch. After release of the tourniquet, patellar tracking is assessed and a lateral release is performed if necessary. A final verification of soft tissue balance is performed following cementing of all implants before placing the final polyethylene insert (Fig. 14.5).

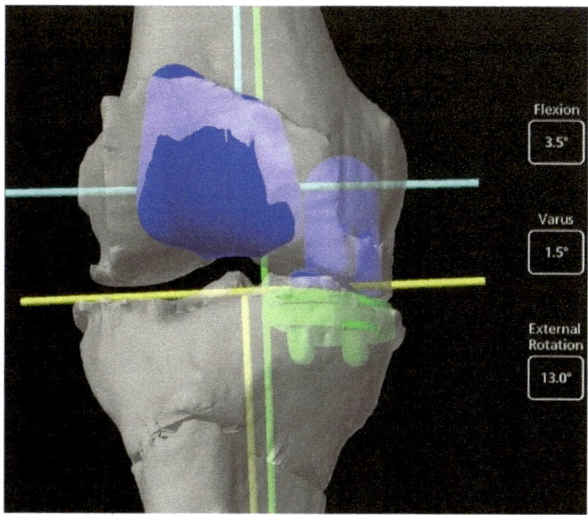

Fig. 14.5 Kinematic tracking to verify alignment, soft tissue balancing, and final poly insert thickness following cementing of implants in MAKO medial bicompartmental knee arthroplasty

Surgical Methods and Considerations for MAKO Lateral BIKA (Off-Label Use)

Many of the considerations and steps taken for the MAKO medial BiKA are carried over to the MAKO lateral BiKA, with some variation necessary to accommodate any valgus alignment of the knee. However, as the MAKO lateral BiKA is an off-label application, the MAKO TGS software is not configured for simultaneous bone registration of the lateral and patellofemoral compartments. Thus, bone registration, balancing, resection, and trial implant placement are completed in the lateral compartment before proceeding with the PFA. The registration points are the same as required for a lateral UKA, as described elsewhere. Similarly, care must be taken to remove any osteophytes prior to soft tissue balancing, and in the case of a valgus knee, any adhesions along the posterior lateral capture must be released. It should be noted that while the author is comfortable allowing some residual (physiologic) varus in MAKO medial BiKA, the author will do additional releases in a valgus knee to achieve neutral alignment (no residual valgus) when performing a MAKO lateral BiKA.

Soft tissue balancing is performed in a manner similar to that described for medial BiKA; however, for a valgus knee, the surgeon will then perform a series of varus stress tests at the minimum of four poses described previously over the full range of motion of the knee joint. In this instance, the varus stress test opens the arthritic lateral compartment joint space to restore tibiofemoral alignment by applying tension on the LCL [8].

Bone resection is performed using the following sequence: first the lateral femoral condyle, then the lateral tibial plateau, and lastly the femoral trochlea. Trial implants are placed and proper soft tissue balancing is confirmed, similar to the method described in the medial BiKA section. Further adjustments can be made as needed; once the desired alignment has been achieved, the final implants are cemented using two separate cement batches. The patellofemoral component is cemented first followed by the tibial component. Once the cement has hardened, the second batch is mixed to cement the femoral component and the patellar button. A final verification of soft tissue balance is performed following cementing of all implants to assess the final polyethylene thickness, and the patella is assessed once the tourniquet is released to allow proper assessment of tracking. Lateral release is performed as needed.

Surgical Methods and Considerations for MAKO Bi-UKA (Off-Label Use)

The MAKO Bi-UKA differs in some respects from the medial and lateral BiKA, as the procedure is essentially two UKAs performed in series, without subsequent PFA. The main goal is to achieve a neutral mechanical axis; therefore, in a slight varus-biased knee the medial compartment is planned slightly tighter, while in a slight valgus-biased knee the lateral compartment is planned slightly tighter to allow for this correction. Similar to the reasoning above, the author will allow a varus knee to remain in physiologic varus but will make every attempt to correct a valgus knee to neutral mechanical axis alignment. This procedure will require two soft tissue balancing steps in sequence and the soft tissue poses must be recaptured once the medial compartment is completed, as we usually start first with the medial compartment. One study detailing Bi-UKA also describes starting with the medial compartment for all involved Bi-UKA cases, as this was the site of greatest deformity [9].

Registration for MAKO Bi-UKA is also based on the same protocol as that for MAKO MCK (medial BiKA) as described earlier, and regardless of varus or valgus alignment, the registration is based on the medial compartment in order to collect as many registration points as possible. This is due to the fact that the software is not configured for simultaneous medial and lateral unicondylar Bi-UKA [5]. Thus, a careful and meticulous registration of these surfaces is imperative for accurate lateral measurements. While this initial step does not include any registration of the lateral compartment, the verification of the registration points of the lateral compartment is completed prior to proceeding with balancing and preparation of the lateral side. However, if registration was done correctly during the preparation of the medial compartment, this re-registration should be redundant [5]. As for BiKA, osteophytes must be removed prior to soft tissue balancing. The medial gutter must be re-established, and any adhesions or contractures along the posterior medial or lateral capsules should be released [5].

As previously discussed, the MAKO Bi-UKA is indicated for patients with either slight varus, valgus, or neutral alignment. The native knee alignment dictates the method to be employed for soft tissue balancing. In cases of varus or neutral knee alignment, a valgus stress is applied during the initial soft tissue capture, followed by a minimally necessary varus stress when capturing the poses for the subsequent lateral compartment reconstruction to assure that the medial trial components make contact throughout the range of motion. However, in cases of valgus knee alignment, a varus stress is applied during both soft tissue capturing events. To avoid a bias toward additional valgus when preparing the medial compartment, the planning of the components of the medial compartment is toward a slightly looser ligament balance. After recapturing the four poses, the lateral compartment is planned to achieve neutral alignment. However, if this cannot be attained the procedure should be converted to TKA.

Both bone resection and trial implant placement are performed in the medial compartment prior to completing the bone resection and trial implant placement of the lateral compartment [5, 9]. New soft tissue balancing poses are obtained once the medial compartment is completed in order to fine-tune the soft tissue balance of the lateral compartment. These should be adjusted until optimal joint alignment and flexion-extension gap balancing is achieved [5]. Once the trial implants have been placed and the joint has been optimally balanced, the trial implants are removed, the bone is irrigated and dried as previously described, and the final implants are placed and cemented in the following order: the lateral tibial plateau followed by the medial tibial plateau with a first batch of cement, followed by lateral femoral condyle and the medial femoral condyle with a second batch of cement [5]. The rationale for placement of the lateral component before the medial component is that there is less room to maneuver instruments in the lateral compartment, and placement of medial components first limits this even further. Once all implants are cemented, a final verification of soft tissue balancing is completed by trialing different thicknesses of trial tibial inserts before determining the final polyethylene thicknesses for the medial and lateral compartment (Fig. 14.6).

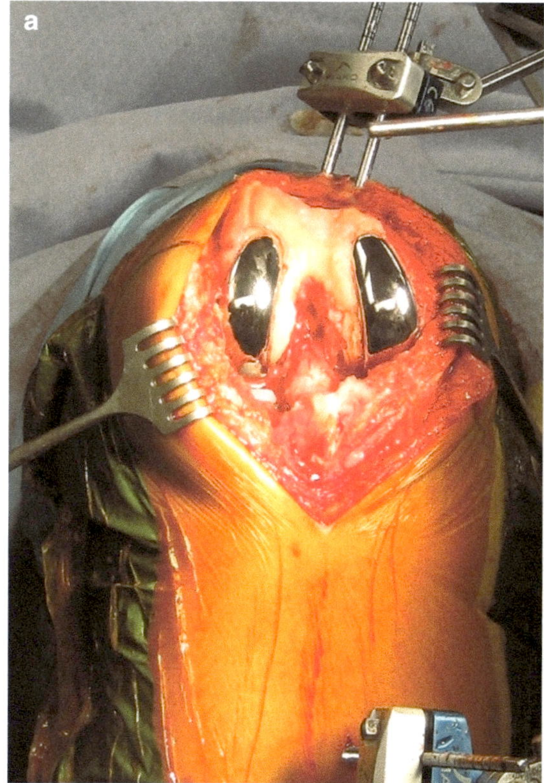

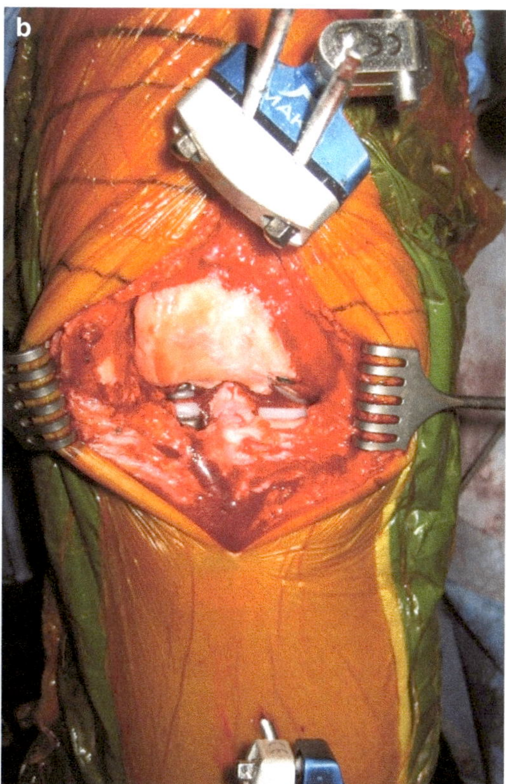

Fig. 14.6 The knee is moved through a range of joint positions, including (**a**) 90° and (**b**) full extension, to verify alignment, soft tissue balancing, and final poly insert thickness in the medial and lateral compartments following cementing of implants in MAKO bi-unicompartmental knee arthroplasty

Clinical Outcomes

To date, there are few studies assessing the outcomes of robot-assisted BiKA, and these have primarily reviewed medial UKA and PFA. Kamath et al. reported on a series of modular BiKAs performed with robotic assistance, with a mean follow-up of 31 months (range, 24–46 months). Outcome measures included Knee Society Knee and Function Scores, KOOS, SF-12, and WOMAC, as well as radiographic assessments and implant survivorship. Mean range of motion (ROM) improved from 122° to 133° ($p < 0.001$). There was a statistically significant improvement across all functional scores. One patient underwent conversion to total knee arthroplasty at 3 years for knee instability. There were no cases of patellar instability, implant loosening or wear, or progressive arthritis [11].

Tamam et al. also reported on outcomes of 30 BiKA's bicompartmental arthroplasty (PFA associated with medial [83%] or lateral [17%] UKA) using the MAKO system [12]. At a mean follow-up of 27 months (range 12 to 54), robotic-assisted BiKA alleviated pain and improved Oxford Knee Scores by 18 ± 6 (range 10–28) points ($p < 0.0001$). There was one patient with a poor functional outcome. Twenty four out of 29 patients (83%) had good to excellent outcome, with no mechanical failures.

Conclusion

MAKO bicompartmental knee arthroplasty is beneficial regarding the preservation of bone tissue unaffected by OA and other tissues, such as ligaments, surrounding the knee joint. With a focus on CT imaging and software-based accurate planning/templating, and the feature of tactile-guided bone preparation, MAKOplasty BiKA represents a viable alternative to other traditional partial or total knee arthroplasty treatments.

References

1. Naal FD, Impellizzeri FM, Leunig M. Which is the best activity rating scale for patients undergoing total joint arthroplasty? Clin Orthop Relat Res. 2009. https://doi.org/10.1007/s11999-008-0358-5.
2. Plate J, Mofidi A, Mannava S, Lorentzen C, Smith B, Seyler T, et al. Unicompartmental knee arthroplasty: past, present, and future. Reconstr Rev. 2012:52–62.
3. Pandit H, Jenkins C, Gill HS, Smith G, Price AJ, CAF D, et al. Unnecessary contraindications for mobile-bearing unicompartmental knee replacement. J Bone Joint Surg B. 2011;93-B:622–8. https://doi.org/10.1302/0301-620X.93B5.26214.
4. Sabatini L, Giachino M, Risitano S, Atzori F. Bicompartmental knee arthroplasty. Ann Transl Med. 2016;4:5. https://doi.org/10.3978/j.issn.2305-5839.2015.12.24.
5. Dettmer M, Kreuzer SW. Bi-unicompartmental, robot-assisted knee arthroplasty. Oper Tech Orthop. 2015;25:155–62. https://doi.org/10.1053/j.oto.2015.03.004.
6. Jacofsky DJ, Allen M. Robotics in arthroplasty: a comprehensive review. J Arthroplast. 2016. https://doi.org/10.1016/j.arth.2016.05.026.
7. Pearle AD, O'Loughlin PF, Kendoff DO. Robot-assisted unicompartmental knee arthroplasty. J Arthroplast. 2010;25:230–7. https://doi.org/10.1016/j.arth.2008.09.024.
8. Conditt MA, Roche MW. Minimally invasive robotic-arm-guided unicompartmental knee arthroplasty. J Bone Joint Surg Am. 2009;91(Suppl 1):63–8. https://doi.org/10.2106/JBJS.H.01372.
9. Confalonieri N, Manzotti A, Montironi F, Pullen C. Tissue sparing surgery in knee reconstruction: unicompartmental (UKA), patellofemoral (PFA), UKA + PFA, bi-unicompartmental (Bi-UKA) arthroplasties. J Orthop Traumatol. 2008;9:171–7. https://doi.org/10.1007/s10195-008-0015-5.
10. Lonner JH. Robotically assisted unicompartmental knee sculpting tool. Oper Tech Orthop. 2015;25:104–13. https://doi.org/10.1053/j.oto.2015.03.001.
11. Kamath AF, Levack A, John T, Thomas BS, Lonner JH. Minimum two-year outcomes of modular bicompartmental knee arthroplasty. J Arthroplast. 2014;29:75–9.
12. Tamam C, Plate JF, Augart M, Poehling GG, Jinnah RH. Retrospective clinical and radiological outcomes after robotic assisted bicompartmental knee arthroplasty. Adv Orthop. 2015;2015:747309.

Total Knee Arthroplasty Technique: NAVIO

15

Ameer M. Elbuluk and Jonathan M. Vigdorchik

Although conventional total knee arthroplasty (TKA) remains a successful intervention for end-stage arthritis, some patients still experience reduced functionality and require revision procedures related to component malposition or soft tissue imbalance [1]. Robotic-assisted TKA has gained increasing popularity as orthopedic surgeons aim to increase accuracy and precision of implant positioning and quantified ligament balance [2]. Postoperative alignment of TKA components may influence clinical outcomes, range of motion, and implant longevity [3]. The use of robotics in orthopedic surgery has helped to minimize human error, which may in turn reduce implant wear and theoretically lead to longer prosthesis survivorship [4, 5]. The following chapter is meant to provide a frame-work of the surgical techniques for using the NAVIO robotic system to perform total knee arthroplasty (TKA).

Traditional surgical instrumentation has been challenged by robotic systems as a method to decrease mechanical alignment outliers, optimize soft tissue balancing, and restore normal knee kinematics [6–9]. Robotic-assisted surgery has been available for nearly 15 years, with current systems using various navigation platforms that typically provide a haptic window that allows the surgeon to conduct a total knee arthroplasty (TKA) based on preoperative planning [10]. NAVIO (Smith & Nephew, Inc., Memphis, TN, United States) is a semiautonomous handheld robotic tool that is held and moved by the surgeon, restricting the bone cutting to within the confines of the planned resection area by providing robotic control of the speed or exposure of the tool. It is intended to assist the surgeon in providing spatial boundaries for orientation and reference information to anatomical landmarks during TKA. In the following chapter, we will provide an overview of our preferred surgical techniques for using the NAVIO surgical robotic system for TKA. We will summarize the NAVIO technique for TKA as follows: (1) patient and system setup, (2) surgical preferences, (3) bone tracking hardware, (4) registration, (5) implant planning, (6) bone cutting and soft tissue balance, and (7) trialing and implantation.

A. M. Elbuluk (✉) · J. M. Vigdorchik
Department of Orthopaedic Surgery, NYU Langone
Medical Center, Hospital for Joint Diseases,
New York, NY, USA
e-mail: ameer.elbuluk@nyumc.org

© Springer Nature Switzerland AG 2019
J. H. Lonner (ed.), *Robotics in Knee and Hip Arthroplasty*,
https://doi.org/10.1007/978-3-030-16593-2_15

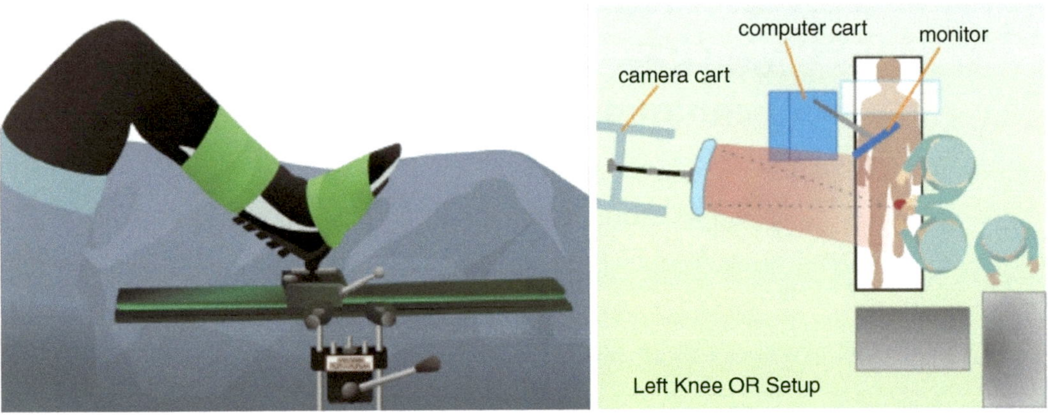

Fig. 15.1 Patient and system setup. (Courtesy of Smith & Nephew, Inc., Memphis, TN, USA)

Patient and System Setup

Proper assembly of the NAVIO system is a critical first step to ensuring unimpeded workflow during surgery. The NAVIO computer should be placed to allow the surgeon to easily operate the graphical user interface during the planning stage and to provide visual feedback and guidance during surgery. After the system is well-positioned and the patient has been properly prepped and draped, sterile drapes should be applied to the monitor to allow the surgeon to manipulate the touchscreen intraoperatively. The NAVIO handpiece should also be assembled according to the surgeon's preference, but the configuration we find most conducive to bone removal is typically 5 mm spherical burr and speed control guard. During patient setup, care should be taken to avoid wrapping the ankle with bulky drapes since this can make it difficult to locate malleolar reference points needed during patient registration. Next, with the help of a leg positioner, elevate the femur to approximately 45°, and flex the knee to 90° (Figs. 15.1 and 15.2). After incision, carefully inspect the joint to remove any prominent spurs or osteophytes. Remove all peripheral osteophytes that can interfere with exposure as this can affect the surgeon's ability to reliably assess joint stability during virtual mapping and gap balancing. Following resection and excision of osteophytes, ensure that the knee is able to achieve approximately 120° of flexion.

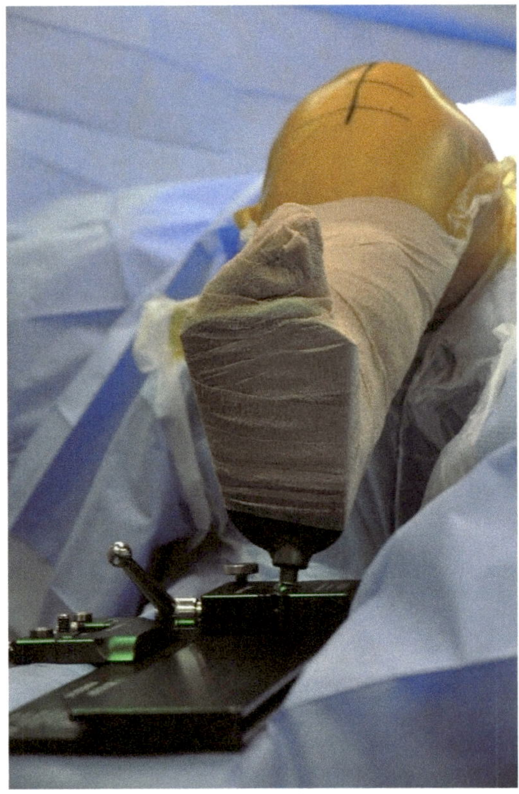

Fig. 15.2 With the help of a leg positioner, the femur is elevated to approximately 45° and the knee is flexed to 90°

Surgical Preferences

The NAVIO system allows the surgeon to decide on a femur-first or tibia-first workflow (Fig. 15.3). In order to define rotational preferences, the

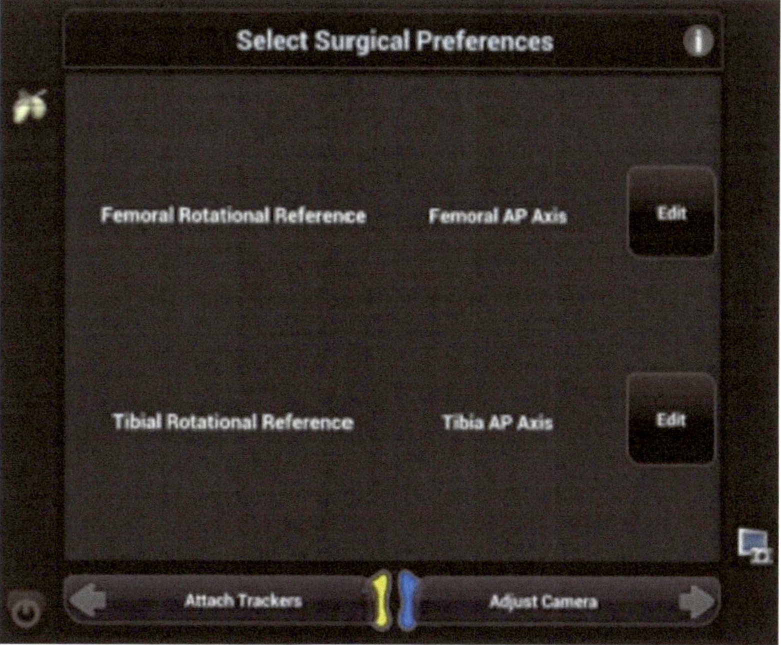

Fig. 15.3 Surgical preferences are set with the NAVIO system. (Courtesy of Smith & Nephew, Inc., Memphis, TN, USA)

application allows the surgeon to choose landmark preferences on the femur and tibia, which calculates the implant component placement and ligament balancing. For the femur, the rotational references can be defined as follows: transepicondylar, femoral anteroposterior (AP), or posterior condylar axis. For the tibia, the reference options for computing its rotation are the tibial AP axis, mediolateral axis, axis rotationally aligned to the femoral mechanical axis, or axis aligned with the medial third of the tibia tubercle. After deciding preferences for rotational references, the collection stage of registration points and surface mapping based on patient anatomy precedes.

Bone Tracking Hardware

A successful NAVIO-assisted surgery is highly dependent on rigid independent fixation of the femoral and tibial tracking frames to the bones. NAVIO utilizes a two-pin bi-cortical fixation system. To place the tibia tracker, percutaneously place the first bone screw approximately one handbreadth inferior to the tibial tubercle on the medial side of the tibial crest. Slowly drill the bone screw into the tibia, perpendicular to the

bony surface, stopping once the opposing cortex has been engaged. Then, use the tissue protector to mark the position of the second bone screw inferior to the initial placement and engage the second screw with the bone. Slide the bone clamps over the two bone screws until the bottom of the clamp is within 1 cm of the patient's skin. Clamp the tibia array, orienting the reflective markers toward the camera, and then slide the array away from the incision site. Next, percutaneously place the first bone screw one handbreadth superior to the patella in the center of the femoral shaft. This can be done after the arthrotomy to ensure the quadriceps tendon is not tethered. If placing the array prior to arthrotomy, ensure the pins are placed laterally to the quadriceps tendon and with the knee in deep flexion to minimize tethering of the quadriceps. Clamp the femoral tracker frame onto the bone clamp. Confirm that the position of the optical tracking arrays is fully in line of sight with the camera through a full range of motion to optimize the flow of the registration and cutting processes (Fig. 15.4). With the leg in deep flexion, then in full extension, advance the camera orientation adjustment screen to confirm the visibility of the femur and tibia tracker frames (Fig. 15.5). Checkpoint pins should also be placed in the

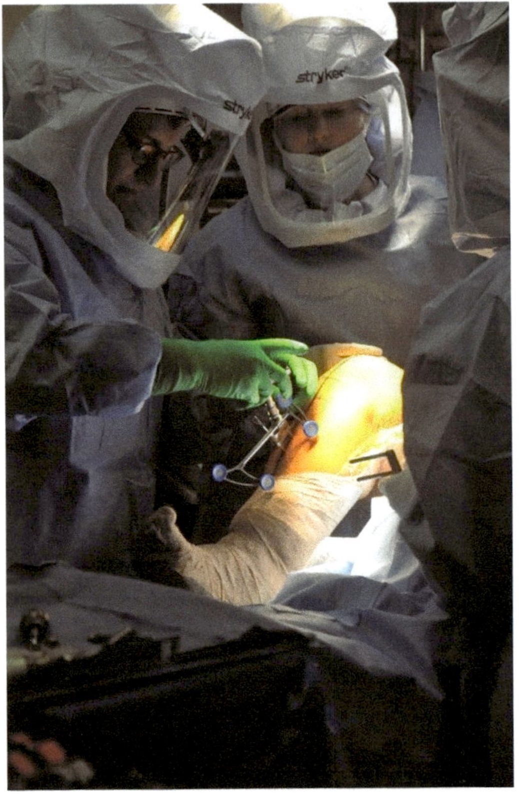

Fig. 15.4 The position of the optical tracking arrays are confirmed to be fully in line of sight with the camera through a full range of motion

femur/tibia so that these points can be used throughout the procedure to determine if bone tracking frames have moved. Be sure to place the checkpoint pins away from the bone surfaces that are to be prepared in order to avoid cutting or shifting them. On the tibial side, this pin must be placed far enough below the resection level; on the femoral side, this pin is placed on the medial condyle, posteriorly toward the epicondyle to avoid being disturbed by the femoral chamfer cuts (Fig. 15.6).

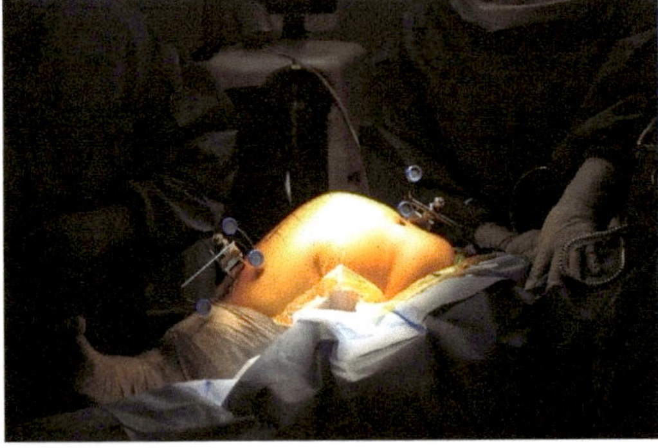

Fig. 15.6 On the tibial side, the pin must be placed far enough below the resection level; on the femoral side, this pin is placed on the medial condyle, posteriorly toward the epicondyle

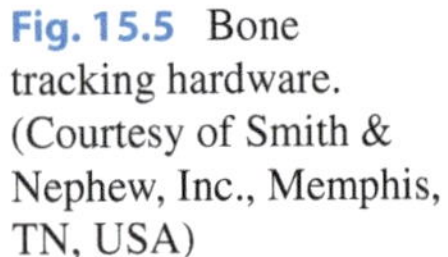

Fig. 15.5 Bone tracking hardware. (Courtesy of Smith & Nephew, Inc., Memphis, TN, USA)

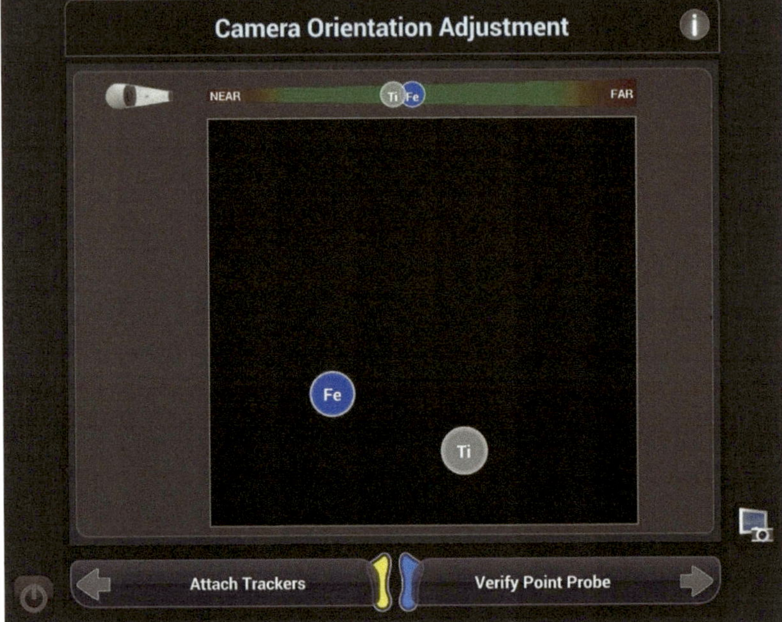

Registration

NAVIO utilizes a CT-free registration process that relies on standard image-free principles to construct a virtual representation of the patient's anatomy and kinematics. The first step in registration is to use the point probe to identify the most prominent points on the medial and lateral malleoli in order to register the ankle center. The next step, hip center calculation, follows the femoral tracker array through circular movements of the hip. A key point at this stage is to avoid pelvic movement, which can serve as a source of error. The femur should start in approximately 20° of flexion (avoid hip flexion greater than 45°), and then slowly rotate the hip until all sectors of the graphic on the screen have turned green (Fig. 15.7). Then place the leg in full extension, press and hold the right foot pedal, which will calculate the patient's varus/valgus alignment. The *Preoperative Knee Motion Collection* screen then allows the user to record

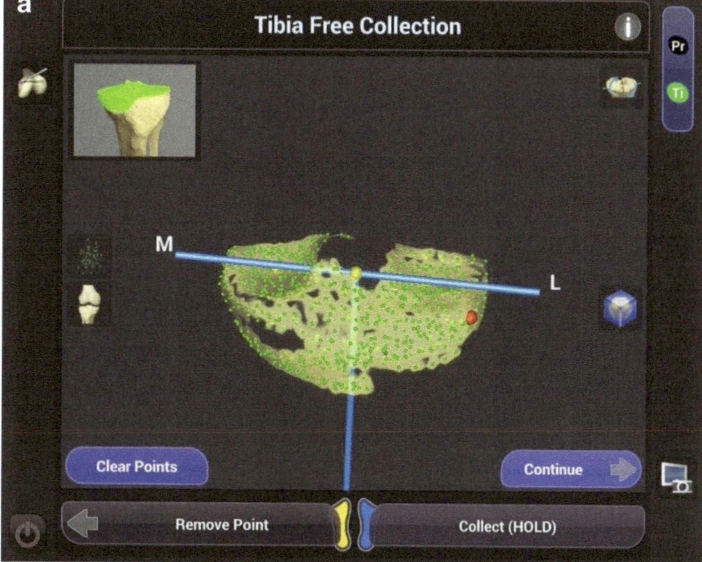

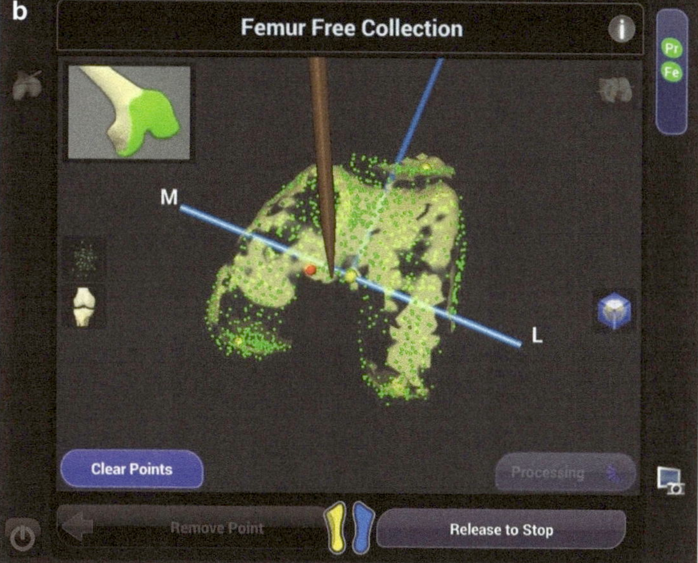

Fig. 15.7 (**a** and **b**) Registration through the NAVIO system. (Courtesy of Smith & Nephew, Inc., Memphis, TN, USA)

normal flexion motion. Move the leg through a normal (unstressed) range of motion to maximum flexion, making sure to collect all possible sectors between 20° and 50° at minimum. Then, apply constant varus and valgus stress to the collateral ligaments and collect data throughout flexion. The system turns orange for the medial compartment and purple for the lateral compartment. This data will be used to identify how much laxity will be built into the respective medial and lateral gaps for proper joint balancing.

In order to register the femoral condylar surfaces, there are four landmark points that must be collected. Using the point probe, collect the knee center, most posterior medial point, most posterior lateral point, and the anterior notch point (Fig. 15.8). Based on surgeon preference, there are three options for defining the femoral reference for rotational alignment: transepicondylar axis, femoral AP axis, or posterior condylar axis. At this stage, femoral condylar surface mapping is performed by "painting" the probe over the entire femoral surface while holding down the foot pedal (Fig. 15.7). After mapping the femoral surfaces, if the surgeon does not feel that the rotational axis is properly established, then femoral axis redefinition can be performed to redefine the rotational axis of the femur.

Following successful femoral registration, there are three tibial landmarks to collect: knee center, medial plateau, and lateral plateau points (Fig. 15.9). Then, as defined during previous surgical preference selection, there are four options to define the tibial rotational axis: tibia AP axis, mediolateral axis, transfer femoral mechanical axis, and medial third of the tibial tubercle collection. The last registration step, tibial condyle surface mapping, offers visualization of the previously collected tibial mechanical and rotational axes. The user should also digitize the tibial condylar surfaces by "painting" the point probe over the surface while holding down the foot pedal until the virtual model is formed. To ensure accuracy, it is encouraged to "paint" over the edges to help with sizing of the model. Similar to above, the rotational axis can be redefined at this stage if the surgeon feels that the axis is not properly defined.

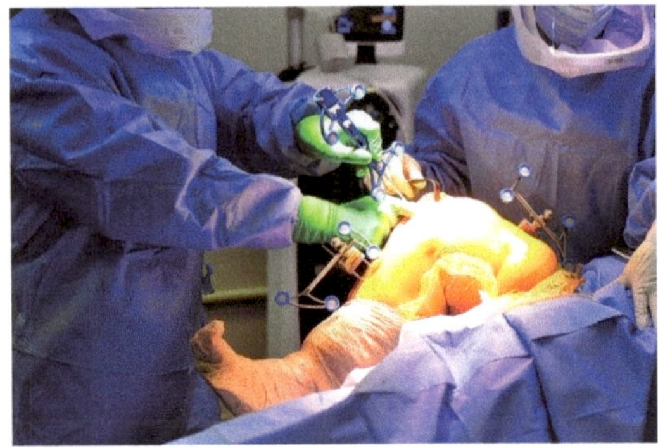

Fig. 15.8 Four landmark points are collected to register the femoral condylar surfaces. (Courtesy of Smith & Nephew, Inc., Memphis, TN, USA)

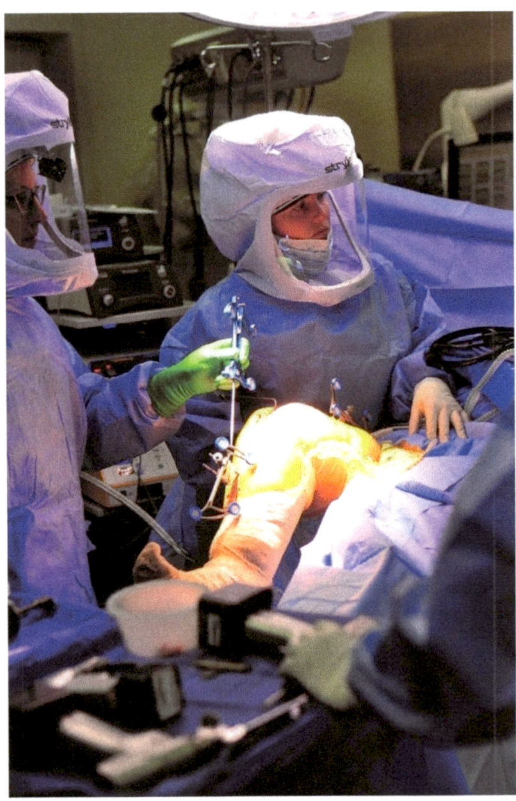

Fig. 15.9 Three tibial landmarks are collected: knee center, medial plateau, and lateral plateau points

Implant Planning

The implant planning stage provides a virtual reconstruction of the patient's femoral and tibial anatomy, soft tissue ligament tension, and joint balance. There are three stages: (1) initial sizing and placement, (2) gap planning/balancing, and (3) cut guide placement (if that is the preferred method of bone preparation). Landmark points collected during registration are used to adjust the size and placement of the components. For the femoral component, using the cross-section mode, first confirm that the component size provides adequate coverage on the digitized femur bone surface. To avoid notching, be sure to assess the transition of the implant's anterior/proximal tip with the bone surface (Fig. 15.10). Then, verify the transition of the implant component in the sagittal view screen and adjust the component in the AP position and flexion to achieve the desired anterior transition. Assess the posterior coverage of the component in both the sagittal and transverse views. The implant components for NAVIO are anteriorly referenced.

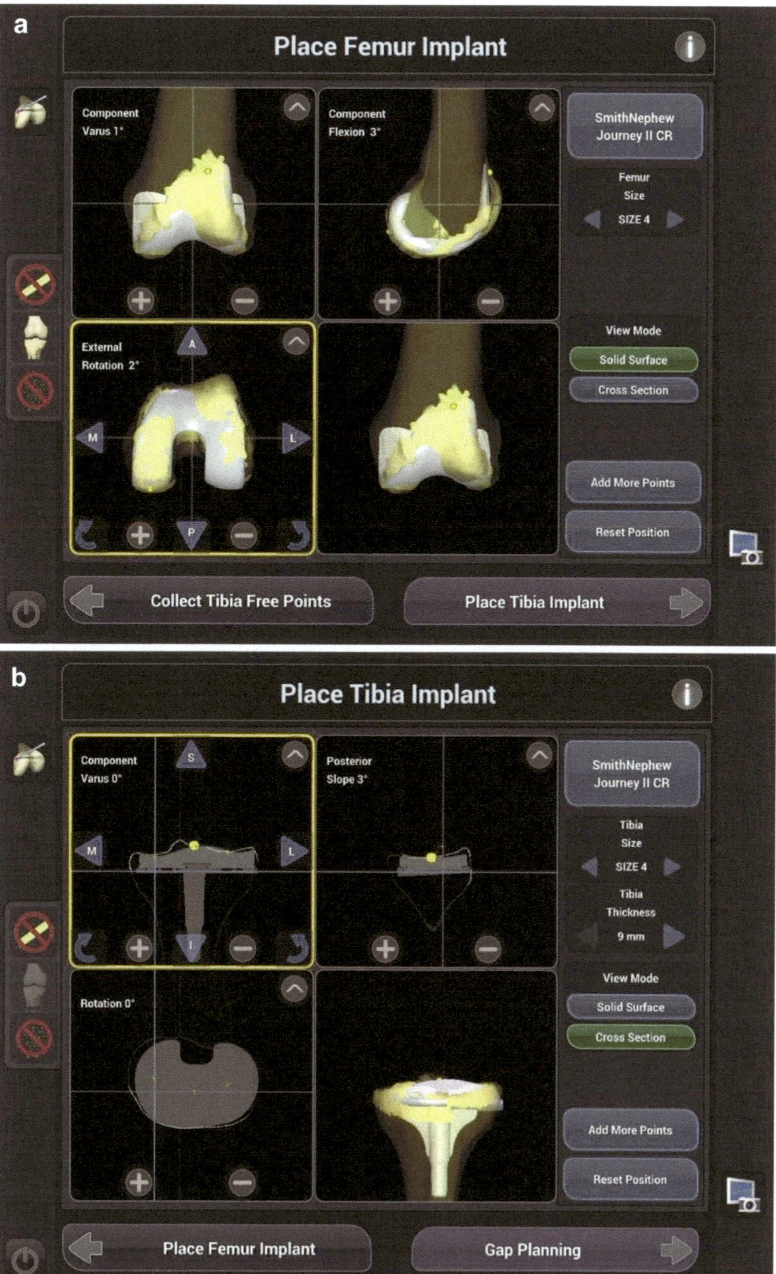

Fig. 15.10 (**a** and **b**) Implant planning with NAVIO

Therefore in order to have greater resection on the posterior bone and to increase the posterior gap, the component may be downsized, without any change to the anterior transition of the component on to the bone. In order to assess size coverage, implant anterior transition, and the bone resection plan, toggle on the virtual cut to visualize the implant component on the bone surface. The user should also confirm that the component is not overhanging medially or laterally.

For the tibial component, the NAVIO software provides a starting size and initial placement based on the tibia free point collection. Begin by confirming and adjusting the implant size using the transverse view. Next, confirm the posterior slope, which reflects the slope of the tibial component with respect to the mechanical axis defined during registration. The rotation of the tibial component is initialized to 0° with respect to the tibial AP axis. Placement of the tibial component is not constrained by NAVIO cut guides since the final implant rotation and placement is performed manually. Initially, the tibial component will default to the thinnest bearing, but thicker inserts can be selected by changing the polyethylene component. The user can also choose to move the component proximally, which will decrease the resection depth based on the two plateau points collected on the tibia during the *Tibia Landmark Point Collection* stage.

The second stage of implant planning allows the user the ability to dial in the virtual soft tissue laxity for the patient through a full range of flexion based on the prior ligament balancing section. There are four interactive views for translating and rotating the components with respect to the patient's virtualized joint. The goal of this stage is to have balanced extension and flexion gaps with no virtual overlap in either the medial or lateral compartments. The surgeon can choose to perform various cruciate or collateral/capsular soft tissue releases and then re-collect laxity information by clicking on the Re-collect Joint Laxity button in order to depict what the joint space will actually look like once the initial balancing is performed. The surgeon can also manipulate the virtual coronal, sagittal, translational, or rotational positions of the implants to adjust gap balance, such that the resulting gap is approximately 2–3 mm above the zero line through a range of motion (Fig. 15.11). Balancing of the flexion gap in the medial and lateral compartments can be performed by rotating the femur component internally or externally. Adjustments to femoral component rotation should be carefully considered relative to prior parameters such as anterior notching and patellofemoral tracking. Adjustments to femoral flexion should also be considered against prior considerations regarding anterior fit and alignment to the intramedullary (IM) axis.

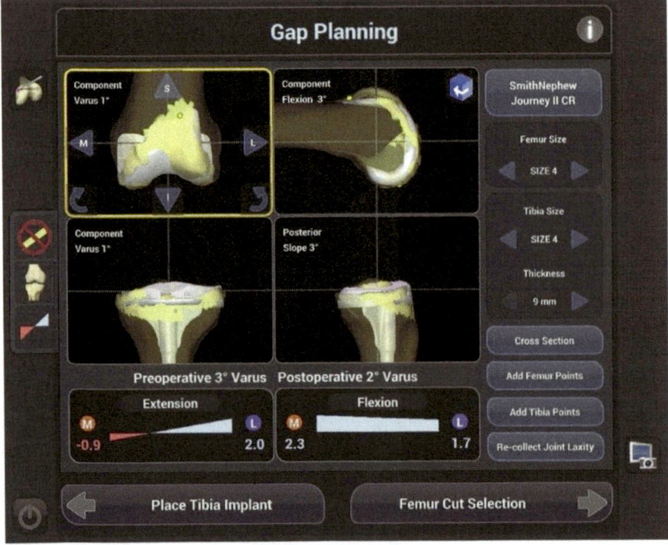

Fig. 15.11 Gap planning with NAVIO. (Courtesy of Smith & Nephew, Inc., Memphis, TN, USA)

The joint laxity assessment consists of collecting information on ligament stress or laxity throughout the full range of knee motion. First, while keeping the operative leg in full extension and maintaining knee flexion between −10° and +10°, apply constant and maximal stress to the contralateral ligaments to collect varus and valgus data. A graph is then generated that depicts the tightness or laxity in the medial or lateral knee compartments based on the stress collections. This graphic illustration allows the user to determine the degree of ligament release that is required to restore equal gaps in the medial and lateral compartments in full extension. Next, flex the operative knee to 90° and apply constant and maximal stress to the contralateral ligaments to collect varus/valgus data within 80°–100° of knee flexion. The surgeon may want to use a Z-retractor or laminar spreader to open up the medial and lateral compartment spaces to capture the maximum joint laxity to varus and valgus stresses in flexion.

Bone Cutting

While the entirety of the bone preparation can be performed with a 5 mm burr, for efficiency purposes, most NAVIO users utilize a hybrid approach, with the use of burrs and saws, for complete bone preparation in TKA. In accordance with the implant placement plan, the robotic handpiece is used to create locking lug slots in the patient's bones that securely position the cutting guides in place (Figs. 15.12 and 15.13). The femoral distal cut guide is then mounted onto the anterior femur via the prepared anterior lug holes and locked into position using a stabilizer block and additional pins. A manually controlled saw is used to resect the distal femur through the robotically positioned cut guide. Based on the virtual preoperative implant sizing plan, the drill guide adapter is attached to the distal cut guide and drill holes made at the predetermined size. The appropriately sized 5-in-1 cutting guide is then impacted and pinned into position. A plate probe can be used to ensure that the cut guide is placed in its intended position prior to resection, and it can also be used after saw cuts are made to confirm precision of the resections. The remaining femoral resections are made through the cutting block (Fig. 15.14).

For tibial resection, precise positioning and mounting of the tibial cutting guide is facilitated by using the robotic tool to make four recipient lug slots on the tibia, as directed based on the virtually modeled plan. The tibia cut guide is

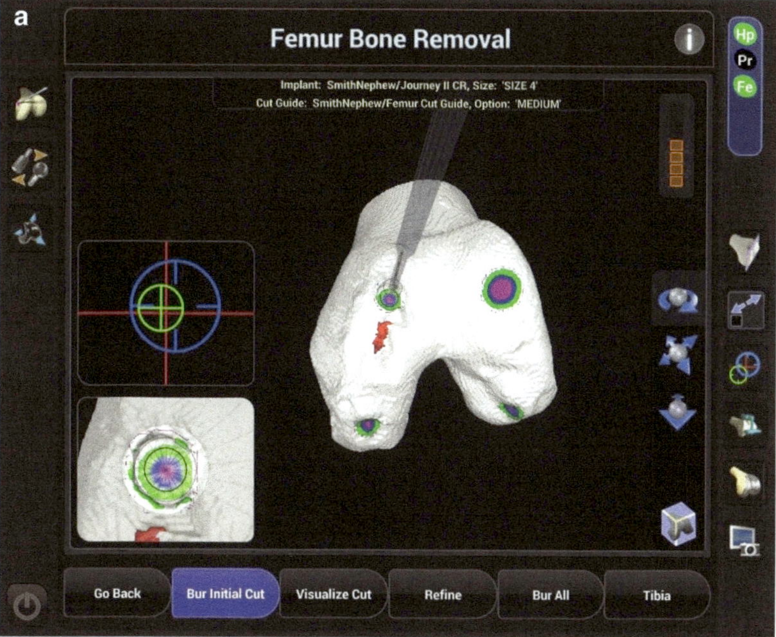

Fig. 15.12 (**a** and **b**) Bone cutting with NAVIO. (Courtesy of Smith & Nephew, Inc., Memphis, TN, USA)

Fig. 15.12 (continued)

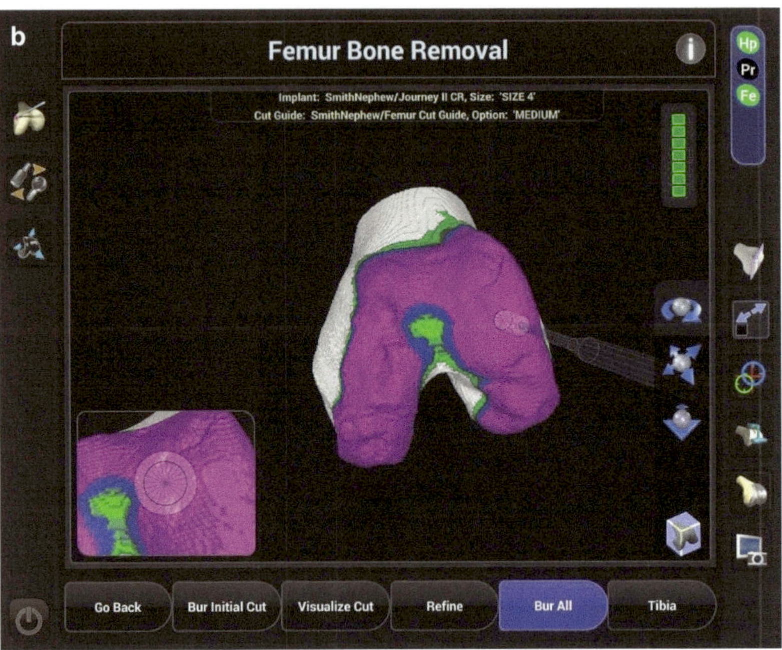

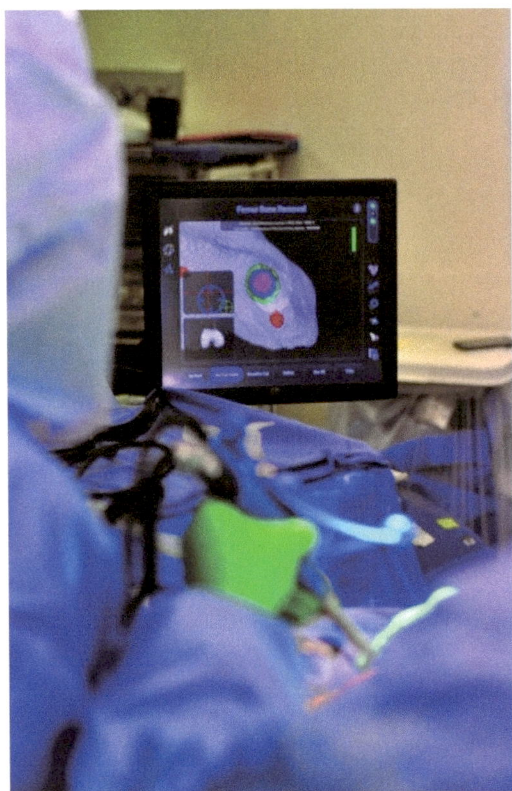

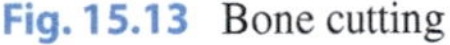

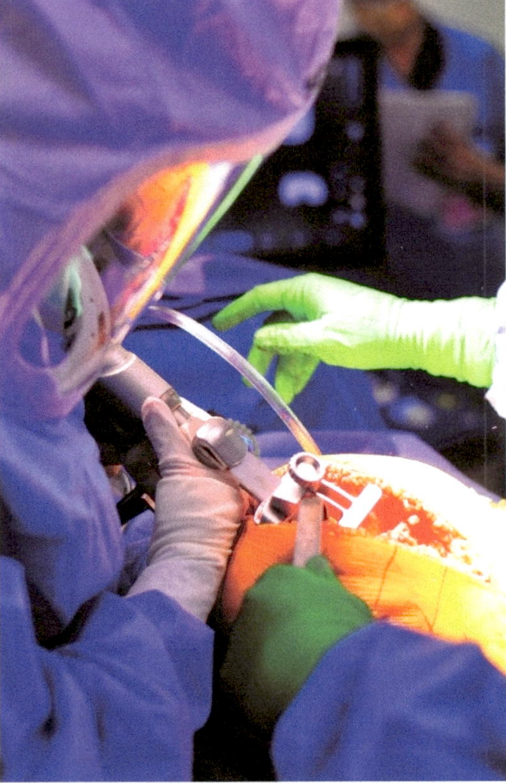

Fig. 15.13 Bone cutting

Fig. 15.14 The remaining femoral resections are made through the cutting block

inserted into the prepared bone lug holes and further secured with additional pins. The tibia is then resected with a saw, with care taken to use soft tissue protectors to prevent the saw (or burr) from causing inadvertent damage to the collateral ligaments and other soft tissues.

Trialing

Leaving the femoral and tibial tracking arrays in place, after completing all bone cuts and adjustments to the final surfaces, the trial components are provisionally implanted, and their positions, limb alignment, range of knee motion, and varus/valgus balance are assessed throughout a full flexion arc both by clinical assessment and virtual quantification (Fig. 15.15). The *Postop Stressed Gap Assessment* screen allows the user to quantifiably assess the post-op laxities throughout flexion in both the medial and lateral compartments. At this point, adjustments in bone resections or soft tissue releases can be made to further optimize position, motion, and soft tissue gap balancing. After the dynamic ROM testing is finalized, final surface preparation is completed for manual implantation of the final components (Fig. 15.16).

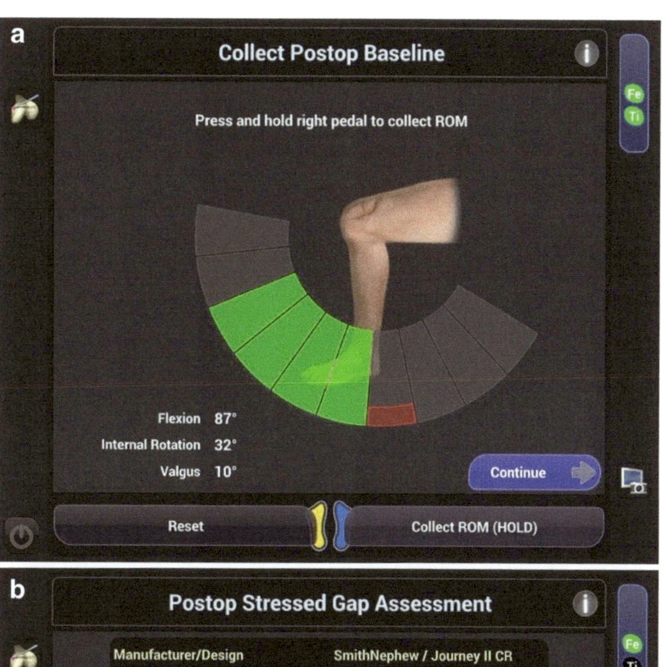

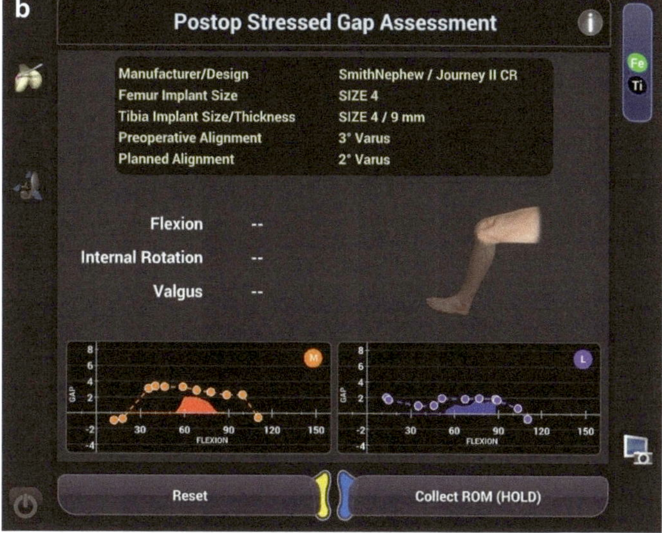

Fig. 15.15 (**a** and **b**) Trial reduction with NAVIO. (Courtesy of Smith & Nephew, Inc., Memphis, TN, USA)

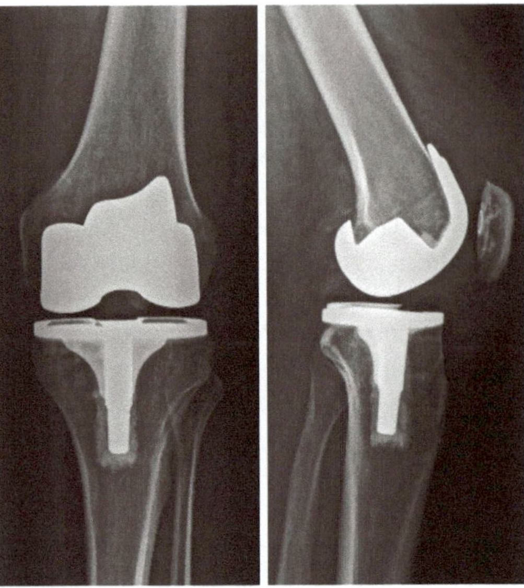

Fig. 15.16 Implantation of the final components

Data/Outcomes

While there are presently no published data on the radiographic or functional outcomes of TKA performed with assistance of the NAVIO robotic system, the preliminary data of our initial 54 unilateral primary TKA cases show promising results. Mean age was 68 ± 7 years, and gender breakdown was 75% female and 25% male. With regard to preoperative comorbidity risk, the majority of patients were ASA 2 (58%) and ASA 3 (42%). The average hospital length of stay was 3 ± 1.4 days. Intraoperatively, average estimated blood loss (EBL) was 292 ± 85 mL, and surgical time was 130 ± 43 min. Postoperative alignment was within ±3° for all cases. There were no intra- or postoperative complications and no reoperation or revision surgeries.

Conclusions

Robotic-assisted surgery for TKA continues to gain popularity as orthopedists seek to enhance their abilities to place implants more precisely and consistently. However, the benefits of robotic assistance must be weighed against factors such as increased surgical time, cost, and learning curve challenges. Furthermore, due to the paucity of data on many of these newer systems, clinical studies have yet to determine their long-term benefits. Robotic-assisted navigation does provide distinct 3D data during preoperative planning that allow the surgeon to increase implant placement accuracy. The use of robotic technology is a valuable technological development that can help to improve surgical technique and potentially clinical results in total knee arthroplasty.

References

1. Kim YH, Kim JS, Kim DY. Clinical outcome and rate of complications after primary total knee replacement performed with quadriceps-sparing or standard arthrotomy. J Bone Joint Surg Br. 2007;89:467–70.
2. Park SE, Lee CT. Comparison of robotic-assisted and conventional manual implantation of a primary total knee arthroplasty. J Arthroplast. 2007;22:1054–9.
3. Matsuda S, Kawahara S, Okazaki K, Tashiro Y, Iwamoto Y. Postoperative alignment and ROM affect patient satisfaction after TKA. Clin Orthop Relat Res. 2013;471(1):127–33.
4. Bellemans J, Vandenneucker H, Vanlauwe J. Robot-assisted total knee arthroplasty. Clin Orthop Relat Res. 2007;464:111–6.
5. Song EK, Seon JK, Yim JH, Netravali NA, Bargar WL. Robotic-assisted TKA reduces postoperative alignment outliers and improves gap balance compared to conventional TKA. Clin Orthop Relat Res. 2013;471:118–26.
6. Borner M, Wiesel U, Ditzen W. Clinical experiences with Robodoc and the Duracon Total knee. In: Stiehl JB, Konermann WH, Haaker RG, editors. Navigation and robotics in total joint and spine surgery. Berlin: Springer; 2004. p. 362–6.
7. Mai S, Lorke C, Siebert W. Clinical results with the robot-assisted Caspar system and the search-evolution prosthesis. In: Stiehl JB, Konermann WH, Haaker RG, editors. Navigation and robotics in total joint and spine surgery. Berlin: Springer; 2004. p. 355–61.
8. Decking J, Theis C, Achenbach T, et al. Robotic total knee arthroplasty: the accuracy of CT-based component placement. Acta Orthop Scand. 2004;75:573–9.
9. Kharwadkar N, Kent RE, Sharara KH, Naique S. 5 degrees to 6 degrees of distal femoral cut for uncomplicated primary total knee arthroplasty: is it safe? Knee. 2006;13:57–60.
10. Paul HA, Bargar WL, Mittlestadt B, et al. Development of a surgical robot for cementless total hip arthroplasty. Clin Orthop Relat Res. 1992;(285):57–66.

Total Knee Arthroplasty Technique: MAKO

16

Kenneth Gustke

The MAKO robotic arm-assisted total knee replacement is performed as a semi-active system in which haptic guidance of a saw is used to precisely and safely position and align components [1]. Component position and alignment is pre-planned after creating a 3-D virtual model from CT imaging and can be modified as needed throughout the procedure. Use of robotics has the potential to obtain the exact alignment and component position target desired by the surgeon, as well as assist with soft tissue balance [2–6].

The knee can be planned to a neutral mechanical alignment. Intraoperatively, the computer will demonstrate compartment gap measurements to assist with soft tissue balancing. Alternatively, preoperative planned limb and component alignment can be modified and accurately adjusted several degrees off the neutral axis to balance the knee and avoid or minimize soft tissue releases. This allows a constitutional alignment, within the alignment parameters accepted by the surgeon.

It is hoped that accurate component positioning, alignment, and soft tissue balance reproducibility will eliminate alignment outliers and less balanced total knees that could contribute to the 15–20% of patients who tend to be unsatisfied with surgical outcomes after total knee arthroplasty (TKA) [7, 8]. Revision for instability is a common reason for early revision, second only to infection [9]. A more stable total knee replacement may lessen manipulations for stiffness and lessen the pain and effusions associated with subtle instability. A total knee aligned within acceptable parameters that the polyethylene, locking mechanism, and supporting bone can tolerate will lessen early and late revision for loosening. Our expectation is that improved surgical technique with robotic assistance should lessen instability and malalignment.

Component position, alignment, and soft tissue balance data can be collected during and at the end of the robotic arm-assisted procedure from which one can potentially correlate to eventual total knee replacement outcomes.

Features of the MAKO Robotic Arm

Tracker arrays are placed on the tibia and distal femur, so that the registered bones can be tracked by an infrared camera (Fig. 16.1). The MAKO rigid arm autonomously places the end effector saw blade at a precise location and within the correct resection plane. The end effect is semiautonomous. Movement of the end effector tool

K. Gustke (✉)
Florida Orthopaedic Institute, Tampa, FL, USA

Department of Orthopaedic Surgery, University of South Florida College of Medicine, Tampa, FL, USA
e-mail: kgustke@floridaortho.com

© Springer Nature Switzerland AG 2019
J. H. Lonner (ed.), *Robotics in Knee and Hip Arthroplasty*,
https://doi.org/10.1007/978-3-030-16593-2_16

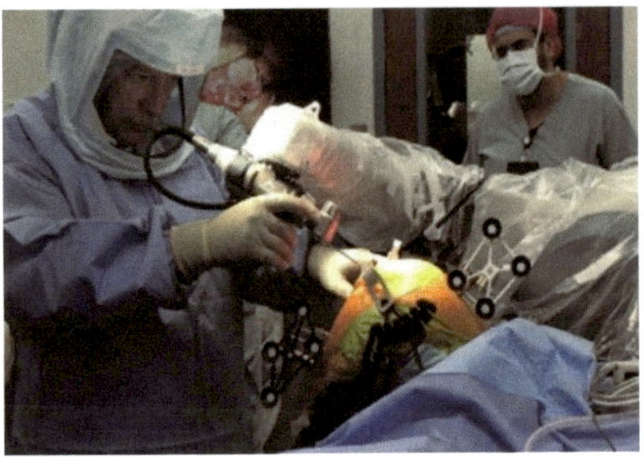

Fig. 16.1 The saw end effector on the MAKO robotic arm is controlled by the surgeon. The straight saw is utilized for the tibial bone resection

requires physician input for initiating oscillation of the saw and guidance of the tool location within the haptic boundaries (Fig. 16.1). The rigidity of the arm and fast computer refresh rate maintain the saw blade precisely in the correct plane even with vibration and minor movements of the limb. The haptic boundaries are determined from preoperative planning of implant locations and translated to the patient via bone registration. The haptic boundaries are designed along with typical soft tissue retraction to avoid potential soft tissue damage from the saw blade.

MAKO Robotic TKA Preoperative Planning

A CT scan of the involved limb from the hip to ankle is obtained preoperatively. The MAKO protocol allows for reduced cuts to reduce radiation risk. The default preoperative plan for alignment and bone resection follows classic bone cuts as would be created while using standard instrumentation. In a typical knee with a varus wear pattern, this would have a 0 degree tibia and femur coronal alignment, femoral rotation following the femoral transepicondylar line, 8-mm bone resection from the distal medial femoral condyle, 7-mm bone resection from the lateral tibial plateau, and 8-mm bone resection from posterior medial femoral condyle (Fig. 16.2).

The surgeon has the option to modify the preoperative plan in order to have an oblique joint line, such as 1 degree tibial coronal varus, 1 degree femoral coronal valgus, and femoral rotation closer to following the posterior condylar line. Preoperative plan will also optimize component size and position to avoid femoral notching, tibial or femoral bony overhang, and incomplete resection of bone surfaces.

Room, Operating Room Table, and Patient Setup

The robot is placed on the operative knee side at the level of the hip. The computer monitor and camera are placed on the contralateral side at the level of the hip. The distal 1/3 of the operating table is dropped down. The non-operative limb is secured on a traditional lithotomy position leg stirrup.

A Stryker leg holder is attached to the distal end side of the operating table on the operative side (Fig. 16.3). The bar should be at least 3 inches lower than the top of the operating table pad. The patient should be distal enough on the table to allow full knee flexion when the foot is attached to the leg holder but not too distal to lessen knee extension while the foot is attached to the leg holder. In very tall patients, full knee extension may not be possible with the foot attached to the leg holder even with the extension. The surgeon stands on the lateral side of the operative knee and an the assistant medial to the operative knee in between the two legs.

Surgical Exposure

The surgeon's standard manual surgical dissection and arthrotomy technique is performed. Osteophytes are not removed until after bone registration.

Tracker Array Placement

Secure the tibial array and clamp to two 3.2-mm bicortical threaded pins with a short stabilizer at

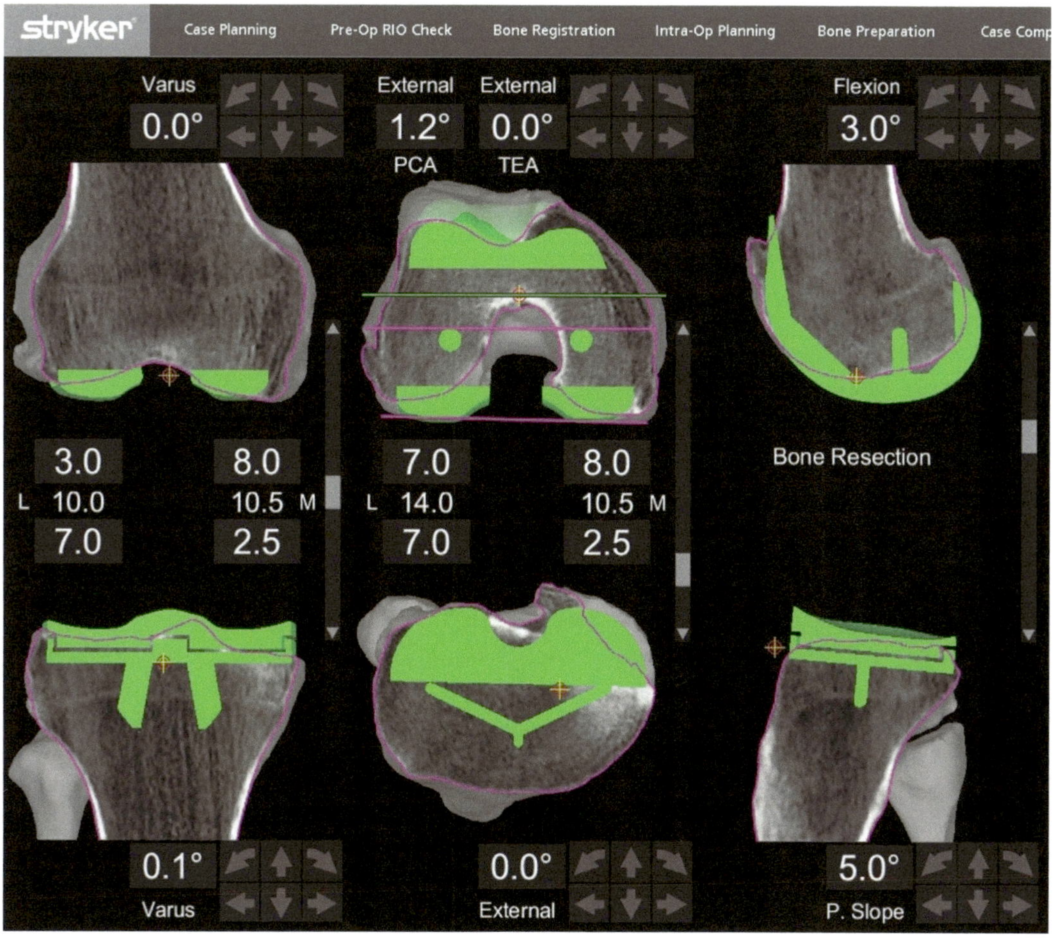

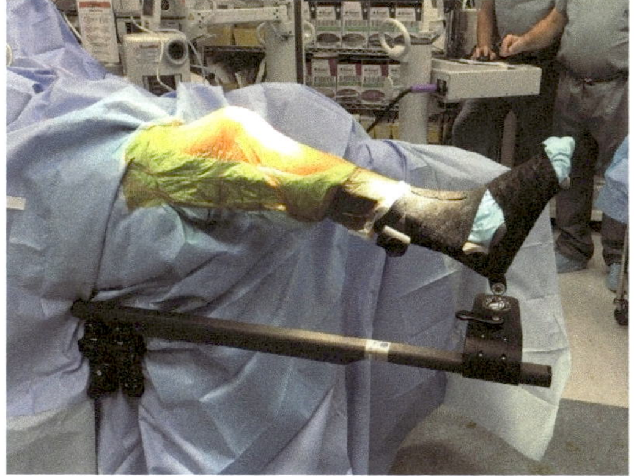

Fig. 16.2 The default preoperative plan calls for a 0 degree of mechanical alignment, 0 degree of distal femoral and proximal tibial bone resections, and femoral rotation parallel to the femoral transepicondylar line

Fig. 16.3 The operative leg is on a leg holder. The contralateral leg is secured to a stirrup and the distal end of the operating table is dropped down. An assistant can stand between the legs

the mid-tibial diaphysis. The pins are inserted perpendicular to the tibial crest. The femoral array and clamp is secured to two 3.2-mm bicortical threaded pins with the long stabilizer in distal femoral diaphysis either inside or outside of the knee incision (Fig. 16.1).

Try to avoid tethering the quadriceps muscle. The pins are inserted at a 30–40 degree angle to the anteroposterior axis of the knee, going anteromedial to posterolateral. This should place the pins within the proximal quadriceps incision and minimize tethering of motion by the muscle or tearing of the muscle while flexing the knee. Verify that the infrared camera visualizes both arrays throughout full knee range of knee motion.

Checkpoint Placement

A checkpoint is placed medial to the tibial tubercle. Another checkpoint is placed slightly proximal and anterior to the medial femoral epicondyle. Make sure that the checkpoints are against bone so they will not move. The checkpoints are used to verify that the trackers have not moved prior to each group of bone cuts.

Registration of the Distal Femur and Proximal Tibia to Link to CT-Determined 3-D Virtual Bone Model

The hip is rotated to register the hip center. The most prominent points on the medial and lateral malleoli are registered with the blunt tip probe. The blunt tip probe is also used to register the tibial and femoral checkpoints. Registration points are obtained with the sharp tip probe by piercing articular cartilage to reference to bone and along bony edges of medial femoral condyle, lateral intercondylar notch, and medial tibial condyles. The registration points are designed to follow an easily memorized pattern. An audible beep confirms that the registration points were recognized by the camera. Overall accuracy of registration is confirmed by touching the bone by the blue registration spheres.

Pose Capture

All osteophytes are removed going as posterior as possible. Manual varus and valgus stress is applied in near full extension to passively correct the coronal deformity. This determines what the medial and lateral compartment gaps and alignment would be after making the bone cuts as determined from the preoperative virtual plan (Fig. 16.4a, b).

Applying manual varus and valgus stress is not as effective in flexion due to the inability to minimize femoral rotation. The surgeon should avoid the instinct to try to prevent limb rotation during ligament tensioning by holding the femoral tracker array, since that could loosen the array pins in the bone. Use of spacer spoons is preferred to distract the medial and lateral compartments at 90 degrees of flexion to determine the flexion gaps. The gap measurements will also demonstrate if the lateral side of a varus worn knee or the medial side of a valgus worn knee has been stretched out.

Modify Preoperative Plan

If one is satisfied that the knee is balanced in extension and flexion as determined by the pose captures, the preoperative plan can be accepted. Also if large posterior tibial or femoral osteophytes are present, the pose capture gap balance may not be reliable, so the preoperative plan should be accepted at this point. Alternatively, based on the gap measurements from the pose capture, the preoperative plan can be modified. The femoral and/or tibia component positions or alignments are changed to more equalize the medial and lateral gaps, both in flexion and extension. This will lessen the need for large soft tissue releases. A modification of the preoperative plan will demonstrate what the final effect will be on alignment with the accuracy that is achieved with the robotic arm-assisted bone cuts. One can keep the component and axial alignments within surgeon's acceptable alignment parameters. In general, the lateral compartment gap can be slightly looser than the medial gap, especially in flexion. The extension and flexion gaps can be equalized by repositioning the femoral component distally or anteroposteriorly. If the medial or lateral gap is more than 2 mm tighter in both flexion and extension, the tibial varus/valgus alignment is changed (or soft tissue releases can be performed). If the medial or lateral gap is tighter only in extension, the femoral varus/valgus alignment is changed. If the medial or lateral gap is tighter only in flexion, femoral rotation is changed. Full correction of gap measurements should be avoided if the less worn compartment gap measures more than 20 mm. This indicates that soft tissues are stretched out. Trying to balance the knee only

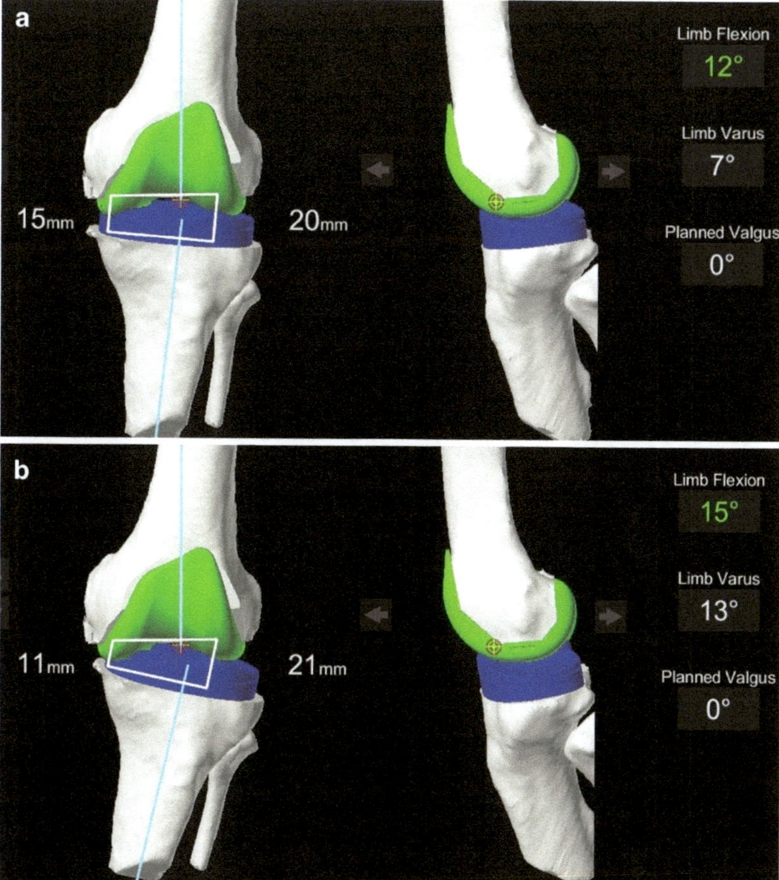

Fig. 16.4 (**a**) Pose capture of the knee with valgus stress applied near full extension. (**b**) Pose capture of the knee with varus stress applied near full extension. The difference in the medial and lateral gaps is 6 mm

with modified bone cuts could result in a significant malalignment. The presence of stretched out soft tissues will usually require an additional soft tissue release.

Robot Base and Robotic Arm Positioning

The position of the robot base is important to facilitate all bone cuts. The robotic arm is locked in position. The knee is placed in the knee holder at 90 degrees of flexion. The robot is moved closer to the patient's ipsilateral hip and oriented such that the base of the saw handle on stabilized arm is located 10 cm above the knee. The robot base is locked in position. The base array position is verified that it is visible to the camera.

Knee Preparation for Femoral Bone Resections

The operative extremity is stabilized in the leg holder with the knee at about 105 to 110 degrees of flexion. Z-shaped retractors are placed at medial and lateral joint lines and secured to leg holder antlers with elastic cords (Fig. 16.5). Use of the leg holder and fixed retractors eliminates the need for the assistant during bone cuts and improves accuracy of saw cuts by not requiring the saw to constantly adjust to moving haptic boundaries. The 90-degree angle saw is used to perform the distal femur and posterior chamfer bone cuts (Fig. 16.5). The straight saw is used for the posterior, anterior, and anterior chamfer femoral bone cuts and for the tibial cut (Fig. 16.1).

The saw blade and femoral checkpoint are verified with the probe before making the cuts.

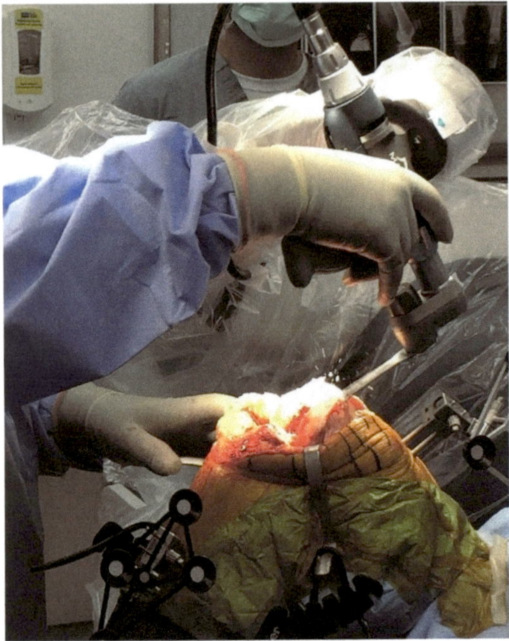

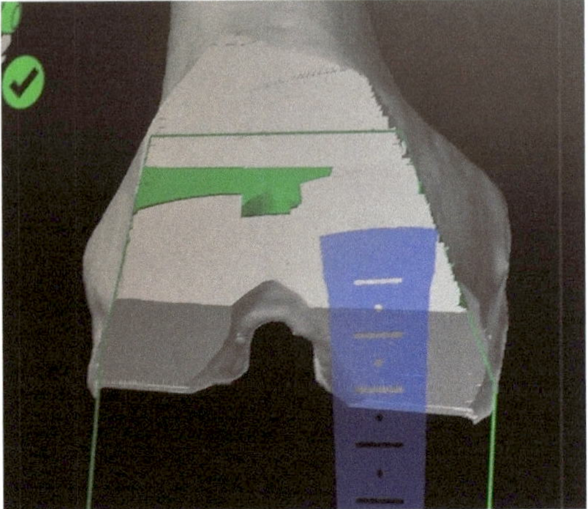

Fig. 16.6 As the saw completes the bone resection, the green area disappears. The green line represents the haptic boundary. Note that the tip of the saw can't migrate outside the haptic boundary

Fig. 16.5 Knee retractors are self-retained to the leg holder. The 90-degree saw is used for the distal femoral bone resection

The saw blade is manually located close to actual cutting plane. The haptic boundaries will become visible on the monitor screen. The saw blade is moved closer to the bone until it appears on the monitor screen within the haptic boundaries. The saw trigger is depressed and the saw blade will automatically rotate into the exact cut plane. Releasing the trigger and depressing it again will now activate the saw. The saw blade is gently moved through the bone. Progression of the saw cut is noted by disappearance of the green surface on the screen monitor (Fig. 16.6).

Since the haptic boundary is based on the implant dimension, occasionally some bone will remain outside the boundary. This extra bone can be removed by extending the haptic boundary temporarily. The alignment and depth accuracy of the saw cut can be verified with the planer probe (Fig. 16.7).

Knee Preparation for the Tibial Bone Resection

The extremity is stabilized in the leg holder with the knee at about 115 degrees of flexion.

A wide MAKO curved retractor is placed along the proximal medial tibial condyle. A MAKO pointed retractor is placed at anterolateral tibia to assist with lateral capsule and patellar tendon retraction. The MAKO retractors are secured to the leg holder antlers with elastic cords. The straight saw is used for the tibial bone cut. The saw blade and tibial checkpoint are verified with the probe before making the bone cuts. The tibial bone cut is robotically guided as noted with the femoral bone cuts (Fig. 16.1). If a posterior cruciate retained implant is planned, an island of bone is retained around the base of the posterior cruciate ligament (Fig. 16.8). Alignment and depth accuracy of the saw cut can be verified with the planer probe.

Soft Tissue Balancing with Trials

The femoral, tibial, and standard insert trials are inserted. Varus and valgus stress is applied near full extension and around 90 degrees of flexion to assess stability. Quantified compartmental gap measurement differences can be visualized on the monitor screen [10].

Assess if extension and flexion gaps are near equal. Also assess if the medial and lat-

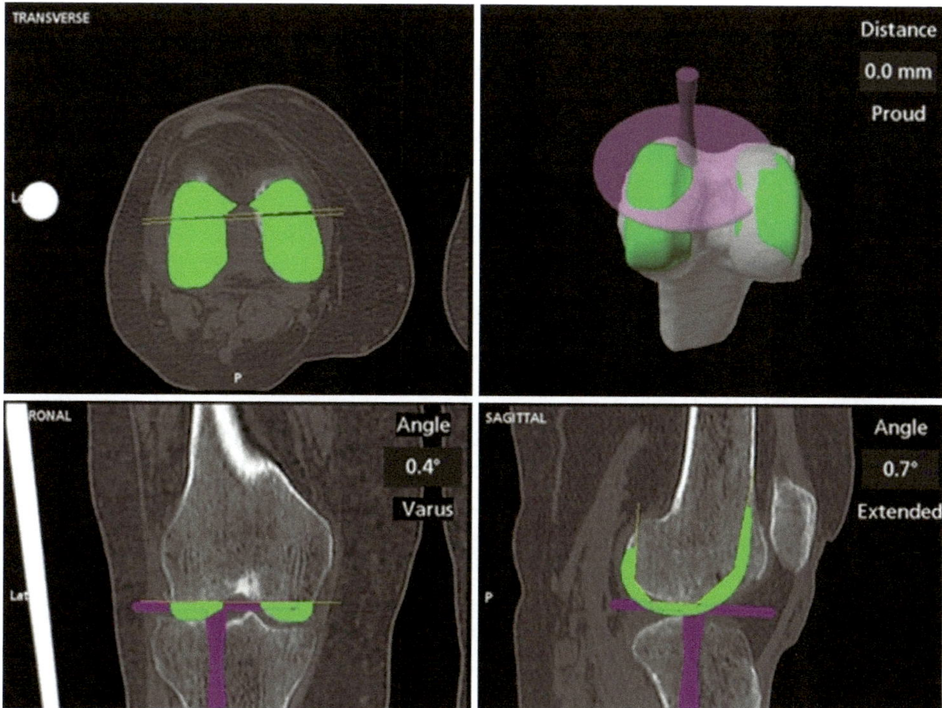

Fig. 16.7 The planner probe is used to check accuracy of bone resections

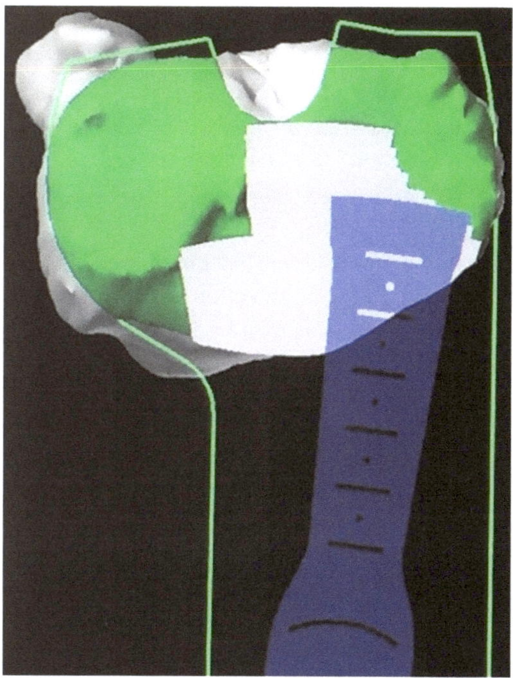

Fig. 16.8 The haptic boundary for the tibial bone resection has cut outs to protect the patellar tendon and maintain a bone island at the base of the posterior cruciate ligament

eral compartment gaps are near equal in extension and flexion. Soft tissue releases can be performed as necessary to balance the gaps.

Alternatively, one can modify the preoperative plan to remove additional bone from the tight compartment by realigning the components (Fig. 16.9). If the extension gap is too tight, change the plan to resect more distal femur, which is then done under robotic guidance. If flexion gap is too tight at 90 degrees of flexion, downsize the femoral component and move the femoral component anteriorly. Alternatively, if the posterior cruciate ligament is also tight, one can modify the plan and increase the tibial slope. A tight posterior cruciate ligament can be visualized as an excessive femoral rollback on the monitor screen. If the posterior cruciate remains too tight despite equal flexion and extension gaps (which can occur with an extensive medial or lateral soft tissue release), either perform a partial soft tissue release or resect it and plan to use posterior stabilized device.

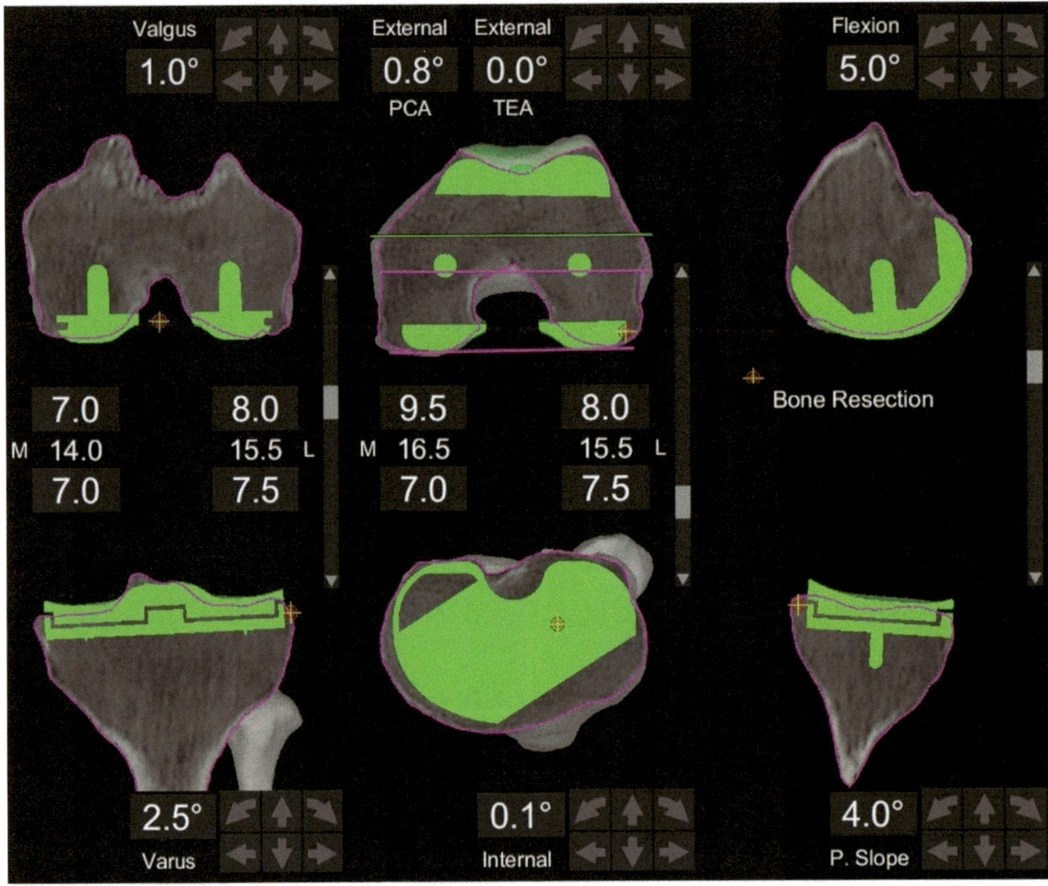

Fig. 16.9 The preoperative plan has been modified, adding an additional 1½ degree of tibial varus to decompress a tight medial compartment in extension and flexion. An overall final varus mechanical alignment of 1½ degree of varus is anticipated and accepted

Soft Tissue Balancing with Tensioner

An alternative check to soft tissue balancing, which can complement the method above which incorporates the computer, is to use a conventional tensioner. After making the bone resections, insert a tensioner device and distract medial and lateral compartments near full extension and around 90 degrees of flexion. Soft tissue releases are performed as necessary to balance the gaps. Alternatively, one can modify the preoperative plan by changing component position or alignment to remove additional bone from the tight compartment. Changes can be made to the preoperative plan as outlined above. A tensioner device can also be used before all bone resections are performed. The tibial resection can be performed first. The tensioner is then inserted with the knee in extension, and soft tissue releases are performed to align the knee in the desired alignment. The distal femoral resection level and alignment can be modified if it is different from the preoperative plan. An alternative work flow is by performing the distal femur and tibial resection first. The tensioner is inserted in extension. Soft tissue releases are performed to equalize the medial and lateral gaps or done in combination with an alignment adjustment to the tibia or femur. Once the extension gaps are equalized, the knee is placed in 90 degrees of flexion. The medial and lateral gaps are distracted with the tensioner. The femoral component rotation is then modified on the preoperative plan if it is not parallel to the tibial resection. One should be careful not to internally rotate the femoral component relative to the posterior condylar line.

Soft Tissue Balancing with Sensor Trial

Another potential device to supplement the computer navigation is a pressure sensor trial. The femoral and tibial trials are inserted along with a sensor spacer trial of appropriate thickness. The patella is reduced and the medial retinaculum approximated with towel clips. Compartment pressures are recorded while holding the knee near full extension and around 90 degrees of flexion, taking care not to apply additional varus or valgus force (Fig. 16.10). Soft tissue releases are performed as necessary to equalize the compartment pressures within 15 pounds [1], with the lateral compartment preferably having less compartment pressure than the medial compartment.

The extension and flexion compartments are assessed for the presence of similar pressures. The flexion space pressures may be a little less than the those of the extension compartment. Alternatively, one can modify the preoperative plan realigning the femoral and/or tibial compo-

nents to effectively remove additional bone from the tight compartment.

Implantation

The patellar preparation and preparation of the femoral box for a posterior stabilized femoral component if needed are currently performed with standard instruments. Once a balanced knee and appropriate knee kinematics are confirmed, the femoral and tibial components are inserted via standard technique. After inserting the final components, medial and lateral gap measurements in extension and flexion, varus/valgus balance, and component and axial alignments are recorded.

Summary

There has been the concern that arthroplasty surgery with robotic assistance will not be safe, allowing inadvertent damage to important ligaments and neurovascular structures. That has not been the case with this system due to the accuracy of the end effector tool and use of haptic boundaries, as well as judicious use of soft tissue retractors. The semi-active nature of this technology also forces the surgeon to be actively involved in the actual cutting of bone. This also adds to the

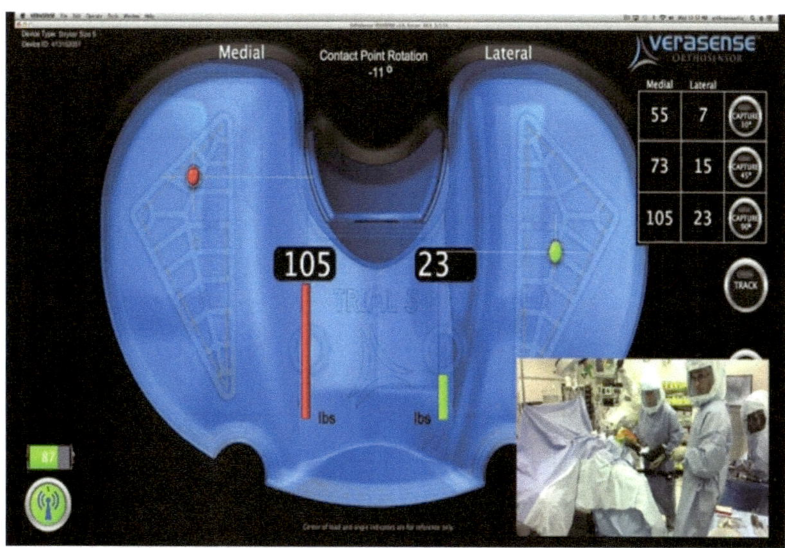

Fig. 16.10 A sensor trial is used to quantify ligament balance as shown by comparing intracompartmental pressures throughout knee range of motion. The location of maximum pressure, the dwell point, is also visualized indicating component rotation and knee kinetics

"fun factor" of the surgery. It is similar to the computer action of video gaming or landing an airplane on a runway. Having the robot perform part of the surgery may also decrease surgeon fatigue and wear and tear on their joints.

Robotic assistance provides the surgeon the ability to accurately place the components and achieve their desired alignment. Having quantifiable data demonstrating actual knee balance and alignment has led to performing more soft tissue releases or bone cuts. Knowing exactly what effect a modification of component alignment will have on the final desired alignment target has led to performing more bone recuts to balance the soft tissues and minimize or eliminate the need for additional soft tissue releases.

A recent cadaver study demonstrated greater accuracy and precision to plan comparing robotic-assisted bone cut alignment to cuts with conventional instruments [11]. The mean robotic bone cuts were 0.3 to 1.1 degree of plan, and conventional instrument bone cuts were 0.8 to 4.7 degrees of plan. Another study showed that the intraoperative knee alignment data are highly accurate when compared to long leg radiographs obtained at 6 weeks [12]. Overall average change in the alignment was only $0.16°$ Recording accurate data on final alignment and balance can be correlated to functional outcomes, so that we may eventually know what balance and alignment provides optimal patient satisfaction. Further study is needed to prove the expected role of this system in impacting implant position, soft tissue balance, and functional outcomes.

Conflict of Interest The author certifies that there is a conflict of interest in connection with the submitted article. He is a consultant and designer for Stryker/MAKO and does receive consulting fees and royalties for the device discussed in this article.

References

1. Urish KL, Conditt M, Roche M, Rubash HE. Robotic total knee arthroplasty: surgical assistant for a customized normal kinematic knee. Orthopedics. 2016;39:e822–7.
2. Sinha RK. Outcomes of robotic arm-assisted unicompartmental knee arthroplasty. Am J Orthop. 2009;38(2 Suppl):20–2.
3. Bell SW, Anthony I, Jones B, MacLean A, Rowe R, Blyth M. Improved accuracy of component positioning with robotic-assisted unicompartmental knee arthroplasty: data from a prospective, randomized controlled study. J Bone Joint Surg Am. 2016;98(8):627–35.
4. Citak M, Suero EM, Citak M, Dunbar NJ, Branch SH, Conditt MA, Banks SA, Pearle AD. Unicompartmental knee arthroplasty: is robotic technology more accurate than conventional technique? Knee. 2013;20(4):268–71.
5. Lonner JH, John TK, Conditt M. Robotic arm-assisted UKA improves tibial component alignment: a pilot study. Clin Orthop Relat Res. 2010;468:141–6.
6. Liow MH, Xia Z, Wong MK, Tay KJ, Yeo SJ, Chin PL. Robot-assisted total knee arthroplasty accurately restores the joint line and mechanical axis. A prospective randomized study. J Arthroplast. 2014;29:2373–7.
7. Noble PC, Conditt MA, Cook KF, Mathis KB. The John Insall Award: patient expectations affect satisfaction with total knee arthroplasty. Clin Orthop Relat Res. 2006;452:35–43.
8. Bourne RB, Chesworth BM, Davis AM, Mahomed NN, Kory DJ, Charron KDJ. Patient satisfaction after total knee arthroplasty: who is satisfied and who is not? Clin Orthop Relat Res. 2010;468:57–63.
9. Sharkey PF, Hozack WJ, Rothman RH, Shastri S, Jacoby SM. Insall Award paper. Why are total knee arthroplasties failing today? Clin Orthop Relat Res. 2002;404:7–13.
10. Gustke KA, Golladay GJ, Roche MW, Elson LC, Anderson CR. A new method for defining balance: promising short-term clinical outcomes of sensor-guided TKR. J Arthroplast. 2014;29(5):955–60.
11. Hampp EL, Chughtai M, Scholl LY, Sodhi N, Bhowmik-Stoker M, Jacofsky DJ, Mont MA. Robotic-arm assisted total knee arthroplasty demonstrated greater accuracy and precision to plan compared with manual techniques. J Knee Surg. 2018. https://doi.org/10.1055/s-0038-1641729.
12. Roche M, Law T, Vakharia R, Wang K, Nevelos J. Does Intraoperative robotic arm assisted total knee arthroplasty alignment correlate with standing long leg postoperative alignment? Unpublished data. Presented at the Florida Orthopaedic Society Annual Meeting, June 2018.

Jan Albert Koenig and Christopher Plaskos

Healthcare providers are under enormous pressure to reduce costs while improving clinical outcome measures. In 2010, the US federal government introduced the Affordable Care Act (ACA), which aimed in part to introduce innovative medical care delivery methods designed to lower the overall costs of healthcare. This initiative led to the Center for Medicare and Medicaid Services Innovation Center, whose objective was to test innovative payment and service delivery models that have the potential to reduce public healthcare expenditures while preserving or enhancing the quality of care for beneficiaries [1]. As a result, the Innovation Center launched the Bundled Payments for Care Improvement (BPCI) initiative, a voluntary model designed to evaluate the efficacy of a single payment structure covering an entire episode of care [2]. Early reports from several centers participating in the BPCI model have demonstrated cost savings to Medicare through the implementation of standardized, evidence-based, coordinated clinical care pathways across the various healthcare service settings [3, 4].

The role of robotic- and computer-assisted orthopedic (RCAOS) technologies in this new paradigm of episodic-based reimbursements and cost-efficiency has yet to be established. RCAOS technologies have the potential to improve outcomes through improved component positioning and soft tissue balance in TKA while reducing blood loss and systemic emboli release [5, 6]. When integrated into a coordinated, evidence-based clinical care pathway, intraoperative robotic assistance may demonstrate increased value through the abovementioned benefits. Resulting improvements in clinical metrics may include further reductions in length of stay, complications, 90-day readmission rates, and higher discharge rates to home versus costly skilled nursing facilities, thus reducing overall episode costs. Additional benefits are expected to extend beyond the 90-day period, including better functional outcomes and higher patient satisfaction rates, improved pain relief, quality of life, and implant survivorship with fewer early failures [7, 8].

In this chapter, we review one commercially available robotic-assisted total knee arthroplasty system (OMNIBotics®) and the clinical and economic results associated with its use in an academic teaching and a community hospital setting. The system was first introduced into a community hospital, and the authors evaluated implant placement and limb alignment accuracy, surgical time and learning curve, and overall system utility in routine and complex cases with significant deformities. The system was subsequently introduced

J. A. Koenig (✉)
Department of Orthopaedic Surgery, NYU Winthrop Hospital, Mineola, NY, USA
e-mail: JKoenigMD@OrthoExcellence.com

C. Plaskos
Technology and Clinical Research,
Omni/Corin-Group, Raynham, MA, USA

© Springer Nature Switzerland AG 2019
J. H. Lonner (ed.), *Robotics in Knee and Hip Arthroplasty*,
https://doi.org/10.1007/978-3-030-16593-2_17

into a teaching hospital that thereafter began participating in the model 2 BPCI initiative, where overall procedure costs over the 90-day episode of care period were evaluated relative to target historical procedure costs at that institution. We evaluated differences in average length of stay, complications, readmissions, and overall cost savings between patients undergoing robotic-assisted surgery versus conventional intramedullary (IM)-based TKA instrumentation.

The OMNIBotics Knee System

The OMNIBotics Knee System is an image-free robotic-assisted TKA surgery (RAS-TKA) platform founded on patented Bone morphing™ technology for 3D anatomical modeling and implant planning. The system includes a miniature robotic cutting guide for guiding femoral bone resections (the OMNIBot™) [9] and a recently introduced robotic ligament tensioning tool called the BalanceBot™ (formerly called the active spacer) [10] (Fig. 17.1). The active spacer is a computer-controlled ligament tensioning and gap spacing tool that allows the surgeon to accurately and reproducibly tension the soft tissues surrounding the knee joint both prior to and after femoral bone cuts. This allows for characterization of the soft tissue envelope throughout the range of knee motion and for femoral bone resection planning integrated with predictive ligament tensioning. The active spacer can also be used to measure tension and balance during the implant trialing phase to adjust for and document final ligament balance and tension.

Bone morphing is a process that uses morphometric modeling to reconstruct the patient's

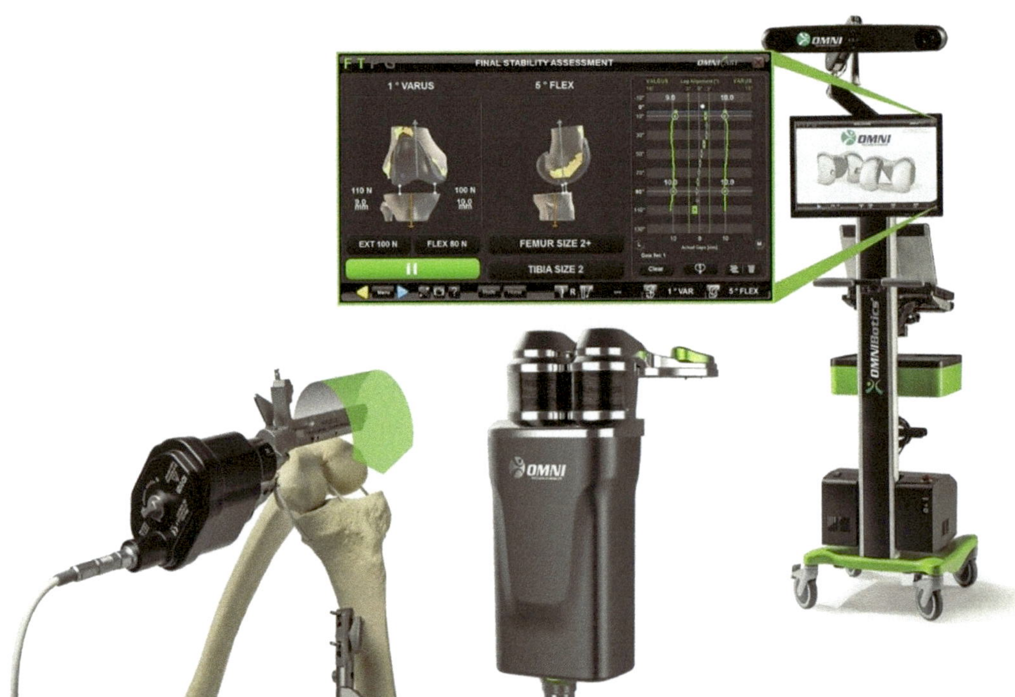

Fig. 17.1 The OMNIBotics® system – an image-free robotic-assisted TKA system that integrates intraoperative 3D anatomical modeling, real-time pre- and postoperative knee alignment and gap kinematics, and miniature robotic systems for bone cutting and ligament balancing. (Courtesy of OMNI, Raynham, MA, USA)

unique anatomy in 3D, where statistical models are deformed to match point clouds acquired intraoperatively on the patients' bone surface [11]. The reconstruction process requires no preoperative CT, MRI, or x-ray imaging modalities, thereby reducing radiation, cost, and time burdens, and is accurate to within 1 mm in all mapped areas (Fig. 17.2a). The

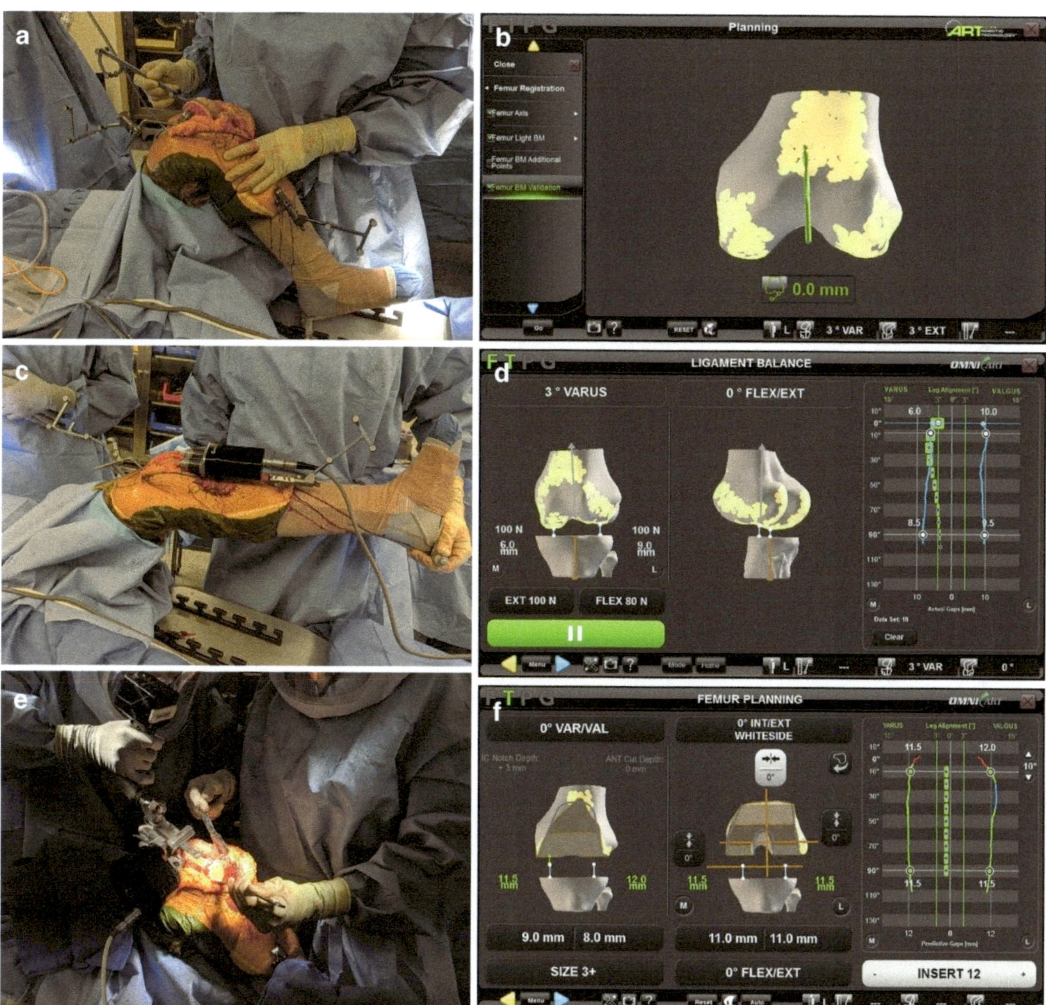

Fig. 17.2 Intraoperative photos and screenshots illustrating the surgical technique steps: (**a**) bone morphing is performed by mapping the cartilage and bone surface with a ball-end tip pointer that glides over the cartilage surface; (**b**) the morphed model is accurate to within 1 mm in all digitized areas and can be verified intraoperatively at any stage of the procedure; (**c** and **d**) in the tibial cut first technique, the active spacer is inserted after performing the tibial resection, prior to femoral resection, and the native gaps are dynamically acquired throughout the range of flexion under active robotically controlled ligament tension; (**e**) bone resections are executed to plan using a miniature bone-mounted robot; (**f**) femoral implant planning with virtual bone resection data (left) and predicted medial and lateral gap data (right); (**g** and **h**) tibial and femoral bone resection are validated using the cut controller; (**i**) final alignment and gap balance can be evaluated using the active spacer in place of a manual tibial insert; (**j** and **k**) screenshot of pre- and postoperative kinematics, illustrating initial limb deformity and overall correction throughout the range of flexion

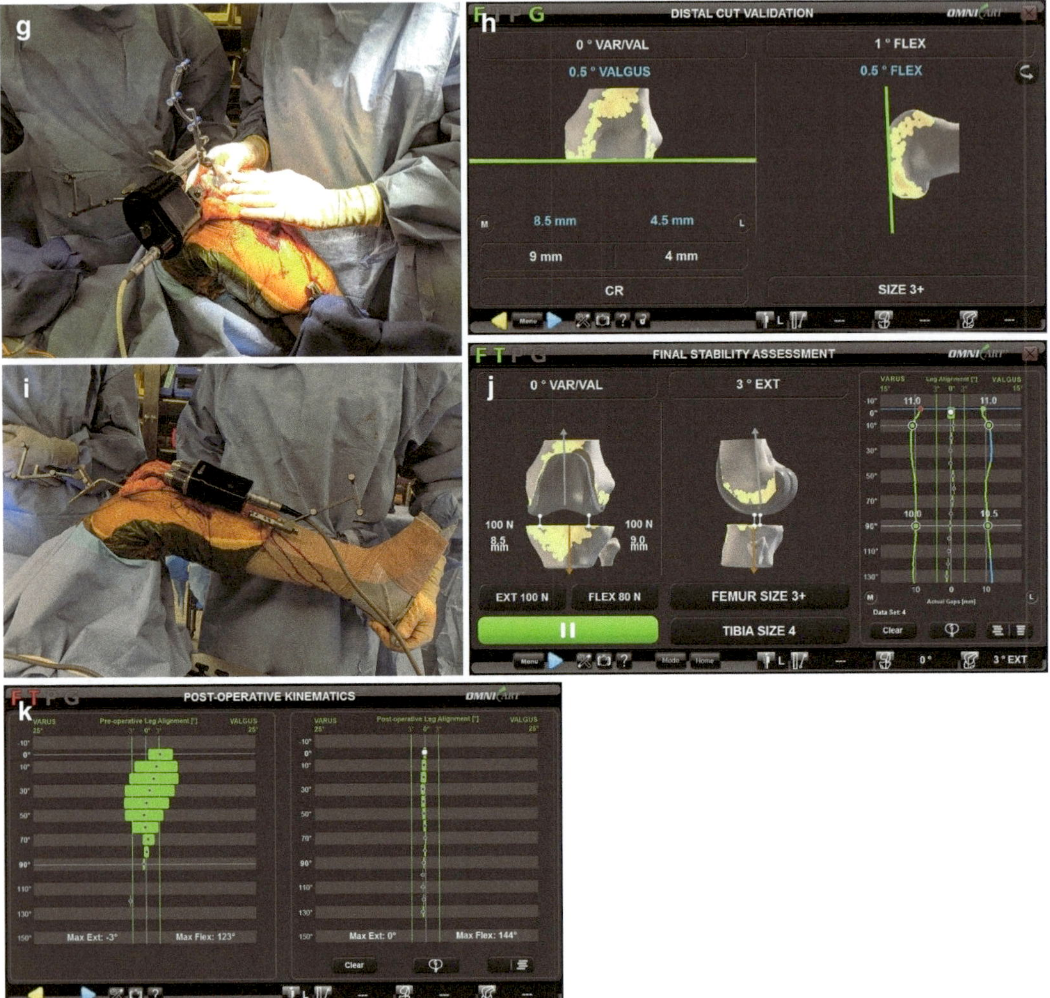

Fig. 17.2 (continued)

duration of the entire intraoperative registration process takes approximately 2–3 min for an experienced user. Flexible customizable workflows permit implant planning based on measured resection and/or gap referencing techniques [12, 13].

Femoral resections are precisely executed by the surgeon to the validated plan using the iBlock™ bone-mounted robotic-assisted cutting guide (Fig. 17.1). Benefits of using a single robotic guide for all femoral implant sizes and resections include a significant reduction in the manual instrumentation that is normally required to perform the procedure. This may help in reducing inefficiencies and potential infection risk associated with instrument tray reprocessing and OR back table clutter. Bone-mounted robotic systems also do not require camera-to-tracker line-of-sight during robotic positioning and resection guidance once the robot is mounted and calibrated to the bone, allowing for greater flexibility for the physician's assistant and soft tissue retractor positioning around the patient and OR table while performing bone resections.

A unique feature of the OMNI robotic system is the ability to adjust the interface fit of the prosthesis with the bone intraoperatively using the ART application software. The anterior and posterior femoral bone resections can be varied in depth and angle in increments of 0.25 mm to achieve progressively higher levels of interference "press" fit with the inner dimensions of the prosthesis. This allows for greater flexibility to accommodate for the variability observed in patient bone quality intraoperatively, as well as for surgeon-specific preferences in prosthesis fixation type (cemented or bone ingrowth) and in trial or implant fit during impaction [11, 14].

Surgical Technique

The surgical technique typically starts with a standard exposure with a medial parapatellar or subvastus approach. Femoral and tibial tracking arrays (Fig. 17.2a) are attached with two bone pins per array. Tibial pins are placed percutaneously from medial to lateral either proximally near the incision or distally so as not to interfere with the active spacer. Femoral pins are placed in the incision anterior to the insertion of the medial collateral ligament (MCL). These two pins support the femoral tracking array as well as the robotic cutting guide such that no other bone pins are required. The registration process starts with a kinematic acquisition of the hip center followed by an anatomic acquisition of the ankle center. Bone morphing is then performed on the femur and tibia using the pointer (Fig. 17.2a, b). The bone and cartilage surface is dynamically "painted" or mapped using the probe tip, which has a spherical ball-shaped tip to facilitate sliding on the bone surface. The medial and lateral condyles and anterior aspect of the distal femur are mapped to produce a complete pre-segmented

3D model of the distal femur that is accurate to within 1 mm in all morphed areas (Fig. 17.2b). The tibia is resected using an adjustable cutting guide that is navigated and pinned into an initial position and then fine-tuned using the adjustment screws to precisely align with the target plane [15, 16]. In the tibia cut first gap balancing protocol, the active spacer is inserted into the knee prior to resecting the femur (Fig. 17.2c). The applied load can be customized to the patient and independently set in extension and in flexion on the medial and lateral sides using the on-screen buttons (Fig. 17.2d). Once the target load is set and the spacer is activated, the limb is taken through a range of flexion while the knee is supported posteriorly, and the software graphs the medial and lateral gaps and alignment with flexion in real-time. The surgeon should avoid introducing a varus or valgus stress or tibial rotation during the gap acquisition and allow the leg to follow its natural path. The amount of applied tension can be evaluated in each patient by switching the active spacer from force mode to gap mode, where the device locks its height at a specific tension and varus/valgus stress can be performed to assess the degree of opening in the knee. The process can be used to predict postoperative ligament tension and to verify that the currently applied tension is suitable for each individual patient. Femoral planning can then be performed using the predicted laxity curves on the right side of the screen (Fig. 17.2f). Femoral component varus or valgus and femoral rotation can be adjusted to achieve balanced gaps mediolaterally in extension and flexion. The femoral component can also be flexed or shifted posteriorly, or the size can be increased, to decrease flexion gap laxity. Similarly, distal resection depth can be increased or decreased to adjust the extension gap, while the predictive laxity curves can be used to evaluate the effects of joint line elevation on mid-flexion laxity. Ligament releases may be performed either before or after femoral planning and bone resecting in cases where adjustments in implant position are not sufficient to achieve balance. However, in our experience the incidence of soft tissue releases appears much less common in the tibial first soft tissue and gap balancing technique which we believe is due to the interactive information the computer provides, allowing the surgeon to plan implant position for both alignment and optimal balance. Once the femoral implant plan is validated, the robot is attached to the femoral fixation base and locked into varus/valgus and internal/external rotation using two adjustment screws and the optical tracking system for position guidance. The robot then automatically aligns a single saw blade to the five femoral resections of the distal femur, and the resections are made by the surgeon in sequence using an oscillating saw and a 1.27 mm thick saw blade (Fig. 17.2e). An advantage of using a single saw guide for all cuts over a 4-in-1 block is the enhanced visibility during the resection process. Additionally, as the robot moves with the knee, line-of-sight with the camera is not required, and the surgeon and assistant can stand on either side of the knee. Distal femoral and proximal tibial resections are validated using the system cut controller and stored in the operative report (Fig. 17.2g, h). Implant trialing is performed with a standard femoral trial, and the active spacer acts as the tibial baseplate and insert trial (Fig. 17.2i), so there is no need for separate trials. Postoperative gaps can be assessed under constant robotically controlled ligament tension throughout the range of motion (Fig. 17.2j). In the femur-first measured resection or in the tibia-first gap balancing protocols, soft tissue releases or recuts can be performed to correct any residual imbalance measured at this stage. However, this is not that common in the tibial cut first technique since soft tissue balance was planned into the bone resections. The active spacer can also be used in "insert" mode at this stage to replicate the height of the tibial insert and to measure the force balance acting on the medial and lateral sides throughout the range of flexion. The height of the insert can be adjusted automatically with the touch of a button, and the medial and lateral pressures acting on the insert can be evaluated as a function of the insert thickness. Finally, the post-op kinematics can be evaluated and compared side-by-side with the pre-op kinematics (Fig. 17.2k). This graphic depiction of the pre- and postoperative kinematics can be a very useful document for the surgeon in the future as it memorializes the pre-op deformity, motion, and instability as well as the post-op mechanical alignment, motion, stability, and soft tissue balance achieved during surgery (Fig. 17.3).

Clinical Studies

Initial Studies on Clinical Accuracy and Learning Curve

In our first clinical study, we retrospectively reviewed our first 100 consecutive cases starting with the first surgery performed with the OMNIBotics system in the USA in June 2010 [11, 17]. At that time (and still today) RCAOS systems were often criticized for adding substantial OR time and having a long learning curve, thereby reducing efficiency. We therefore evaluated the learning curve for surgical time and accuracy and found that the learning phase required only an additional 7 minutes of tourniquet time on average over the first 25 cases as compared to the subsequent 75 cases (56 vs 49 minutes). Final leg alignment was within 3° of neutral to the mechanical axis in 98.7% of cases as measured by the computer intraoperatively and 90.9% as measured radiographically postoperatively (Fig. 17.4, Table 17.1), and accuracy was not affected during the learning curve period. In a subsequent study in 128 consecutive patients, the authors reported that severe varus and valgus deformities could be corrected to within 3.5° of neutral in all cases, while these more difficult cases added only 3–5 minutes of surgery time [12].

We are currently studying our 5–7-year follow-ups of our first 150 patients, including our learning curve patients, and have not performed any revisions in this group for aseptic loosening, chronic pain, or instability. By reducing the number of

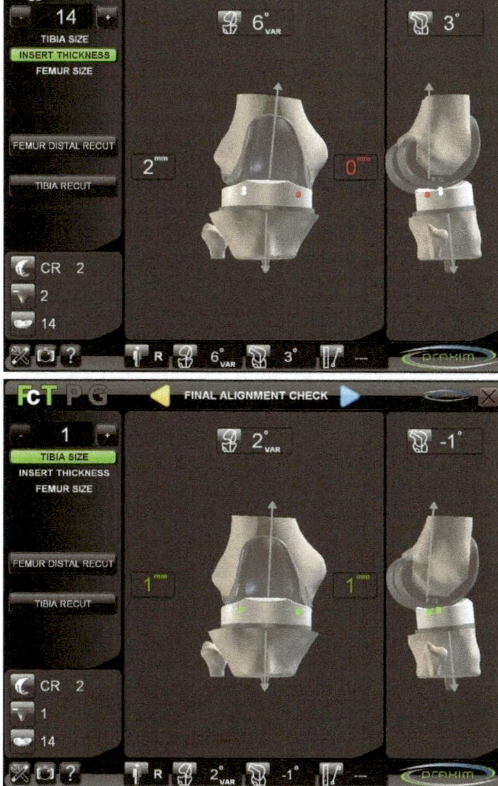
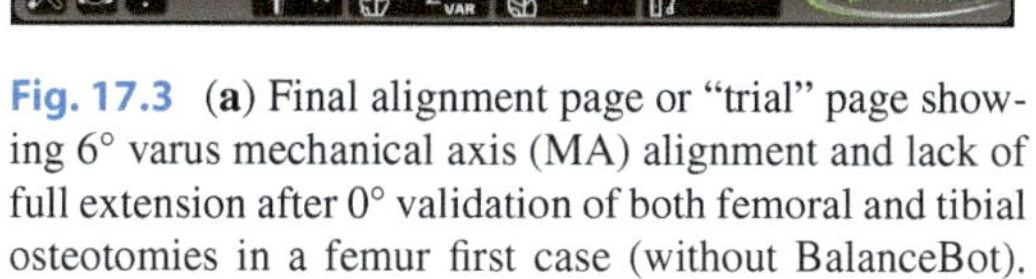
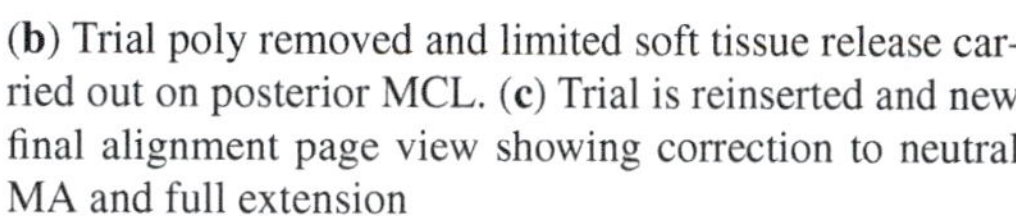

Fig. 17.3 (**a**) Final alignment page or "trial" page showing 6° varus mechanical axis (MA) alignment and lack of full extension after 0° validation of both femoral and tibial osteotomies in a femur first case (without BalanceBot). (**b**) Trial poly removed and limited soft tissue release carried out on posterior MCL. (**c**) Trial is reinserted and new final alignment page view showing correction to neutral MA and full extension

mechanical axis and soft tissue balance outliers, we believe we have lowered the early failure rate. Future long-term studies are needed to evaluate whether the longevity of TKR implantations is improved.

Prospective Study on Patient-Reported Outcomes and Implant Survivorship

One prospective study entitled *Patient Reported Outcomes and Implant Survivorship Using the Apex Knee™ and the OMNIBotics System for Robotic-Assisted TKR* of 105 patients undergoing robotic- and computer-assisted TKRs (RCAS-TKRs) using the OMNIBotics system and a femur-first approach (these data were collected prior to clinical use of the active spacer) has been presented [18] (Table 17.2).

Changes in the five KOOS subscales (pain, symptoms, activities of daily living (ADL), sport and recreation function (Sport/Rec), and knee-related quality of life (QOL)) were compared to available literature data from FORCE-TJR [19, 20], a large, prospective, national cohort of TJR patients enrolled from diverse high-volume centers and community orthopedic practices in the USA, as well as to individual studies reporting on conventional (CONV-TKA) and computer-assisted (CAS-TKA) at 3 M [21] and on conventional TKA at 6 M [22]. RCAS-TKA PROs significantly improved at 3, 6, and 12 M from preoperative baseline values (Tables 17.3 and 17.4). When compared to the FORCE registry cohort data, the improvement in KOOS subscales were generally higher for RCAS for pain at 6 M [19], and for pain, ADL, and QOL at 1Y when compared with FORCE 2Y data [20] (Table 17.3). Higher improvements were also seen at 3 M [21], except for Sports/Rec, and at 6 M for symptoms and QOL [14] when compared with the smaller cohort studies (Table 17.3).

Sustained improvement in the 2011 KSS patient satisfaction and functional scores were also seen throughout the first post-op year (Table 17.4). A mean of 31 points for the patient satisfaction score at 6 months and 1 year indicates that on average patients were "satisfied" with their knee function and pain level. A mean pre-op "patient expectation" score of 14 out of 15 points indicates that patients had an extremely high level of expectation that the surgery would provide a great degree of pain relief and help with carrying out normal ADL and performing leisure, recreational, or sports activities. A mean of 10 points for the expectation score at 6 months indicates that on average patients felt their expectations for pain relief, ADL, and leisure, sports, and recreational activities were between "just right" or "too low." The patients hence were reporting that they were doing better than they thought they would at that given point in time after their RCAS-TKR. Our femur-first, measured resection outcomes study indicates continued improvement in both function and pain levels (Table 17.3) and patient satisfaction (Table 17.4) during the first postoperative year and that our 1.0% patient dissatisfaction rate at 1 year compares well to the rates reported in the literature, which range from 7 to 20% dissatisfaction after total knee replace-

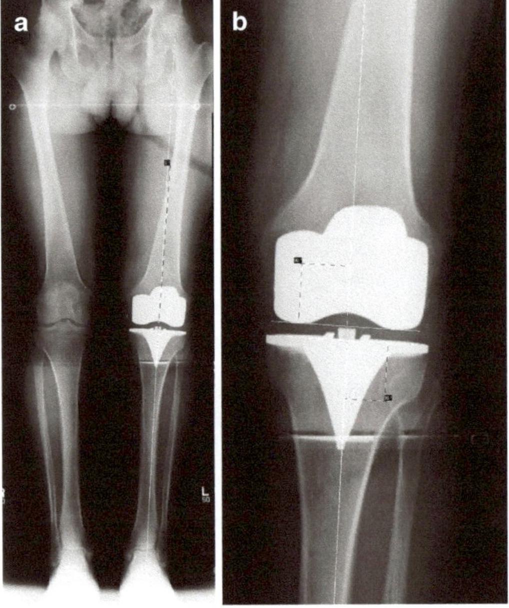

Fig. 17.4 Example postoperative radiograph of a RAS-TKR. Postoperative overall alignment (**a**) and individual femoral and tibial alignment (**b**) in the coronal plane were measured relative to the mechanical axis on standing long-leg radiographs

Table 17.2 Patient demographic, operative time, and length of stay ($n = 105$)

Gender	72 Female	
	Mean	Std Dev
Age (years)	69	± 8.4
BMI (kg/m²)	29.8	± 4.1
Tourniquet time (mm:ss)	42:52	± 7:15
Skin-to-skin time (h;mm)	1:09	+0:10
Time in operating room (h:mm)	1:54	± 0:14
LOS (days)	2.5	± 1.0

Table 17.1 Intraoperative computer data and radiographic data for component and leg alignment from our first 108 OMNIBotic cases

% of cases within 3° [Range]	Intraoperative computer data	Radiographic alignment data
Femoral component alignment	**100% (103/103)** [2.0° valgus to 2.0° varus]	**98.7% (76/77)** [2.0° valgus to 3.5° varus]
Tibial component alignment	**99% (102/103)** [3.5° valgus to 1.5° varus]	**98.7% (76/77)** [4.0° valgus to 2.5° varus]
Final limb alignment	**97.2% (104/107)** [2.0° valgus to 3.5° varus]	**90.9% (70/77)** [4.5° valgus to 4.5° varus]

Table 17.3 KOOS subscale scores for NYU Winthrop's OMNIBotics Study as compared with literature data

	WUH RAS-TKA							Literature data									
								Gøthesen [21]				Roos [22]		Li [19]		Lyman [20]	
	Pre-Op	3 M	6 M	1Y	Δ Pre-op and 3 M	Δ Pre-op and 6 M	Δ Pre-op and 1Y	Δ Pre-op and 3 M		P value 3 M	P value 3 M	Δ Pre-op and 6 M	P value 6 M	Δ Pre-op and 6 M	P value 6 M	Δ Pre-op and 2Y	P value 1-2Y
KOOS subscale	$n=105$	$n=104$	$n=101$	$n=101$	$n=104$	$n=101$	$n=101$	Conv. $n=90$	CAS $n=92$	ΔRAS vs ΔConv.	ΔRAS vs ΔCAS.	Conv. $n=97$	ΔRAS vs ΔConv.	Reg. $n=2792$	ΔRAS vs ΔReg	Reg. $n=1114$	ΔRAS vs ΔConv
Pain	42.6	75.3	82.8	85.5	32.6	40.5	43.8	19.7	27.4	**<0.001**	0.06	41	0.86	31.1	**<0.001**	38.2	**0.002**
Symptoms	45.2	72.4	78.0	80.1	27.1	32.8	35.5	7.0	13.1	**<0.001**	**<0.001**	25	**0.01**	–	–	32.1	0.087
ADL	45.3	78.6	83.8	86.1	32.9	38.5	41.5	20.9	26.3	**<0.001**	**0.01**	36	0.38	–	–	31.1	**<0.001**
Sport/Rec	20.5	40.7	49.7	59.7	20.0	29.0	39.0	7.6	21.1	**0.02**	0.84	32	0.57	–	–	33.9	0.13
QOL	21.1	62.2	67.5	72.4	40.9	46.6	52.2	27.8	35.0	**0.01**	**0.01**	40	**0.01**	–	–	42.8	**<0.001**

Table 17.4 2011 Knee Society Scores (KSS) for NYU Winthop's OMNIBotics Study

2011 KSS	RCAS-TKA					
	Pre-op	3 M	6 M	1Y	Δ Pre-op and 3 M	Δ Pre-op and 6 M
	$n = 105$	$n = 104$	$n = 101$	$n = 101$	$n = 104$	$n = 101$
Expectation (15 points)	14.0	10.2	10.2	10.5	–	–
Satisfaction (40 points)	12.1	29.4	31.2	32.3	17.3	19.2
Functional (100 points)	36.7	62.2	67.3	70.5	25.3	30.5
Objective	22.0	72.9	72.3	74.7	50.9	50.3

Table 17.5 Overall rates of dissatisfaction and satisfaction in robotic-assisted (RCAS) TKA and in the literature

RCAS-TKA with OMNIBotics	n	f/u time	Dissatisfied or very dissatisfied	Neutral	Satisfied or very satisfied
Current study (femur-first measured	104	3 M	5.8%	18.3%	76.0%
resection, without active spacer)	101	6 M	3.0%	13.9%	83.2%
	101	1Y	1.0%	10.9%	88.1%
Literature data	n	f/u time	Dissatisfied or very dissatisfied	Neutral	Satisfied or very satisfied
Turcot et al. [26]	78	3 M	9.0%	15.4%	75.6%
Bourne et al. [27]	1703	1 yr	11.6%	7.7%	80.6%
Heck et al. [28]	330	>2 yr	9.0%	3.0%	88.0%
Baker et al. [29]	8095	>1 yr	7.0%	11.2%	81.8%
Noble et al. [30]	253	>1 yr	14.0%	11.0%	75.0%
Robertsson et al. [31]	27,372	2-17 yr	8.0%	11.0%	81.0%

ment (Table 17.5). We feel this is because the knee implants have been precisely fit and fixed to the bone in neutral alignment and with good balance with very few outliers, which has been supported by other studies [23–25].

BPCI and RCAS-TKR at NYU Winthrop Hospital 2014–2015

In January 2013, NYU Winthrop began its participation in BPCI Model 2 initiative, which includes a retrospective bundled payment arrangement where actual expenditures for a defined episode of care are reconciled against a target price [32]. In this model, Medicare continues to make fee-for-service payments to providers for all costs incurred during the TJR episode, starting 72 hours prior to admission through to 90 days post discharge. The total cost for each episode is then reconciled against a target price that is determined by CMS. Medicare then issues either a payment or a recoupment amount to the provider depending on whether the total costs for the episode are above or below the target price. Physician-specific target prices were established from institutional historical payment data over a prior 3-year period.

Prior to implementing bundled payments, NYU Winthrop developed and implemented a standardized clinical pathway for each care episode to improve quality and reduce variance. Coordinated evidence-based clinical pathways were established by multidisciplinary teams to standardize treatment across service departments and physicians, starting from patient education 6 weeks prior to surgery to post-discharge rehabilitation. Anesthesia, pain management, blood management, and physical/occupational therapy throughout the length of stay were standardized for all TKR patients. All surgeons used a medial parapatellar approach and were assisted by the same OR and RN/CST teams, with the only differences in care being variations in surgical technique and instrumentation used (robotic or conventional).

In a retrospective review of NYU Winthrop's first seven consecutive quarters of BPCI participation beginning January 2014 through October 2015, we compared average LOS, 90 readmission rates, discharge disposition, and gains per episode versus target prices for sur-

Table 17.6 NYU Winthrop BPCI 90-Day Bundle Data – RCAS-TKR vs conventional TKR (7 Quarters 2014–2015)

	Gain/episode	Total gain	LOS (days)	90-Day readmit	% Home	% SAR
RCAS-TKR group (3 surgeons, 147 cases)						
Surgeon A	$ 7603	$ 927,616	3.4	5%	66%	31%
Surgeon D	$ 8838	$ 159,084	3.3	11%	39%	61%
Surgeon F	$ 4292	$ 30,046	4.7	0%	43%	57%
Group average	$ 7600	$ 1,116,746	3.4	5.4%	62%	37%
CONV-TKR group (3 surgeons, 85 cases)						
Surgeon B	$ 6629	$ 245,263	3.5	14%	57%	38%
Surgeon C	$ 6639	$ 212,444	4.1	9%	56%	41%
Surgeon E	$ 1033	$ 16,523	3.6	12%	12%	88%
Group average	$ 5579	$ 474,249	3.8	11.7%	48%	51%

geons performing RCAS with OMNIBotics to those performing TKR with conventional instruments. There were three surgeons in each of two the groups, the RCAS-TKR group (147 cases in total) and the Conv-TKR group (85 cases in total). The analysis included all Medicare TKR patients (DRG 470) from all TJR surgeons who had performed at least 7 cases in the 7 quarter period. It was found that patients undergoing RCAS-TKR using the OMNIBotic system had almost a half day shorter LOS, less than half of the 90-day readmission rates, a 10% higher rate of discharge to home coupled with a lower rate of discharge to subacute rehabilitation facilities (SARs), as compared to the patients undergoing conventional TKR (Table 17.6). The RCAS-TKR cases also exhibited a 36% increase in profitability per case or a gain of over $2000 per case as compared with conventional TKR. The average total cost per episode was $2059 lower across the patients receiving robotic-assisted TKR compared to conventional instrumentation ($28,943 versus $31,002, Fig. 17.5), with the majority of the cost savings being a result of reduced readmissions and skilled nursing facility (SNF) usage [33].

Implementation of a standardized care pathway across all service departments and physicians at NYU Winthrop resulted in overall reductions in LOS, readmissions, discharge to inpatient rehab, and episode costs in general, with a reduced number of readmissions in the RCAS-TKA group. A higher percentage of patients were being discharged to homecare ver-

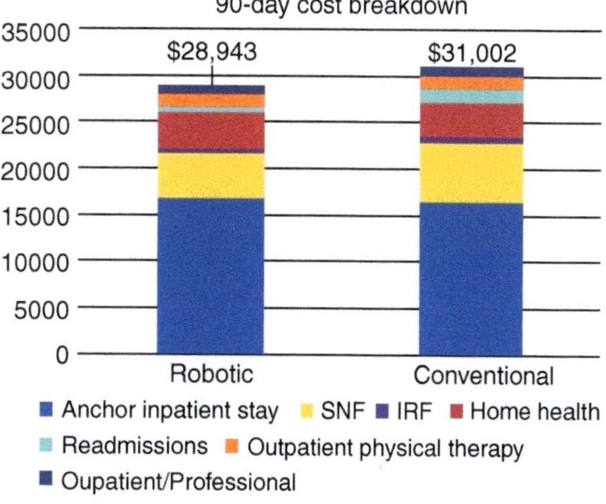

Fig. 17.5 Robotic-assisted TKR demonstrated an average total cost savings per 90-day episode of $2059 when compared with conventional instrumentation

sus SARs (subacute) and inpatient rehab (acute), which contributed to overall cost savings (Fig. 17.6). Additionally, the LOS in subacute care has reduced from up to 30 days to approximately 5–7 days on average. Patient education plays a key role in preparing patients for discharge to home. All patients and either a family member or a friend became an integral part of NYU Winthrop's *Joints in Motion program*, which is a patient-centered and family-/friend-focused approach to the continuum of joint replacement care. The group attends a preoperative educational program where they meet and are taught by representatives of the *Joints in Motion* multidisciplinary team. This education encompasses the period from the 6 weeks preop where patients are medically optimized and

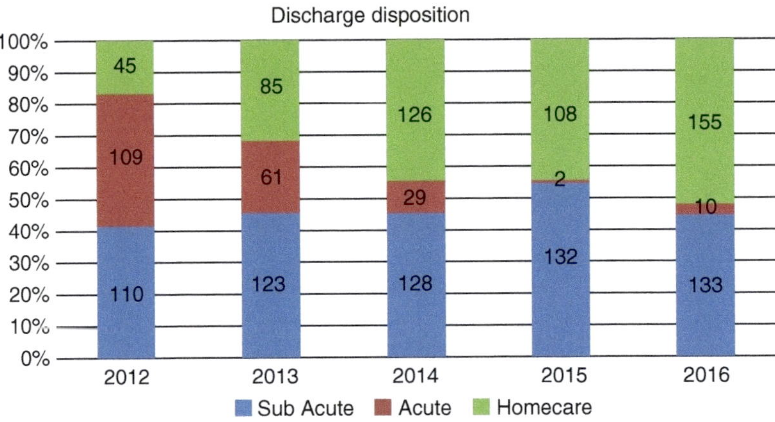

Fig. 17.6 Implementation of a stanwdardized care pathway resulted in more patients being discharged to homecare versus skilled nursing facilities (subacute) and inpatient rehab (acute)

prepared for their surgical intervention to the hospitalization and mutually agreed post-op care pathways and what to expect post-op after discharge including discharge planning, homecare physiotherapy arrangements, and contacts for support. All patients in this group underwent the same perioperative in-patient early mobilization physical therapy protocols as individually tolerated. Both groups (RAS and Conv) used the same pre-op orthopedic clinical care coordinators throughout the continuum. Finally, all the patients were part of NYU Winthrop's and CMS's 90-Day Bundled Payment Initiative. The Joint in Motion team meets at least monthly as part of our own continuing quality review; new initiatives are presented such as patient shadowing or evidence-based advances in pain management. There was no NYU Winthrop "dashboard" for real-time review of patient data metrics at this time. All data was retrospectively collected and sent to NYU Winthrop from CMS via the BPCI initiative with at least 3 to 4 quarter lag time from the time of the index intervention to receiving the data from CMS.

Discussion

The goal of successful TKR is having well-fixed and fitted components in a neutral mechanical axis with well-balanced soft tissues [34, 35]. We believe that RCAS-TKR with real-time validation is an excellent tool to help the surgeons attain these goals. Early failure rates may occur in TKR

when the final alignment is outside of the 3° window of the neutral mechanical axis, particularly in the setting of postoperative instability [36–38]. Compared with traditional methods, RCAS-TKR helps reduce the incidence of TKR outliers that may lead to early aseptic loosening and failure [17]. Soft tissue balancing and malalignment complications currently account for most early revisions. Revisions for stiffness, instability, and chronic pain currently outnumber those performed for infection. Recent studies have shown that these complications can significantly impact patient outcomes and satisfaction [39].

Our results have shown that introducing a RCAS-TKA system in a bundled payment model can help further reduce overall 90-day episode of care costs when integrated into an evidence-based care pathway. We believe the reduction we observed in overall TKR episode costs with RCAS versus conventional TKA at NYU Winthrop is a result of the improved reproducibility in knee alignment and soft tissue balance and reduced blood loss and systemic embolic release which are associated with RCAS-TKA. Those patients discharged to SAR after RAS-TKR had a shorter LOS in the SAR than the Conv-TKR group. We are not aware of any other published studies that have demonstrated reduced care episode costs when introducing RCAS-TKA in a bundled payment model.

In our hands the use of RCAS-TKR with virtual planning and robotic assistance has made it easier to consistently perform extremely accurate and efficient TKR's in cases from the smallest to the largest deformities. It does so by acting as a constant global positioning unit (GPS) for the leg that gives continuous feedback and instant validation to the surgical team so that they can formulate an individualized intraoperative TKR plan and base their many intraoperative decisions on real-time dynamic data. Moreover the consequences of very small 1–2 mm or 1–2° bone resections or soft tissue releases are instantly quantified, displayed, and validated to the surgical team in an easy-to-understand graphic fashion. We did find that knees with a preoperative valgus deformity of 10° or more were corrected significantly closer to neutral postoperatively than pre-op varus knees and even pre-op "neutral" knees. It is probable that bias toward mild varus is not because of the bone cuts which were validated to within the neutral mechanical axis range ± 3° but has more to do with the preoperative deformity and resulting state of a contracted stiff soft tissue envelope we often see in a varus knee. Also the author's (JAK) goal was to correct to within a 3° window of a neutral mechanical axis and not a goal of 0° alignment so that limited soft tissue releases were performed with that goal in mind.

RCAS-TKR that features virtual planning and robotic assistance not only helps to assure accuracy but can also save time and stress in difficult deformity cases. Our study showed that in one surgeon's hands, managing severe deformities in the coronal and sagittal planes only added 3–5 minutes of time on average [12]. This was achieved by intraoperatively assessing the patient's own pre-resection kinematics, formulating a virtual plan, and executing and validating in real time that plan's execution. Important intra-op corrections large or small are achieved easily and quickly, such as resecting more distal femur or proximal tibia, adding slope, or releasing soft tissues with real-time computer feedback and data not just "blind" visual confirmation and "feel" commonly used in traditional methods. The final alignment page (Fig. 17.2j) and graphical analysis quantify the final intra-op coronal and sagittal alignments as well as the soft tissue balance of the TKR, assuring the surgeon that he or she achieved what they originally planned: good correction of the pre-op deformity, restora-

tion of the proper mechanical alignment, and having a well-balanced knee with an improved arc of motion.

Many studies have documented improvements in achieving mechanical alignment to within 3° of neutral, with reported success rates in the ranges of 89–99% [40–42]. RCAS-TKR not only offers this degree of extreme accuracy but also delivers this to a now quantifiable higher level of efficiency. In the author's (JAK) current series now over 1000 successful implantations with OMNIBotics, the current average tourniquet time is 41 minutes with a >99.0% level of accuracy of achieving a neutral mechanical axis as we have improved our limited soft tissue balancing techniques. Ritter et al. [36] have published their retrospective results on over 5300 consecutive traditional TKR surgeries. They found knees with a preoperative deformity ≥8° varus or 11° valgus had a 4.3X> risk of early failure (aseptic loosening) than knees within the neutral range. They also found that knees with large deformities corrected to the neutral range had the lowest risk of early failure as compared with those under or over corrected. Ritter also found that knees regardless of preoperative deformity that were corrected to the neutral range (2.5°–7.5° of anatomic valgus) had the lowest risk of failure. Finally this prolific surgeon, teacher, and researcher of TKR reported that only 70% of all their knees were corrected to within the neutral range. This means that 30% of his TKR population were outliers that were subject to higher risk and rates of early failures from aseptic loosening and probably malalignment and instability or stiffness. In our current series now out over 1000 consecutive surgeries with OMNIBotics RCAS-TKR, we only report an outlier rate of <1% and never out by more than 1° varus or 1.5° valgus. We have no revisions in this group for aseptic loosening or instability; we have had 4 late infections ≥9 months post-op that did require one or two stage revision surgery. We have only seen 1 or 2 lateral releases in this 1000 case series, and we feel that is because we are doing a better job of getting the proper femoral rotation planned and executed. We conclude that using RCAS-TKR significantly lowers the rate of TKR alignment outliers and thus the rate and percentage of early failures and complications associated with malalignment, early loosening, stiffness, and pain.

Klima and Josten [43] reported longer femoral guide positioning times in their navigation techniques than we observed in our study: 11 minutes average for freehand navigation and 6 minutes for positioning of adjustable blocks (what JAK calls increased fiddle factor time). With our robotic cutting guide, we have demonstrated that femoral robotic guide positioning and preparation (boney cuts and validation) has been reduced to 5 minutes which is comparable if not more efficient than traditional TKR showing that the OMNIBotics system and RCAS-TKR are both more accurate and efficient as compared with traditional techniques and manual navigation without automation. Our study has also shown that, after 20–25 cases, we were able to consistently perform accurate and efficient RCAS-TKR's in about 49 minutes of tourniquet time, even when we were teaching other surgeons on the use of the system [17]. Moreover the small increases of minutes of surgical time we observed for severely deformed knees and for obese patients were not due to longer computer or robotic times as that stayed constant under $\leq$ 5 minutes. The slight increase in surgery times was rather related to more intensive soft tissue exposures, going back and performing limited soft tissue releases and validating them real time, or careful removal of posterior osteophytes to re-establish the posterior recess and extension, which are all inherent to the more complex cases. It is likely we have saved time via more accurate planning of increased bone resections and soft tissue and ligament releases, and not having to go back and recut and rebalance later. Most importantly the improved level of accuracy achieved as compared with traditional techniques was there from the first case to the last case in the series.

This is unlike previous studies published on patient-specific instruments (PSI) that report an accuracy level similar to traditional TKR [44, 45]. The combination of an individually programmable streamlined workflow, easy-to-interpret intuitive GUIs, virtual planning with constant intra-op feedback, and robotic precision with fine surgical control has certainly led to this extreme level of accuracy, precision, and efficiency.

Traditional TKR and PSI cannot provide this highly accurate and valuable intraoperative feedback as they both leave the computer out of the OR where you need it most. It is important to not only consider surgery time when comparing PSI techniques against other surgical techniques as there is additional time associated with the surgeon logging on to a computer to do his or her surgical plan statically outside of the operating room or confirming pre-op planning from an off-site software engineer. There is additional time and effort and cost associated with the office arranging and authorizing the scans as well as the patients' time and effort going for them and the co-pays associated with these scans. Using these static technologies such as PSI appears to remove one of the biggest benefits that this technology affords us; without RCAS-TKR, one loses the dynamic feedback and the instantaneous intraoperative validation associated with the steps of planning, bone resecting, soft tissue balancing, and final implant placement. It is our observed belief that RCAS-TKR maximizes the technological benefits helping to make surgeons better by providing constant feedback on bone resections and soft tissue envelope balancing.

Future Perspectives

We believe the next significant advancement in RCAS-TKA technologies will be directed toward intelligent active guidance systems for knee soft tissue balancing. We have recently introduced the active spacer, a novel active tensioning system that can be used for predictive stability-based implant planning as well as for assessment of final soft tissue balance after bone resections have been performed (Figs. 17.1 and 17.2) [46, 47]. Preliminary results in cadavers have demonstrated that when using active computer-controlled ligament tensioning, we are able to predict the effects of implant placement on the soft tissue envelope throughout the range of motion with a root-mean-square accuracy of approximately 1.6 mm [48]. Thus, the trade-off between boney alignment and soft tissue balance can be assessed before making cuts such that the knee is balanced throughout the ROM once the implants are in place, minimizing the amount of soft tissue releases required. Additionally, use of an active spacer that can precisely adjust its height to replicate the range of trial insert sizes and heights can significantly reduce the amount of trialing instrumentation required in the OR, thereby reducing costs and intraoperative complexity. It can also provide quantitative tension data to help the surgeon select the optimum tibial insert height and provide a record of the final tension the implant was left in which would allow us to correlate surgical techniques and balance to outcomes. Early clinical data has demonstrated that the system is accurate in predicting postoperative laxity in vivo [49] and that the angle at which the knee is balanced at in extension (i.e., at 0° or at 10° flexion) can significantly affect the shape of the knee laxity profile in early extension and in mid-flexion, suggesting that the implications of planning at 0° or at 10° flexion should be taken into consideration depending on the clinical circumstances of the case [50].

Conclusions

RCAS-TKA technologies have advanced significantly since their first introduction in TJR over 25 years ago [51]. More cost-effective, time-efficient, extremely accurate, versatile systems are now available that do not require preoperative imaging and work in synergy with the surgeon to achieve an optimally balanced and aligned knee with high reproducibility and short learning curve. Clinical data on the OMNIBotics system has demonstrated accurate and reproducible implant placement and leg alignment, high patient satisfaction, and knee functional outcomes, along with a shortened length of stay and reduced 90-day readmission rates when compared with conventional manual instrumentation. By integrating RCAS-TKA into a standardized,

coordinated evidence-based clinical care pathway, we have demonstrated that coupled with excellent quality indicators and short-term results, a further reduction in the overall cost per episode of care is attainable in a bundled payment reimbursement model.

References

1. CMS Innovation Center. https://innovation.cms.gov
2. Bundled Payments for Care Improvement (BPCI) Initiative: General Information. https://innovation.cms.gov/initiatives/bundled-payments/. 5 Apr 2017.
3. Siddiqi A, White PB, Mistry JB, Gwam CU, Nace J, Mont MA, Delanois RE. Effect of bundled payments and health care reform as alternative payment models in total joint arthroplasty: a clinical review. J Arthro. 2017. pii: S0883-5403(17)30263-2. https://doi.org/10.1016/j.arth.2017.03.027. [Epub ahead of print].
4. Iorio R, Clair AJ, Inneh IA, Slover JD, Bosco JA, Zuckerman JD. Early results of medicare's bundled payment initiative for a 90-day total joint arthroplasty episode of care. J Arthroplast. 2016;31(2):343–50. https://doi.org/10.1016/j.arth.2015.09.004. Epub 2015 Sep 9
5. Licini DJ, Meneghini RM. Modern abbreviated computer navigation of the femur reduces blood loss in total knee arthroplasty. J Arthroplast. 2015;30(10):1729–32.
6. Church JS, Scadden JE, Gupta RR, Cokis C, Williams KA, Janes GC. Embolic phenomena during computer-assisted and conventional total knee replacement. J Bone Joint Surg Br. 2007;89(4):481–5.
7. Choong PF, Dowsey MM, Stoney JD. Does accurate anatomical alignment result in better function and quality of life? Comparing conventional and computer-assisted total knee arthroplasty. J Arthroplasty. 2009;24(4):560–9.
8. de Steiger RN, Liu YL, Graves SE. Computer navigation for total knee arthroplasty reduces revision rate for patients less than sixty-five years of age. J Bone Joint Surg Am. 2015;97(8):635–42.
9. Koulalis D, O'Loughlin PF, Plaskos C, Kendoff D, Cross MB, Pearle AD. Sequential versus automated cutting guides in computer-assisted total knee arthroplasty. Knee. 2011 Dec;18(6):436–42.
10. Shalhoub S, Moschetti WE, Dabuzhsky L, Jevsevar DS, Keggi JM, Plaskos C. Laxity profiles in the native and replaced knee-application to robotic-assisted gap-balancing total knee arthroplasty. J Arthroplast. 2018. https://doi.org/10.1016/j.arth.2018.05.012.
11. Plaskos C, Koenig JA, Ponder CE. Robotic-assisted knee replacement surgery. In: Gomes P, editor. Medical robotics: minimally invasive surgery. Cambridge: Woodhead Publishing Ltd; 2012. p. 113–58.

12. Koenig JA, Plaskos C. Influence of Pre-Operative Deformity on Surgical Accuracy and Time in Robotic-Assisted TKA. Bone Joint J. 2013;95-B(S-28):62.

13. Dabuzhsky L, Neuhauser-Daley K, Plaskos C. Post-operative manipulation rates in robotic-assisted TKA using a gap referencing technique. Bone Joint J. 2017;99-B(Supp 3):87.

14. Ponder CE, Plaskos C, Cheal EJ. Press-fit total knee arthroplasty with a robotic-cutting guide: proof of concept and initial clinical experience. Bone Joint J. 2013;95-B(SUPP 28):61.

15. Koulalis D, O'Loughlin PF, Plaskos C, Kendoff D, Pearle AD. Adjustable cutting blocks for computer-navigated total knee arthroplasty: a cadaver study. J Arthroplast. 2010;25(5):807–11.

16. Suero EM, Plaskos C, Dixon PL, Pearle AD. Adjustable cutting blocks improve alignment and surgical time in computer-assisted total knee replacement. Knee Surg Sports Traumatol Arthrosc. 2012;20(9):1736–41.

17. Koenig JA, Suero EM, Plaskos C. Surgical accuracy and efficiency of computer-navigated TKA with a robotic cutting guide–report on the first 100 cases. J Bone Joint Surg Br. 2012;94-B((S)-XLIV):103.

18. Koenig JA, Neuhauser-Daley K, Shalhoub S, Plaskos C. Early patient outcomes and satisfaction of robotic-assisted total knee arthroplasty. 31st annual congress of the International Society for Technology in Arthroplasty (ISTA), 2018.

19. Li W, Ayers DC, Lewis CG, Bowen TR, Allison JJ, Franklin PD. Functional gain and pain relief after total joint replacement according to obesity status. J Bone Joint Surg Am. 2017;99(14):1183–9.

20. Lyman S, Lee YY, Franklin PD, Li W, Cross MB, Padgett DE. Validation of the KOOS, JR: a short-form knee arthroplasty outcomes survey. Clin Orthop Relat Res. 2016;474(6):1461–71.

21. Gøthesen Ø, et al. Functional outcome and alignment in computer-assisted and conventionally operated total knee replacements, a multicentre parallel-group randomised controlled trial. Bone Joint J. 2014;96-B:609–18.

22. Roos EM, Toksvig-Larsen S. Knee injury and osteoarthritis outcome score (KOOS) – validation and comparison to the WOMAC in total knee replacement. Health Qual Life Outcomes. 2003;1:17.

23. Choong PF, Dowsey MM, Stoney JD. Does accurate anatomical alignment result in better function and quality of life? Comparing conventional and computer-assisted total knee arthroplasty. J Arthroplast. 2009;24(4):560–9.

24. Gustke KA, Golladay GJ, Roche MW, Jerry GJ, Elson LC, Anderson CR. Increased satisfaction after total knee replacement using sensor-guided technology. Bone Joint J. 2014;96-B(10):1333–8.

25. Kayani B, Konan S, Tahmassebi J, Pietrzak JRT, Haddad FS. Robotic-arm assisted total knee arthroplasty is associated with improved early functional recovery and reduced time to hospital discharge compared with conventional jig-based total knee arthroplasty. Bone Joint J. 2018;100-B:930–7.

26. Turcot K, Sagawa Y Jr, Fritschy D, Hoffmeyer P, Suvà D, Armand S. How gait and clinical outcomes contribute to patients' satisfaction three months following a total knee arthroplasty. J Arthroplast. 2013;28(8):1297–300.

27. Bourne RB, Chesworth BM, Davis AM, Mahomed NN, Charron KD. Patient satisfaction after total knee arthroplasty: who is satisfied and who is not? Clin Orthop Relat Res. 2010;468(1):57–63.

28. Heck DA, Robinson RL, Partridge CM, Lubitz RM, Freund DA. Patient outcomes after knee replacement. Clin Orthop Relat Res. 1998;356:93–110.

29. Baker PN, van der Meulen JH, Lewsey J, Gregg PJ, National Joint Registry for England and Wales. The role of pain and function in determining patient satisfaction after total knee replacement. Data from the National Joint Registry for England and Wales. J Bone Joint Surg Br. 2007;89(7):893–900.

30. Noble PC, Conditt MA, Cook KF, Mathis KB. The John Insall Award: patient expectations affect satisfaction with total knee arthroplasty. Clin Orthop Relat Res. 2006;452:35–43.

31. Robertsson O, Dunbar M, Pehrsson T, Knutson K, Lidgren L. Patient satisfaction after knee arthroplasty: a report on 27,372 knees operated on between 1981 and 1995 in Sweden. Acta Orthop Scand. 2000;71(3):262–7.

32. CMS. BPCI model 2: retrospective acute & post acute care episode, 2017. https://innovation.cms.gov/initiatives/BPCI-Model-2/. Accessed 5 Dec 2017.

33. Koenig JA, Plaskos C. 90-day costs and clinical results of robotic-assisted and conventional TKA. 31st annual congress of the International Society for Technology in Arthroplasty (ISTA), 2018.

34. Insall JN. Total knee replacement. In: Insall JN, editor. Surgery of the knee. New York: Churchill Livingstone; 1984. p. 587–695.

35. Laskin RS, Denham RA, Apley AG. Replacement of the knee. New York: Springer-Verlag; 1984.

36. Ritter MA, Davis KE, et al. Preoperative malalignment increases risk of failure after total knee arthroplasty. J Bone Joint Surg Am. 2013;95:126–31.

37. Dalury DF, Mason JB, et al. Why are total knee arthroplasties being revised? J Arthroplast. 2013;28(8 suppl):120–1.

38. Schroer WC, Berrand KR, Lombardi AV, et al. Why are total knees failing today? Etiology of total knee revision in 2010 and 2011. J Arthroplast. 2013 Sep;28(8 Suppl):116–9.

39. Sharkey PF, Hozack WJ, et al. Why are total knees failing today—has anything changed after 10 years? J Arthroplast. 2014;29:1774–8.

40. Mason FA, Fehring TK, et al. Meta-analysis of alignment outcomes in computer-assisted total knee arthroplasty surgery. J Arthroplast. 2007;22(8):1097–106.

41. Ritschl P, Machacek J, et al. The Galileo System for implantation of total knee arthroplasty: an integrated

solution comprising navigation, robotics and robot assisted ligament balancing. In: Stiehl JB, Konermann W, Haaker R, editors. Navigation and robotics in total joint and spine surgery. Berlin: Springer-Verlag; 2004. p. 281–361.

42. Stulberg SD, Loan P, Sarin V. Computer-assisted navigation in total knee replacement: results of initial experience in thirty-five patients. J Bone Joint Surg Am. 2002;84-A((suppl)2):90–8.

43. Klima S, Zeh A, Josten C. Comparison of operative time and accuracy using conventional fixed navigation cutting blocks and adjustable pivotal cutting blocks. Comput Aided Surg. 2008;13(4):225–32.

44. Gonzales FB, Engh CA Jr, et al., Accuracy of CT-based patient specific total knee arthroplasty instruments. AAHKS 2010 Poster 7.

45. Nunley RM, Ellison BS, et al. Are patient specific cutting blocks cost-effective for total knee arthroplasty? Clin Orthop Relat Res. 2012;470(3): 895–902.

46. Plaskos C, Dabuzhsky L, Gill P, Jevsevar DS, Keggi J, Koenig JA, Moschetti WE, Sydney SV, Todorov A, Joly C. Development of an active ligament tensioner for robotic-assisted total knee arthroplasty: concept feasibility and preliminary cadaver results. Bone Joint J. 2017;99-B(SUPP 5):86.

47. Moschetti W, Keggi J, Dabuzhsky L, Jevsevar DS, Plaskos C. Dynamic robotic-assisted ligament tensioning and gap balancing in total knee arthroplasty: a cadaver study. Bone Joint J. 2017;99-B(SUPP 5):30.

48. Shalhoub S, Moschetti WE, Dabuzhsky L, Jevsevar DS, Keggi JM, Plaskos C. Laxity profiles in the native and replaced knee – application to robotic-assisted gap-balancing TKA. J Arthroplast. 2018;33(9):3043–8.

49. Shalhoub S, Randall AL, Lawrence JM, Keggi JM, Plaskos C. Validation of a Laxity Prediction Algorithm for gap-balancing total knee arthroplasty. Orthopaedic Research Society Annual Meeting. New Orleans, March 2018.

50. Shalhoub S, Plaskos C, Randall AL, Keggi JM, Lawrence JM, The effect of gap balancing at 0° versus 10° of flexion on extension and mid-flexion laxity in TKA. Orthopaedic Research Society Annual Meeting. New Orleans, March 2018.

51. Bargar WL, Bauer A, Borner M. Primary and revision total hip replacement using the Robodoc® system. Clin Orthop Relat Res. 1998;354:82–91.

Gregg R. Klein, Dugal James, and Jess H. Lonner

Conventional wisdom from decades of scrutiny regarding the mechanisms of failure in total knee arthroplasty (TKA) has been that precise bone resections within 2 or 3 degrees of variability from a neutral mechanical axis are of paramount importance to ensure implant durability and limit mechanical failures. Twenty years ago, component malalignment, malposition, and instability were common reasons for failure [1]. Despite a better understanding of the importance of achieving acceptable component alignment and soft tissue balancing during TKA, as well as improvements in instrumentation, implant materials, and designs that make them more durable

and accommodating of even subtle "errors," the incidence of failures related to instability, malalignment, or malposition is between 2.9% and 20.7% [2–4]. Some now suggest that a narrow range of component or limb alignment is less important than soft tissue balancing for success and durability in TKA [5, 6]. Still others have argued that positioning the limb and components in alignment with the native anatomy may better restore kinematics and soft tissue balance [7]. To be clear, however, despite the newer tolerances of "imprecision" or "malalignment," positioning the components or limb beyond some acceptable range, particularly when coupled with soft tissue imbalance, can lead to failure and thus must be mitigated [8].

Robotic tools were developed explicitly to optimize bone preparation and enhance limb and component alignment and position. Furthermore, semiautonomous robotic systems provide the additional and important vehicle for quantifying soft tissue balance in TKA, with the expectation that these elements, in concert, will improve kinematics, stability, functional outcomes, and durability [9]. At this time, the preponderance of data shows that compared to conventional manual methods of bone preparation, robotics shows greater precision and less variability in component alignment, with fewer outliers [10–14]. Additionally, robotic assistance can effectively quantify resection orientation in kinematic alignment methods for TKA, with commensurate

G. R. Klein
Hartzband Center for Hip and Knee Replacement,
Paramus, NJ, USA

Department of Orthopedic Surgery, Hackensack
University Medical Center, Hackensack, NJ, USA

Department of Orthopaedic Surgery, Hackensack
Meridian School of Medicine at Seton Hall,
Hackensack, NJ, USA

D. James
Bendigo Orthopaedic & Sports Medicine Practice,
Bendigo, VIC, Australia

J. H. Lonner (✉)
Department of Orthopaedic Surgery,
Rothman Orthopaedic Institute, Sidney Kimmel
Medical College, Thomas Jefferson University,
Philadelphia, PA, USA
e-mail: jess.lonner@rothmanortho.com

© Springer Nature Switzerland AG 2019
J. H. Lonner (ed.), *Robotics in Knee and Hip Arthroplasty*,
https://doi.org/10.1007/978-3-030-16593-2_18

alterations in the need for, or extent of, soft tissue releases [15] while minimizing the misjudgments and the frequency of errors of tibial and femoral coronal plane resections and femoral rotational resections in the so-called "kinematic" approach to TKA [16]. Notwithstanding the above-mentioned controversies on optimal alignment in TKA, robotic assistance should be able to deliver on a particular surgeon's preferences regarding targeted alignment [8]. Ongoing study is paramount to track functional outcomes and durability with newer robotic systems that combine precision of bone preparation and quantified soft tissue balancing. This chapter will review the early experience with the ROSA Knee robotic system (Zimmer Biomet, Warsaw, IN) for TKA.

ROSA Knee Robot System Description

First used in Australia in 2018, ROSA Knee robot (Fig. 18.1) received 510K clearance for use for TKA by the US Food and Drug Administration in January 2019. While some orthopedic robotic systems require the integration of additional advanced preoperative imaging studies, such as CT scans, for planning and integration for bone preparation [9, 10], ROSA Knee does not. ROSA Knee is unique in that it has two options for case

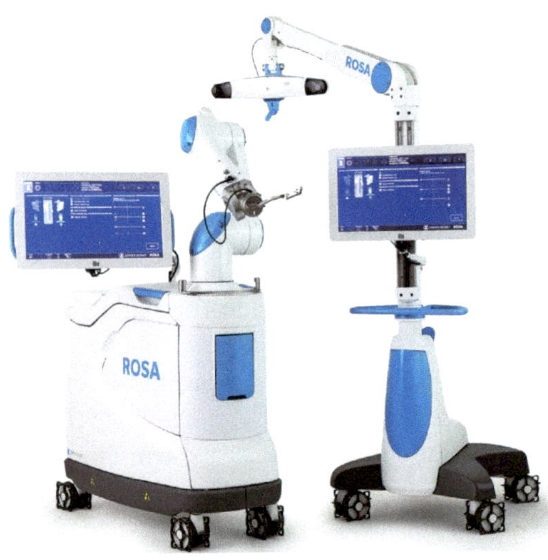

Fig. 18.1 The ROSA Knee Robot system

creation and plan development. One option is the morphing of a three-dimensional virtual model derived from the synthesis of data from preoperative plain radiographs with discrete surface bone and cartilage landmarks registered by the surgeon intraoperatively, serving as a check and balances approach to minimize inaccuracies from use of erroneous data. Compared to CT scans, the use of plain radiographs is less costly, requires less radiation exposure, and is less inconvenient to the patient, as no additional visits are required. The second option, which appears to be equally accurate, does not require any preoperative imaging and uses exclusively intraoperative bony and cartilage landmark acquisition as the guiding data input for three-dimensional modeling, intraoperative decision-making, and resection plans.

ROSA Knee is a robotically assisted semiautonomous surgical system that provides a continuum of data analysis derived from integration of the 3D model, intraoperative bone surface mapping and landmark registration, and soft tissue laxity measurements to augment the ability of surgeons to position surgical instruments, perform bone resections, and assess the balance of the soft tissue envelope in TKA surgery. It uses a captured resection model to precisely execute the preoperatively and intraoperatively determined patient specific plan. There is no constraint of the saw blade, in order to allow the surgeon to maintain the tactile "feel" of cutting the bone, although the resection guides are robotically constrained.

The ROSA Knee robot system has two main components which are positioned on opposite sides of the operating table. A robotic unit which consists of a robotic unit (robotic arm and touch screen) and an optical unit (the camera, positioning arm and touchscreen). The robotic arm contains three unique robotic modes to facilitate ease of use and provide safety during the procedure. In the automatic mode (orange color screen frame), the robotic arm will move to a predetermined position as directed by the computer system. In the collaborative mode (green color screen frame), the robotic arm will move if the surgeon applies a gentle force to the arm so the surgeon can manually move the arm to a desired position. In the stationary mode (gray color screen frame), the robotic arm will lock in place, other than allowing translation of the block tangential to the planned resections, as it is otherwise robotically constrained.

At the end of the robotic arm is the ROSA Knee TKA cut guide, which can be used with any of the Zimmer Biomet TKA implants (Persona®, NexGen®, and Vanguard ®). The robot unit, optical unit, instruments, and patient are linked by optical reference frames.

ROSA Preoperative Planning

While preoperative modeling is unnecessary, some surgeons will prefer the option of using preoperative radiographs to begin planning the surgery. In those circumstances, preoperative X-rays using conventional radiographic equipment are taken. X-ray technologists, trained on the technique, secure a re-usable calibrated X-ray marker to the patient's thigh and calf via a Velcro strap. Standing long leg AP and lateral radiographs are performed from the hip to the ankle. Most conventional radiographic systems can perform this procedure. The two-dimensional radiographic data is then uploaded to as secure portal, and a three-dimensional virtual model of the patient's bony structure and articular surfaces is created. If the surgeon prefers entirely image-free planning, without supplemental radiographs, then the surgeon can also effectively model, plan, and carry out surgery with ROSA Knee with precision.

ROSA Knee Procedure

OR Setup

The patient is placed supine on the operating table. The surgeon and the robot are positioned on the same side of the patient, and the optical system is positioned on the other (Fig. 18.2). The ROSA Knee system will allow the surgeon to stand on either side of the patient as per their standard surgical technique. The robot is positioned at the level of the patient's hip and is

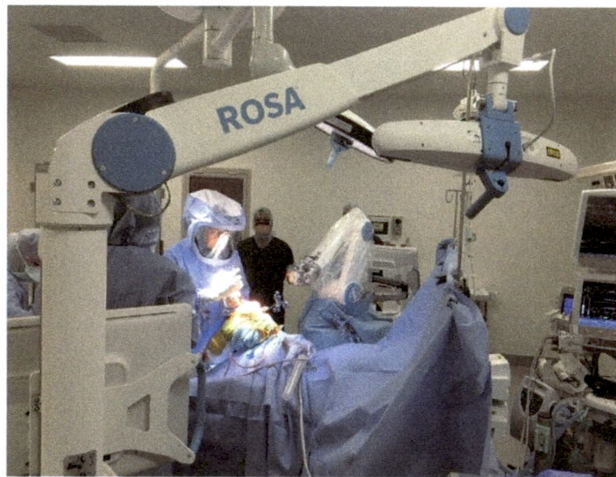

Fig. 18.2 View of the setup of robot within the operating room

angled approximately 45° relative to the table. A leg holder is not required to perform a ROSA Knee robotic procedure but can be helpful in stabilizing the leg.

Draping and calibrating the robot are performed by the surgical technologist and operating room staff either prior to or during the surgical exposure. This is guided on screen in a step-by-step fashion.

Tracker Placement

The trackers should be installed prior to, or after, arthrotomy and surgical exposure. The femoral tracker is placed approximately 4 fingerbreadths proximal to the skin incision parallel to the long axis of the bone. Pins can be inserted percutaneously or through a small incision. It may be helpful to flex the knee during tracker insertion to avoid tethering the quadriceps. Two self-drilling and self-tapping fixed fluted pins (3.2 × 150 mm) are inserted on power in the center of the femur achieving bicortical fixation. The femoral reference tracker is secured to the pins, as close to the bone as possible without impinging on the skin, roughly 1–2 cm from the skin.

The tibial tracker is placed roughly 4 cm distal to the skin incision. The tibial pins must be placed distal enough not to interfere with the keel preparation of the tibial component but at the same time trying to insert the pins in

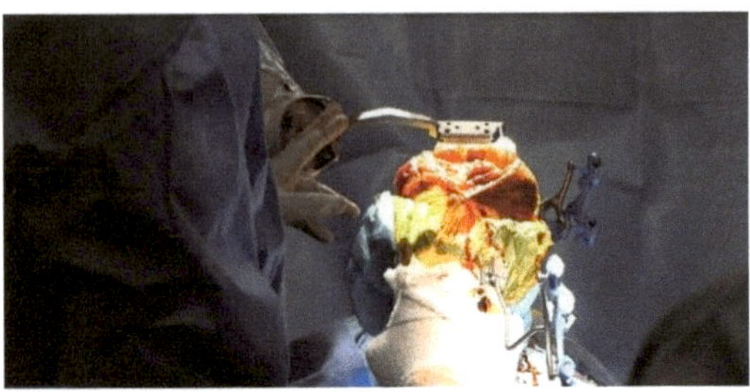

Fig. 18.3 Position of tracking arrays to avoid interference with the robotic arm

metaphyseal bone to minimize risk of pin site fracture. Two self-drilling and self-tapping fixed fluted pins (3.2 × 150 mm) are inserted bicortically along the long axis of the tibia angled toward the optical camera. The tibial reference tracker is placed as close to the bone as possible without compressing the skin. The stability of the pins and reference trackers should be confirmed, as movement during the procedure could result in errors in cuts or positioning. These tracker positions will ensure visualization by the optical camera during the surgical procedure through a full range of knee motion without interfering with, or being interfered by, the robotic arm (Fig. 18.3).

Landmark Registration

Once the trackers are placed, it is necessary to map, register, and digitize a series of bony and surface cartilage landmarks of the knee and limb. Again, this information can be morphed with the preoperative radiographs at the surgeon's discretion. The femoral head center is established by capturing 14 distinct positions of the hip during circumduction. The distal femoral canal entry point is obtained next, and the mechanical axis of the femur is thus determined. Further landmark registration points of the distal femur includes the posterior condyles, anterior trochlear groove, posterior trochlear groove, medial and lateral distal condyles, the medial and lateral epicondyles, and the anterior cortex. The posterior condyles are used to determine the posterior condylar axis, and the

anterior and posterior trochlear groove is used to determine the A/P axis. The anterior cortex is used for femoral sizing and A/P translational positioning and to determine if notching will occur. When landmarking articular surfaces, the ROSA Knee registration Pointer tip should not pierce the cartilage.

Landmarking of the tibia includes capturing the medial and lateral malleoli distally, the medial third of the tibial tubercle, the tibial canal entry point, the PCL insertion, and the medial and lateral plateau resection references. The system then determines the mechanical and rotational axes of the tibia.

Knee Evaluation

Once the landmarks are registered, the surgeon has the option to perform a Knee Evaluation. This is performed at three time periods during the procedure: initial, intraoperative, and postoperative after the implants are inserted. The knee is moved through a range of motion and ROSA Knee will quantify and save the following characteristics of the knee: range of motion, alignment, and medial, and lateral compartment gaps (Fig. 18.4). The values obtained can then be used to guide implant position, size, orientation, and soft tissue balancing.

The Laxity test is performed by either continuously moving the knee through a range of motion while applying varus and valgus stresses or bringing the knee to a series of discrete angles while applying a varus or valgus stress. The system defaults to recording values at 0° and 90°; however, an option exists to also record gap laxities at 30, 45, 60, and 120°, based on the surgeon's preferences.

The *Initial* state is the status of the knee prior to significant soft tissue releases and osteophyte removal. At this time, flexion contractures and coronal deformities can be quantified. The *Intra-Op* state is the same evaluation procedure after the knee has been balanced and prepared, including soft tissue balancing and osteophyte resection. This can be repeated multiple times to evaluate the effect soft tissue releases will have

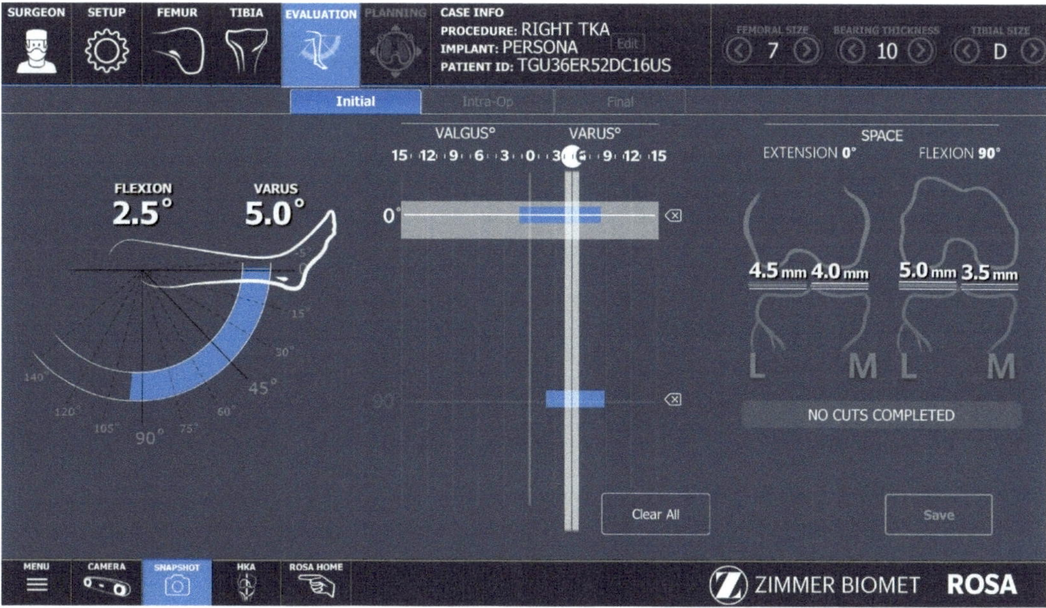

Fig. 18.4 The knee is brought through a range of motion without stressing the ligaments and then with varus and valgus stress to determine range of motion, as well as medial and lateral gap laxity or tightness

on the balance of the knee. The *Final* state is assessed after resections have been made and trials or final implants are inserted. Based on stability and positioning parameters at this point, further releases or adjustments in bone resections can be made to improve flexion or extension, coronal compartmental balance, sizing, etc. In addition, this test can be done at any time to see if specific surgical changes will influence the results.

Planning Panel

The planning panel is used intraoperatively to set the femoral and tibial component sizes and positions and orientations of bone resections (Fig. 18.5a, b). All parameters of the bone cuts and implant sizing and positions can be manipulated on screen to give a "virtual" understanding of the balance of the knee based on the planned implant positions. Manipulation of the implants will give "live" feedback on alignment and gaps (Fig. 18.6). Ultimately ROSA Knee will assist the surgeon in carrying out the cuts, precisely following the plan of resection.

Resection Panel

The Resection panel is where ROSA Knee software will guide the surgeon to perform the distal femoral resection, proximal tibial resection and femoral rotation resections by guiding the robotic arm with the cut guide to the appropriate position to perform the cuts and prepare the bone.

The sequence of bone cuts – either tibia or femur first – can be individualized based on the surgeon's preference. If the surgeon chooses to use the ROSA Knee femoral rotation soft tissue tensioning algorithm, it is necessary to perform the distal femoral and proximal tibial resection prior to making the anterior, posterior, and chamfer femoral cuts with application of the 4-in-1 cutting block. If the surgeon chooses to use standard measured resection protocol, the femoral rotation can be determined by the posterior condylar axis or the A/P axis.

Proximal Tibial Resection

The proximal tibial resection tab is selected. The foot pedal is pressed to bring the robotic arm to the

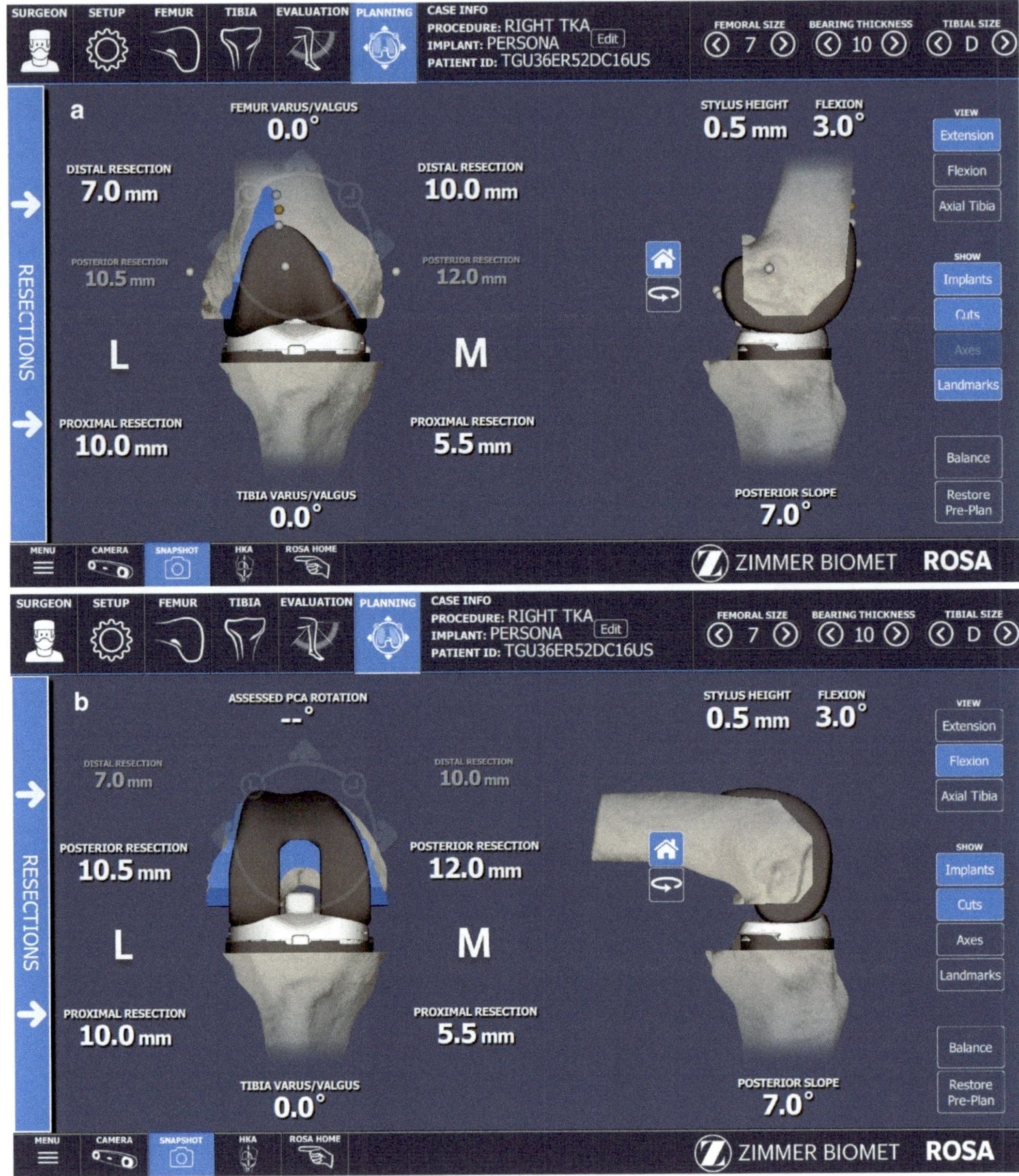

Fig. 18.5 After registering points on the knee surfaces and limb, planning of implant sizing, position, orientation of resections, and gap balancing are performed (in both extension (**a**) and flexion (**b**))

tibial cut plane in automatic mode. This will bring the arm in the appropriate cut plane close to the bone. The ROSA Knee arm will then stop, enter collaborative mode, and the surgeon will need to apply a gentle force to the cut guide to move it to contact the anterior tibial cortex. In collaborative mode, the guide's cut orientation, depth, and slope will be robotically constrained, although the guide remains free to move medially and laterally. With the foot pedal pressed, a pin is placed through the cut guide into bone. On screen, data will show live cut values. If values are acceptable, the second pin can be placed. A standard manual saw cut through the robotically constrained guide is performed,

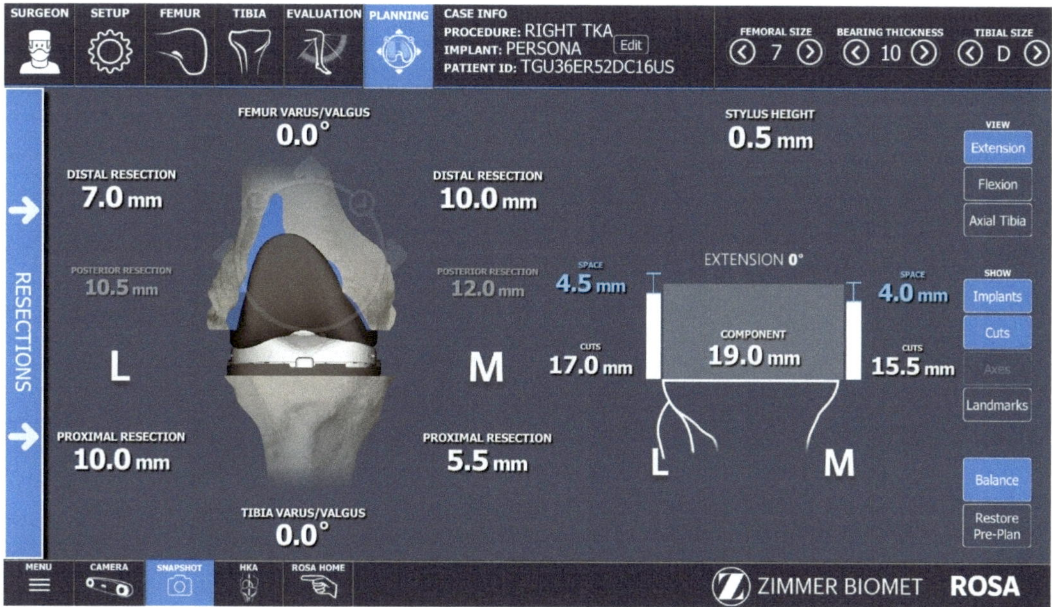

Fig. 18.6 Virtual assessment of gap balancing can inform the orientation of resections, implant positioning, and sizing, as well as soft tissue releases

without any constraint of the saw itself, in order to enhance ergonomics. The pins are removed, and the foot pedal is pressed to move the arm away from the bone. The validation tool is placed on the tibial resection to confirm the cut values correspond with the plan.

Distal Femoral Resection

Once the screen tab for distal femoral resection is selected, the foot pedal is pressed to bring the robotic arm to the femoral cut plane in automatic mode. This will bring the arm in the appropriate cut plane close to the bone. The arm will then stop and ROSA Knee will enter collaborative mode, after which the surgeon will apply a gentle force to the cut guide to move it to the bone. In collaborative mode, the cut plane, slope, volume, and orientation are robotically maintained, but medial and lateral movement will be possible until the guide is pinned. With the foot pedal pressed, a pin is placed through the cut guide into bone. On screen, data will show live cut values. If values are acceptable, the second pin can be placed. Again, a

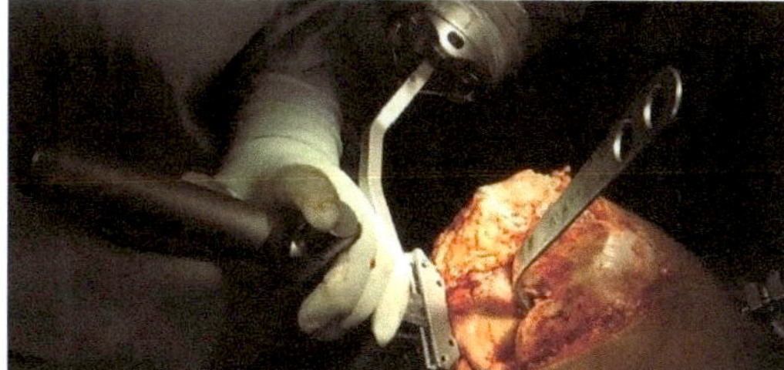

Fig. 18.7 ROSA Knee robot stabilizing the tibial cutting guide on the anterior tibia for the proximal tibial resection

manual saw cut is then made through the robotically constrained guide (Figs. 18.7 and 18.8). The pins are removed, and the foot pedal is pressed to move the arm away from the bone. The validation tool is placed on the distal femur to confirm the cut values correspond with the plan.

Femoral Rotation Using ROSA Knee Rotation Tool

An optional feature of ROSA Knee is the Femoral Rotation Tool, which guides the anterior and posterior rotational cuts of the femur

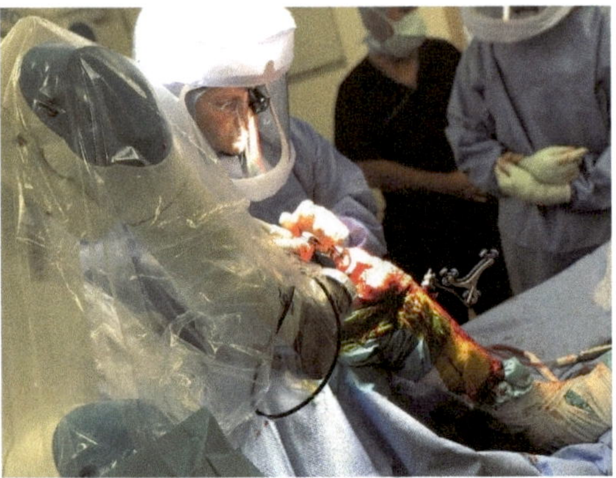

Fig. 18.8 Resection through the distal femoral cutting guide

based on a balanced flexion gap. If this option is selected, the ROSA Knee system will provide quantitative information about ligament laxity in flexion and extension after the surgeon performs a "pull" or distraction test. With the knee in approximately 90 degrees of flexion, a manual pull test is performed. Lamina spreaders or a Zimmer FuZion® instrument can be used to equally tension the medial and lateral compartments in flexion. ROSA Knee will record the flexion gap values and assess femoral component rotation. The 4-in-1 femoral resection can now be performed based on the data obtained by the ROSA Rotation tool.

Femoral 4-in-1 Measured Resection Method

The 4-in-1 resection tab is selected, and the foot pedal is depressed to move the robotic arm to the distal femur. The robot enters the collaborative mode, and the guide is placed on bone, aligning it according to the predetermined parameters as described above (referenced from the AP axis of the femur, posterior femoral condyles, or based on ligament tension with the knee in 90 degrees of flexion). The distal femur is drilled through the robotic cut guide. The robotic arm is removed from the field, and the 4-in-1 cut is performed using the cutting block.

Implantation

The trial implants are then manually provisionally implanted, and the postoperative knee state evaluation can be performed to assess the knee balance and range of motion. If the results are approved, proceed with final manual implantation. If alignment, range of motion, or balance is not satisfactory, the surgeon can return to the planning tool to adjust surface preparations or redo component position as desired.

Results

The early data in 30 TKAs performed with the ROSA Knee robot shows a high level of precision of tibial and femoral bone resection orientations and alignment. Compared to historical controls using conventional manual techniques or computer navigation in TKA, ROSA Knee has fewer outliers [17]. When using ROSA Knee robot for TKA, 99.9% of limb hip-knee-angles were within ±3 degrees of the plan, as compared to 87.2% when using conventional computer navigation or 69.9% with manual instrumentation [17]. Additionally, with ROSA Knee, 99% of coronal, sagittal, and rotational alignment parameters were within 3 degrees of the plan when using ROSA Knee, compared to the substantially greater percentage of outliers that have been reported with computer navigation and manual instrumentation (Table 18.1). Further analysis of quantified soft tissue balance and functional outcomes with ROSA Knee is not yet available.

Summary

Despite recent debate regarding tolerable levels of "imprecision" in TKA, malalignment beyond some acceptable range (particularly when coupled with soft tissue imbalance) can lead to failure and is thus undesirable. Early evidence with ROSA Knee robotic system suggests that not only is the technology effective at restoring or achieving the planned orientation of femoral and tibial bone

Table 18.1 Percentage of alignment parameters within ±3 degrees of plan

Alignment Parameters	ROSA Knee	Computer Navigation [17]	Manual Technique [17]
Femur var/val	100	93	83.6
Femur flex/ext	98.9	82.7	65.7
Tibia var/val	100	94.2	87.6
Tibia slope	99.9	84.2	74.6
Femur rotation	99.2	81.2	85.5
Coronal HKA	99.9	87.2	69.9

resections, but also quantifying soft tissue balance, with a rapid learning curve and acceptable surgical efficiencies. Further clinical follow-up will be needed to corroborate our expectation that intraoperative, real-time mapping of a patient's anatomy and motion, coupled with augmented precision of bone resection, implant position and soft tissue balance provided by ROSA Knee will facilitate personalization of TKA procedures and improve functional outcomes and durability.

References

1. Sharkey PF, Hozack WJ, Rothman RH, Shastri S, Jacoby SM. Insall award paper. Why are total knee arthroplasties failing today? Clin Orthop Relat Res. 2002;7:13.
2. Schroer WC, Berend KR, Lombardi AV, Barnes CL, Bolognesi MP, Berend ME, et al. Why are total knees failing today? Etiology of total knee revision in 2010 and 2011. J Arthroplast. 2013;28(8 Suppl):116–9.
3. Dalury DF, Pomeroy DL, Gorab RS, Adams MJ. Why are total knee arthro- plasties being revised? J Arthroplast. 2013;28(8 Suppl):120–1.
4. Thiele K, Perka C, Matziolis G, Mayr HO, Sostheim M, Hube R. Current failure mechanisms after knee arthroplasty have changed: polyethylene wear is less common in revision surgery. J Bone Joint Surg Am. 2015;97:715–20.
5. Parratte S, Pagnano MW, Trousdale RT, Berry DJ. Effect of postoperative mechanical axis alignment on the fifteen-year survival of modern, cemented total knee replacements. J Bone Joint Surg Am. 2010;92(12):2143.
6. Ritter MA, Davis KE, Meding JB, Pierson JL, Berend ME, Malinzak RA. The effect of alignment and BMI on failure of total knee replacement. J Bone Joint Surg Am. 2011;93(17):1588.
7. Howell SM, Howell SJ, Kuznik KT, Cohen J, Hull ML. Does a kinematically aligned total knee arthroplasty restore function without failure regardless of alignment category? Clin Orthop Relat Res. 2013;471:1000–7.
8. Lonner JH, Fillingham YA. Pros and cons: a balanced view of robotics in knee arthroplasty. J Arthroplast. 2018;33:2007–13.
9. Jacofsky DJ, Allen M. Robotics in arthroplasty: a comprehensive review. J Arthroplast. 2016; https://doi.org/10.1016/j.arth.2016.05.026.
10. Bargar WL. Robots in orthopaedic surgery: past, present, and future. Clin Orthop Relat Res. 2007;463:31–6.
11. Urish KL, Conditt M, Roche M, Rubash HE. Robotic total knee arthroplasty: surgical assistant for a customized normal kinematic knee. Orthopedics. 2016;39:e822–7.
12. Liow MH, Xia Z, Wong MK, Tay KJ, Yeo SJ, Chin PL. Robot-assisted total knee arthroplasty accurately restores the joint line and mechanical axis. A prospective randomized study. J Arthroplast. 2014;29:2373–7.
13. Dabuzhsky L, Neuhauser-Daley K, Plaskos C. Postoperative manipulation rates in robotic-assisted TKA using a gap referencing technique. Bone Joint J. 2017;99-B(SUPP 3):87.
14. Koenig JA, Suero EM, Plaskos C. Surgical accuracy and efficiency of computer-navigated TKA with a robotic cutting guide–report on the first 100 cases. J Bone Joint Surg Br. 2012;94-B(S)-XLIV:103.
15. Calliess T, Ettinger M, Savov P, Karkosch R, Windhagen H. Individualized alignment in total knee arthroplasty using image-based robotic assistance: video article. Orthopade. 2018;47(10):871–9. https://doi.org/10.1007/s00132-018-3637-1.
16. Cinotti G, Ripani FR, Ciolli G, La Torre G, Giannicola G. The native coronal orientation of tibial plateaus may limit the indications to perform a kinematic aligned total knee arthroplasty. Knee Surg Sports Traumatol Arthrosc. 2018; https://doi.org/10.1007/s00167-018-5017-0. [Epub ahead of print].
17. Hetaimish BM, Khan MM, Simunovic N, Al-Harbi HH, Bhandari M, Zalzal PK. Meta-analysis of navigation vs conventional total knee arthroplasty. J Arthroplast. 2012;27:1177–82.

Total Knee Arthroplasty Technique: TSolution One (Robodoc)

Ming Han Lincoln Liow, Pak Lin Chin, and Seng Jin Yeo

Background

The Robodoc system (Curexo Technology, Fremont, CA) was the first robotic system to be used in orthopedic surgery in 1992 [1]. Robodoc is an active-autonomous, image-based, robotic milling system that enables the surgeon to attain a consistently accurate implant component positioning [2]. It was developed originally to improve bony ingrowth and address the high intraoperative fracture rates associated with the use of cementless total hip arthroplasty (THA). Initial human trials were conducted in 1992, and Germany was an early adopter of this technology in 1994 [3]. The technology and accompanying software was relatively immature, resulting in high rates of complications in early trials. This was a significant setback to the advancement of robotic technology, and the United States Food and Drug Administration (FDA) only approved Robodoc 14 years later in 2008 [4]. However, the technology continued to evolve and improve to overcome the initial setbacks. In September 2014, Curexo Technology Corporation changed its name to Think Surgical Inc.

Although initially designed solely for femoral canal preparation, Robodoc can be used today for total knee arthroplasty (TKA) surface preparation through active-autonomous milling. This has expanded the orthopedic surgeon's armamentarium for TKA, enabling the surgeon to reproduce technical excellence via accurate component placement and attain an ideal hip-knee-ankle (HKA) mechanical axis (MA) reliably [2]. The Robodoc system is capable of achieving these technical feats through an image-based preoperative planning system which allows the surgeon to create, view and analyze the surgical outcome in 3D. These 3D rendered images allow the surgeon to anticipate optimum resection depth, restore HKA MA through deformity correction and select predetermined component sizes. This capability is particular important in TKA as component positioning is paramount to the success of the procedure. The ability to have a surgical endpoint prior to the surgery is a unique capability o Orthopedic robotic-assisted surgery [5].

Restoration of the mechanical axis (MA) within $3°$ has been reported to be associated with better clinical outcomes and implant survivorship [6–8]. Robodoc has been shown to achieve reduction of MA outliers through precise and accurate component implantation [9]. The accuracy and precision of component positioning have been attributed to the following factors. First, a customized distal femoral resection angle is used as opposed to a fixed resection angle $(5–6°)$ used in

M. H. L. Liow (✉) · S. J. Yeo
Department of Orthopaedic Surgery, Singapore General Hospital, Singapore, Singapore

P. L. Chin
The Orthopaedic Centre, Mount Elizabeth Medical Centre, Singapore, Singapore

© Springer Nature Switzerland AG 2019
J. H. Lonner (ed.), *Robotics in Knee and Hip Arthroplasty*,
https://doi.org/10.1007/978-3-030-16593-2_19

conventional TKA. A fixed resection angle has been associated with coronal plane mechanical axis deviation [10]. Second, accurate preoperative determination of the rotational alignment of the femoral component can be achieved with robotic-assisted TKA. In contrast, estimation using either the transepicondylar axis, Whiteside's line or posterior condylar axis has only 65–80% accuracy [11]. Third, robotic-assisted milling of bone surfaces results in errors of 0.15–0.29 mm versus 0.16–0.42 mm in a conventional procedure using an oscillating saw [9]. This is important as a maximum distance of 0.3–0.5 mm between bone and the implant may impair osseous integration in noncemented femoral implants [12]. The inaccuracies in hand-held bone sawing may also result in implant alignment variability by up to 1.1° of varus/valgus and 1.8° of flexion/ extension, even if the cutting guides are placed perfectly [13]. Lastly, temperature of bone is maintained within the threshold of 44–47 °C with constant irrigation and control of the robotic milling speed. Temperatures beyond this threshold result in bony injury and compromised implant fixation and are frequently encountered during the use of an oscillating saw in conventional surgery [14].

Despite all these advantages, there is still a paucity of long term, high-quality data that demonstrates the efficacy of Robodoc TKA. Majority of existing literature has demonstrated improvements in radiological outcomes with no significant differences in functional scores [2, 15, 16], with only one study reporting subtle improvements in health-related quality of life measures in Robodoc patients [17]. Questions regarding radiation risks, prolonged surgical duration and cost-effectiveness remain unanswered. The objectives of this chapter are to describe: (1) Robodoc surgical technique; (2) limitations and complications; and (3) clinical and radiological outcomes.

Robodoc Surgical Technique

Indications for robotic-assisted TKA using the Robodoc system are similar to conventional TKA. Ideal patients should be older than 60 years old, have body mass index <25 kg/m², end-stage osteoarthritis, mild to moderate coronal deformity, a fixed flexion deformity less than 15° and intact neurovascular status of the affected limb. Relative contraindications include obese patients with severe coronal deformity >15°, fixed flexion deformity >15°, inflammatory arthropathy and ligamentous laxity.

Preoperative radiography (anteroposterior, lateral, skyline, long-leg films) and computed tomography (CT) of the affected lower limb are performed. A fine-cut (<3 mm) CT scan is essential for the preoperative "virtual surgery." The CT images are imported into the ORTHODOC workstation (Curexo Technology Corp, Seoul, Korea) for image-based preoperative planning (Fig. 19.1). The data enables the creation of hip/ knee/ankle joints surface models, allowing the surgeon to identify anatomical landmarks and definition of the HKA MA. The desired mechanical axes are determined for the femur and tibia separately. Robodoc is an "open" platform which allows the surgeon to select virtual femoral and tibial implants based on the type / size of implant required (posterior-stabilized or cruciate-retaining). The virtual implants are matched onto the surface models to attain a virtual HKA axis of 180° with a sagittal, posterior tibial slope in accordance with prosthesis manufacturer's instrumentation guide. Femoral component rotation is parallel to the transepicondylar axis. Tibial component rotation in the axial plane is based off the posterior cruciate insertion point and a point marking the medial 1/3 width of the tibial tuberosity. Time taken for "virtual surgery" is approximately 15–20 minutes. The preoperative image-based plan is finalized generated for each patient and saved onto a compact disc.

This preoperative image-based plan is uploaded to Robodoc prior to surgery. Robodoc is draped and prepared in a sterile manner. A thigh tourniquet is applied and the leg is fixed using a custom foot holder and thigh support (Fig. 19.2). A midline, conventional incision followed by a standard medial parapatellar approach, with patella eversion and patelloplasty, was performed. Stabilization pins, navigation markers and bone movement monitors were put in place and work-

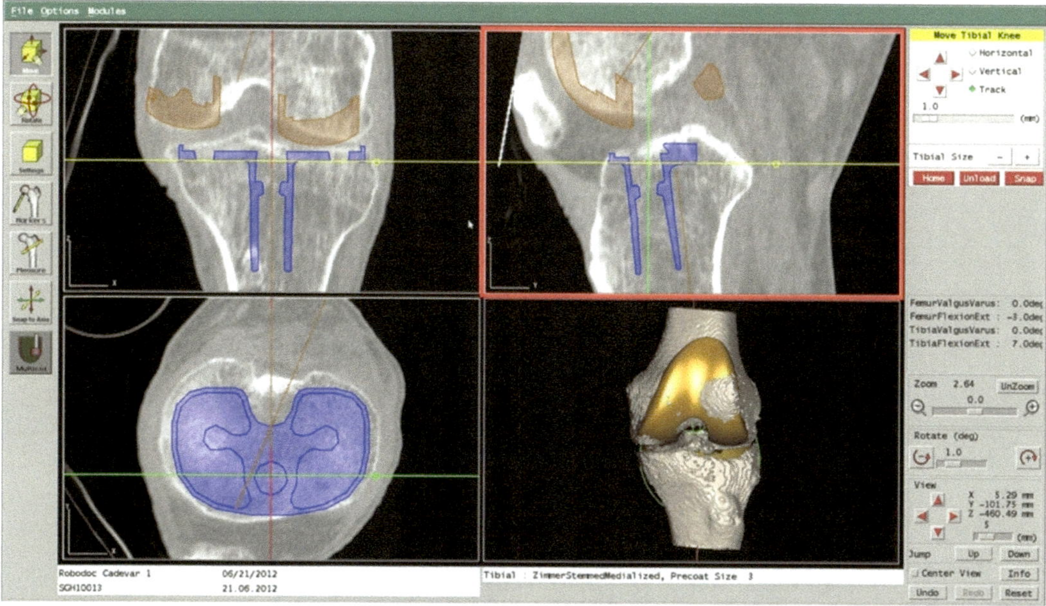

Fig. 19.1 Virtual surgery conducted using ORTHOdoc workstation

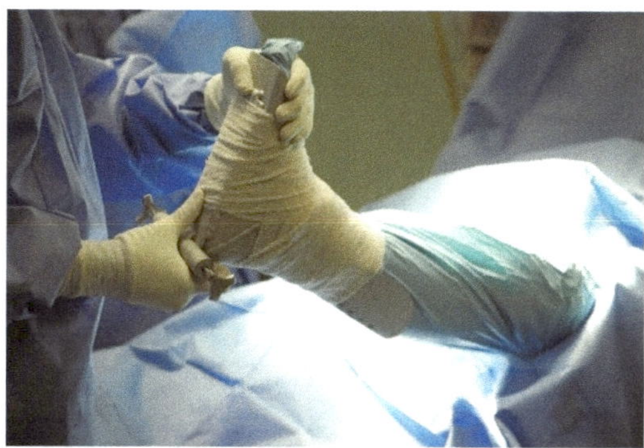

Fig. 19.2 Customized foot and thigh holder

space checks conducted prior to the rigid mating of the patient to Robodoc. Upon completion of workspace checks, the patient is rigidly connected to Robodoc via two transverse stabilization pins in the distal femur and proximal tibia. These two pins are connected to a special fixation frame mounted on Robodoc (Fig. 19.3). The surgeon will identify anatomic landmarks on the femur (Fig. 19.4) and the tibia (Fig. 19.5) and digitize these points as part of the registration process. Upon completion, Robodoc will match the preoperative image-based plan with the intraoperative registration, thereby formulating a milling work-

space for the femur and tibia in three dimensional space.

The surgeon activates Robodoc which proceeds to complete all femoral and tibia bone cuts via the robotic miller (Fig. 19.6). The surgeon maintains control over the milling cutter via a manual override safety button. This process is aided by constant water irrigation for cooling and the removal of milling debris. Soft tissue balancing and a trial of the predetermined femur and tibia components are performed once the milling process is completed. Finalized components were cemented, and stability, patellar tracking and range of motion were assessed. Patella can be selectively resurfaced based on the degree of cartilage wear. An intrasynovial and intramuscular analgesic injection is given if there are no contraindications. Wound closure is performed in a routine fashion via layered closure with absorbable monocryl skin sutures. Postoperatively, all patients received standard mechanical and pharmacologic thromboprophylaxis. Rehabilitation in accordance with the integrated care pathway was prescribed. Weight-bearing radiographies (anteroposterior, lateral, skyline, long- leg films) are performed at the specialist outpatient clinic at one-month follow-up.

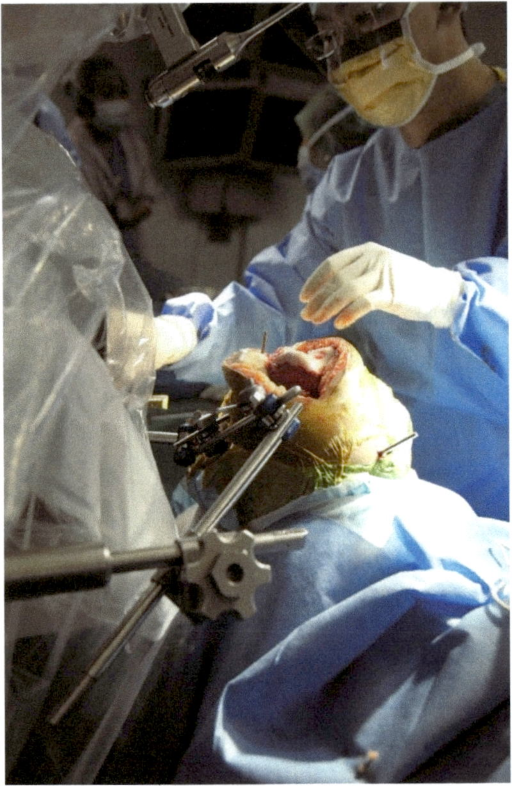

Fig. 19.3 Rigid mating of the patient to Robodoc

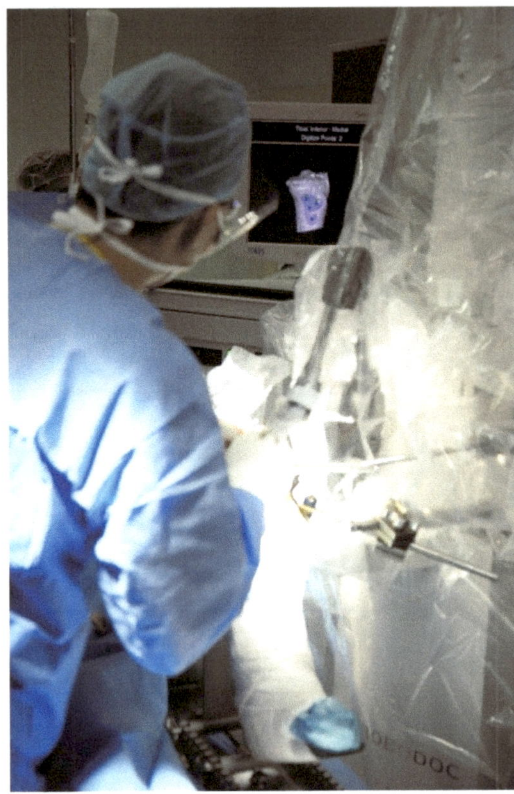

Fig. 19.5 Digitization of tibial landmarks

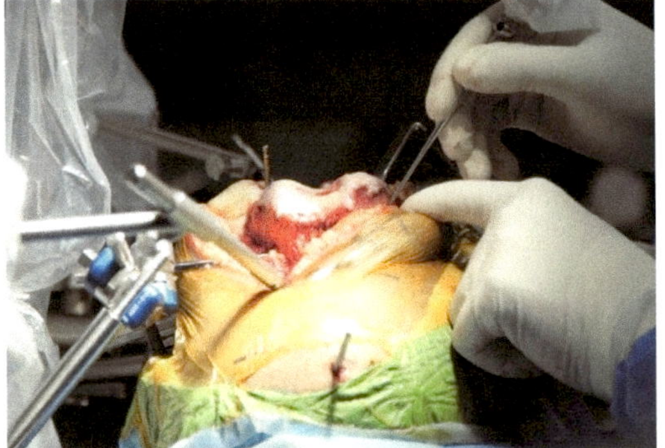

Fig. 19.4 Digitization of femoral landmarks

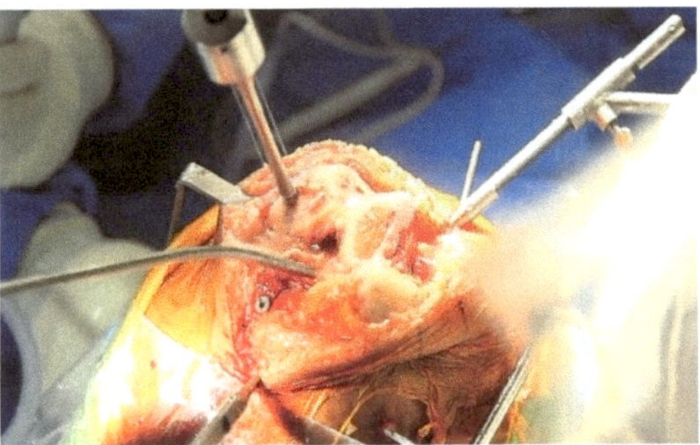

Fig. 19.6 Robotic miller working on femur

Limitations and Complications of Robotic-Assisted TKA

Robodoc TKA has not been proven to be cost-effective due to the lack of long-term survivorship and outcome data. In addition, Robodoc is an image-based system and a preoperative CT scan is required for all patients undergoing Robodoc TKA, exposing patients to avoidable radiation that is not required in conventional procedures [18, 19]. Of note, there are other robotic TKA systems such as which are imageless, however, these systems lack preoperative planning data and are unable to verify the registration points with preidentified anatomic landmarks. In addition, they frequently rely on optical markers which suffer from line of sight issues. Both imaged-based and imageless systems still rely heavily on accurate identification of bony landmarks to ensure that the preoperative strategy is carried out as planned. Regardless, incorrect registration will result in execution of the preoperative plan in a wrong plane, which can be catastrophic.

Workspace related errors are common for Robodoc and occur when Robodoc perceives that the knee is outside the miller's working range. The current system performs planned cuts within the predetermined 3D workspace and does not have fail-safes or the ability to differentiate between difference tissue types. This requires the surgeon to move soft tissues away from the path of the miller, or stop Robodoc to prevent damage to soft tissues during the procedure. New system updates need to address the possibility of soft tissue detection to prevent iatrogenic injury, capability to perform soft tissue balancing and allow modification of the preoperative plan during surgery if there is a need for augments or constraint [20]. Attention to proper positioning of the patient and Robodoc prior to rigid coupling and strict compliance with Robodoc-led workspace checks will reduce the risk of such errors.

Related to workspace errors, the lack of intraoperative versatility while using Robodoc results in abandonment and conversion to a conventional procedure, resulting in time and monetary losses, as well as unnecessary radiation. Such cases have been reported to be as high as 22%, and it is essential to understand, anticipate and prevent such occurrences [21].

Procuring a Robodoc system (Fig. 19.7) does not guarantee better outcomes or a return of the investment. A high capital (USD 800,000) and recurring cost per patient (USD 1500) are required to operate a robotic surgical system in our institution. Cost and other regulatory hurdles including government and insurance companies continue to resist adoption of expensive, new technology which has not demonstrated definite cost-effectiveness [22]. In addition, initial unfamiliarity and the inevitable learning curve for surgeons who opt to use Robodoc will result in prolonged surgical duration, which will add to indirect costs.

However, it has been reported that arthroplasty centers with robotics may experience greater market growth when compared to centers without robotics [23]. A recent study has also used a Markov decision analysis model to demonstrate that robotic-assisted unicompartmental knee arthroplasty is more cost-effective than conventional surgery when there is less than 1.2% failure rates at 2 years and more than 94 cases are performed annually [24]. Based on advances in robotics in other fields, cost-effectiveness and efficacy of robotic-assisted TKA will continue to improve over time and allow it to be adopted as a mainstream TKA procedure.

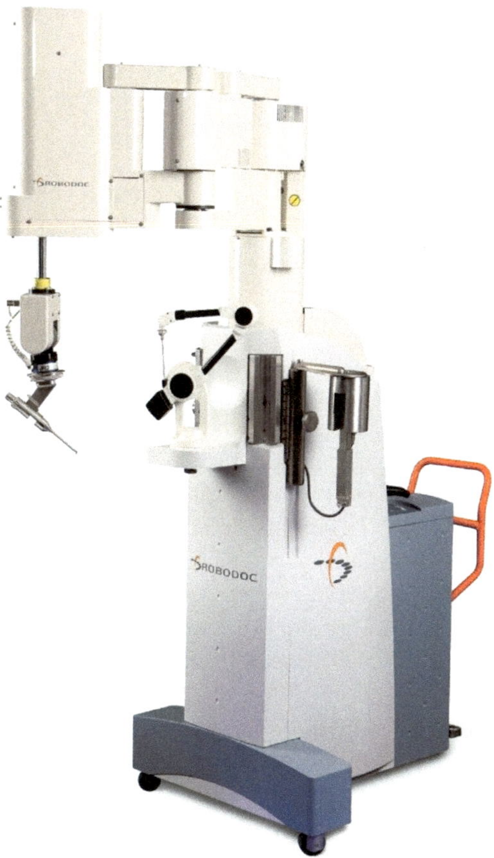

Fig. 19.7 Robodoc system. (Courtesy of Curexo, Seoul, Korea)

Robodoc is an open platform which allows different manufacturer implants to be used in accordance to surgeon's preference or patient's individualized needs. Open platforms such as Robodoc provide surgeons with the convenience of inbuilt 3D implant data for multiple designs but may theoretically lack the depth of biomechanical kinematic data present in closed platforms which use proprietary implants.

In our institution's experience, rigid positioning of the lower extremity during Robodoc procedure may have resulted in two cases of soleal

vein thrombosis. This has prompted us to ensure sufficient wool padding when applying the Robodoc surgical leg holder. Though widely reported in Computer Assisted Surgery, we did not experience any pin-site related complications such as pin site infections or periprosthetic fractures. In addition, we did not have any cases of periprosthetic infection which were attributed to prolonged surgical duration.

Clinical Outcomes

Robotic-assisted TKA has demonstrated clinical success and excellent radiological outcomes. Multiple studies comparing Robodoc assisted TKA and conventional TKA have reported 0% outliers in the Robodoc assisted group [2, 9, 16]. Kim et al. recently demonstrated good radiological and clinical outcomes of Robodoc TKA in end-stage hemophilic arthropathy with severe bony deformity and destruction [25]. However, there is a paucity of long-term clinical outcomes of Robodoc TKA, with short and mid-term studies demonstrating no significant difference in functional outcomes when compared to conventional TKA. Park and Lee compared outcomes of robotic-assisted TKA with conventional knees and reported no differences in Knee Society Scores at a mean follow-up of 4 years [26]. Interestingly, Song et al. reported higher but non-statistically significant HSS and Western Ontario and McMaster Universities (WOMAC) health-related quality-of-life (HRQoL) scores in the Robodoc cohort in 2 studies [15, 16]. Similarly, our institution reported subtle improvements in HRQoL measures, noting significantly larger percentage of Robodoc patients attaining Minimal Clinically Importance Differences (MCID) in SF-36 HRQoL scores [17]. This may represent an early indication of improved functional outcomes associated with accurate joint alignment restoration after robotic-assisted TKA.

Conclusion

Current literature indicates that robot-assisted TKA consistently improves overall mechanical alignment and reduces variability with some emerging evidence supporting definite improvements in clinical outcomes. Will the improved component positioning, enhanced mechanical alignment and correction of joint-line lead to better long-term functional outcomes, higher satisfaction rates and implant longevity? Should surgeon remain cautious and delay adoption of robotic-assisted TKA until the day it demonstrates cost-effectiveness and provides better value for patients than conventional TKA?

We are at the 'preindustrial' phase of the robotic surgical evolution and it is difficult to predict the type of technological innovation that will continue to transform robotic-assisted TKA. Future innovations include improvements of robotic TKA workflow, advanced intraoperative gap balancing sensors, new biomimetic implant designs which can replicate prearthritic knee kinematics and robotically controlled instrumentation and soft tissue balancing.

In conclusion, robotic TKA technology will continue to grow and revolutionize Orthopedic surgery. Robotic technology is advancing rapidly today and will gradually become an indispensable adjunct to the Orthopedic surgeon, allowing optimization of patient-specific arthroplasty.

References

1. Paul HA, et al. Development of a surgical robot for cementless total hip arthroplasty. Clin Orthop Relat Res. 1992;(285):57–66.
2. Liow MH, et al. Early experiences with robot-assisted total knee arthroplasty using the DigiMatch

ROBODOC(R) surgical system. Singap Med J. 2014;55(10):529–34.

3. Bargar WL. Robots in orthopaedic surgery: past, present, and future. Clin Orthop Relat Res. 2007;463:31–6.

4. Jakopec M, et al. The first clinical application of a "hands-on" robotic knee surgery system. Comput Aided Surg. 2001;6(6):329–39.

5. Siebert W, et al. Technique and first clinical results of robot-assisted total knee replacement. Knee. 2002;9(3):173–80.

6. Jeffery RS, Morris RW, Denham RA. Coronal alignment after total knee replacement. J Bone Joint Surg Br. 1991;73(5):709–14.

7. Ritter MA, et al. The effect of alignment and BMI on failure of total knee replacement. J Bone Joint Surg Am. 2011;93(17):1588–96.

8. Berend ME, et al. Tibial component failure mechanisms in total knee arthroplasty. Clin Orthop Relat Res. 2004;(428):26–34.

9. Bellemans J, Vandenneucker H, Vanlauwe J. Robot-assisted total knee arthroplasty. Clin Orthop Relat Res. 2007;464:111–6.

10. Kharwadkar N, et al. 5 degrees to 6 degrees of distal femoral cut for uncomplicated primary total knee arthroplasty: is it safe? Knee. 2006;13(1):57–60.

11. Miller MC, et al. Optimizing femoral component rotation in total knee arthroplasty. Clin Orthop Relat Res. 2001;392:38–45.

12. Bellemans J. Osseointegration in porous coated knee arthroplasty. The influence of component coating type in sheep. Acta Orthop Scand Suppl. 1999;288:1–35.

13. Plaskos C, et al. Bone cutting errors in total knee arthroplasty. J Arthroplast. 2002;17(6):698–705.

14. Eriksson RA, Albrektsson T. The effect of heat on bone regeneration: an experimental study in the rabbit using the bone growth chamber. J Oral Maxillofac Surg. 1984;42(11):705–11.

15. Song EK, et al. Simultaneous bilateral total knee arthroplasty with robotic and conventional techniques: a prospective, randomized study. Knee Surg Sports Traumatol Arthrosc. 2011;19(7):1069–76.

16. Song EK, et al. Robotic-assisted TKA reduces postoperative alignment outliers and improves gap balance compared to conventional TKA. Clin Orthop Relat Res. 2013;471(1):118–26.

17. Liow MH, et al. Robotic-assisted total knee arthroplasty may lead to improvement in quality-of-life measures: a 2-year follow-up of a prospective randomized trial. Knee Surg Sports Traumatol Arthrosc. 2017 Sep;25(9):2942–51.

18. Karthik K, et al. Robotic surgery in trauma and orthopaedics: a systematic review. Bone Joint J. 2015;97-B(3):292–9.

19. Smith-Bindman R, et al. Radiation dose associated with common computed tomography examinations and the associated lifetime attributable risk of cancer. Arch Intern Med. 2009;169(22):2078–86.

20. Urish KL, et al. Robotic total knee arthroplasty: surgical assistant for a customized normal kinematic knee. Orthopedics. 2016;39(5):e822–7.

21. Chun YS, et al. Causes and patterns of aborting a robot-assisted arthroplasty. J Arthroplast. 2011;26(4):621–5.

22. Davey SM, et al. Surgeon opinion on new technologies in orthopaedic surgery. J Med Eng Technol. 2011;35(3–4):139–48.

23. Jacofsky DJ, Allen M. Robotics in arthroplasty: a comprehensive review. J Arthroplast. 2016;31(10):2353–63.

24. Moschetti WE, et al. Can robot-assisted unicompartmental knee arthroplasty be cost-effective? A Markov decision analysis. J Arthroplast. 2016;31(4):759–65.

25. Kim KI, et al. Robot-assisted total knee arthroplasty in haemophilic arthropathy. Haemophilia. 2016;22(3):446–52.

26. Park SE, Lee CT. Comparison of robotic-assisted and conventional manual implantation of a primary total knee arthroplasty. J Arthroplast. 2007;22(7):1054–9.

Total Hip Arthroplasty Technique: Mako

Douglas E. Padgett, David J. Mayman, and Seth A. Jerabek

The era of the modern day hip replacement was heralded by the seminal work of Sir John Charnley and the Low Friction Arthroplasty. Charnley recognized the importance of load transfer across the joint and that for THA to remain durable, the need for implant fixation [1] and appropriate materials [2]. The early results of THA have been nothing less than spectacular. At 20-year follow-up, the results of the original cemented total hip cohort demonstrated a 6% loosening rate of the acetabular component and a 2% loosening rate on the femoral side [3]. Unfortunately, with longer term follow-up as younger cohorts entered the 3rd decade, loosening rates on both the femoral and acetabular side increased significantly [4]. In this concise report on cemented Charnley implants in patients under the age of 50, only 46% of patients were revision-free, suggesting the limitations of cement fixation. What has evolved over the ensuing 2 decades has been the gravitation toward cementless fixation which has greatly improved survivorship even in the group of younger, more active patients. McLaughlin [5] reported his results of minimal 20 years of follow-up on patients under 50 years of age demonstrating a 0% loosening rate on the femoral side. These data clearly suggest that fixation of hip arthroplasty is becoming more predictable.

Unfortunately, failure remains an issue in THA. Bozic and investigators [6] using aggregated United States inpatient sample data found that the most common cause for revision was instability (22.5%) followed by mechanical loosening (19.7%). While these data represent sampling from 2005 through 2006, mechanical loosening includes both failure of cemented implants, failure of first generation uncemented implants, and osteolysis-driven loosening. What is clear from this study is that instability and bearing related failure poses a risk for the long-term success of THA.

Instability has been suggested to be multifactorial including patient factors, implant factors, and surgical factors including implant position [7]. It has a long held orthopedic tenet that implant alignment has an effect upon the risk of instability after THA [8]. Lewinnek described what has long been an accepted concept of a "safe-zone" for acetabular position to mitigate the risk of instability. His concept of approximately 40° of abduction and 15° of anteversion appeared logical and has been the desired alignment goal. While recently some have questioned this "static" picture of optimized implant position [9], in general most surgeons agree that this target position appears reasonable to achieve a stable articulation.

In addition to reducing the risk of instability, reducing acetabular positioning outliers also has

D. E. Padgett (✉) · D. J. Mayman · S. A. Jerabek
Department of Orthopaedic Surgery, Hospital for Special Surgery, New York, NY, USA
e-mail: padgettd@hss.edu

© Springer Nature Switzerland AG 2019
J. H. Lonner (ed.), *Robotics in Knee and Hip Arthroplasty*,
https://doi.org/10.1007/978-3-030-16593-2_20

an impact on bearing wear. Kligman [10] and coauthors were able to demonstrate that higher abduction angles were clearly associated with increased polyethylene wear in a cohort of primary THA. The mechanism of this added wear has been suggested to be the result of the vector of loading attributable to the joint reaction force. In addition, poor composite implant position can lead to prosthetic implant impingement. Impingement has been demonstrated in retrieved implants and may have a profound impact on both articular as well as backside wear [11, 12]. From these data, it is readily apparent that optimized implant position is crucial to ensuring long-term survivorship as well as minimizing risk of instability and bearing wear. The question has been how best to ensure predictable implant positioning.

Reproducible implant positioning unfortunately remains elusive using unaided instrumentation. In a critical review of a series of over 2000 THAs performed at a high-volume center by experienced arthroplasty surgeons, Callanan [13] found that only 50% of acetabular components were within the desired range of abduction and anteversion using a modification of the Lewinnek "safe-zone" as their target. Even with mechanical guides, the range of implant position is quite variable. In a series of primary THA that I performed using one of these instruments, the range of implant abduction spanned from 22° to 57° with a target goal of 40 [14]. While variations in patient positioning on the operating table in the lateral decubitus position may have certainly played a role in this wide range, it is clear that these results are not acceptable. These observations have stimulated many surgeons to pursue alternative strategies to improve implant alignment.

There was and remains an interest in enabling technologies to accomplish this goal and began initially with computer navigation. Navigation – whether using image-guided or imageless techniques – was greeted with some level of enthusiasm and adoption into routine practice. One of the limitations of navigation however has been the inconsistent reproducibility of acetabular component anteversion.

In a study looking at minimally invasive THA using free-hand versus imageless navigation, Sendtner observed an improvement in implant positioning, however there was a fairly wide variability in acetabular anteversion and more consistency in achieving the desired abduction angle [15]. It has been these observations that have led to the interest in robotic assistance as a tool for enabling improvement in total hip positioning.

Robotic-assisted total hip arthroplasty (rTHA) was first introduced as an active robotic system over 25 years ago [16]. Active robotics can be thought of as self-driven. The basics of this robotic system was based upon the principles of computer-aided design and manufacturing. Once the preoperative plan is derived, computer-driven mechanical burrs and reamers are enabled to accurately prepare bone for prosthetic implantation. These investigators were able to validate the precision and accuracy of this process for bone preparation and implantation. While embraced by many centers, detractors of active robotics cite a lack of direct control during surgical procedures. As a result of this, alternatives to active robotics has evolved.

In the late 1990s, researchers at Z-KAT Inc. began working on a novel robotic system for medical applications. The unique approach to computer-assisted surgery focused upon the use of haptics to guide the surgeon in performing medical tasks. The field of haptic guided robotics relates to the sense of touch and proprioception. The haptic guidance defines the boundaries within which the surgeon can "operate" thus retaining control during the procedure. Z-KAT's original technology was based upon the "Whole Arm Manipulator" or WAM which was developed in conjunction with researchers from Massachusetts Institute of Technology (MIT), USA. In 2004, Z-KAT became Mako Surgical and its team led by Rony Abovitz and Arthur Quaid demonstrated proof of concept in the use of haptically guided technology in the field of orthopedics. The first clinical application was utilized in performing partial knee arthroplasty. Its use in total hip arthroplasty was a logical extension of the technology.

Technique

Haptically guided total hip arthroplasty using the Mako system (Stryker, Fort Lauderdale, FL) originates with preoperative computerized tomographic imaging of the patient's pelvis and proximal femur, including select sectioning of the distal femur to determine condylar axis which allows calculation of version. From these images, pelvic and hip anatomy are precisely measured and a team of segmentation specialists confirm the patient's bony architecture. Regions of interest include hip length, offset, as well as femoral version (Fig. 20.1). Length and offset can be compared to the contralateral side if desired. 3-D planning for total hip arthroplasty is then undertaken.

Default acetabular component position is placement in the anatomic position, defined at the level of the inter-teardrop line, with cup abduction of 40° and anteversion of 20°. Anteversion is relative to the plane of the CT gantry. In determining sizing of the acetabular component, the planning boundaries are the medial extent of "Kohlers line," inferior to the obturator foramen

and the superolateral boundary of the subchondral plate. The "planned" cup position can be modified in all three planes: medial-lateral / cephalad-caudad / and anterior-posterior. The "planned cup" position often results in a change in the location of the center of rotation and this should be accommodated for by appropriate adjustments on the femoral side (Fig. 20.2).

At this time, 3-D planning for the femoral component is performed. Using implants whose CAD models have been incorporated into the planning software, an accurate determination of the optimal stem can be determined. Factors to note include the impact of stem geometry upon length, offset and version. Femoral version must be taken into account in determining the degree of desired acetabular version (Fig. 20.3a). The concept of combined version as described by Dorr [17] is useful in adjusting version accordingly. Recognizing that there is often little latitude in adjusting version on the femoral side, especially when utilizing uncemented fixation, socket version adjustments should be made in order to achieve the desired combined effect. At this point, preoperative planning is complete.

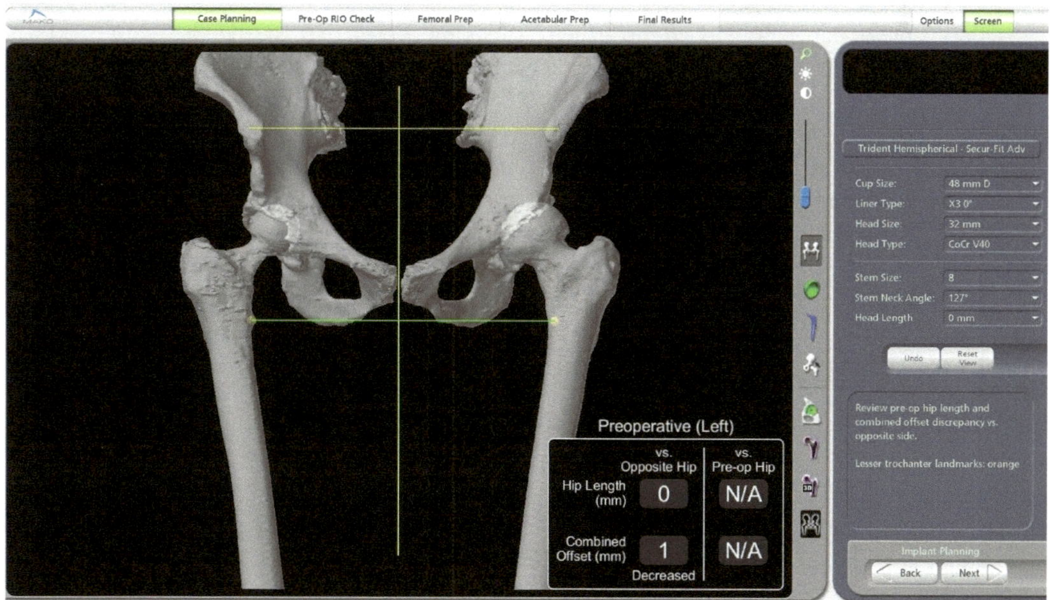

Fig. 20.1 Haptically guided total hip arthroplasty using the Mako system (Courtesy of Stryker, Fort Lauderdale, FL) originates with preoperative computerized tomographic imaging of the patient's pelvis, including hip length, offset, as well as femoral version

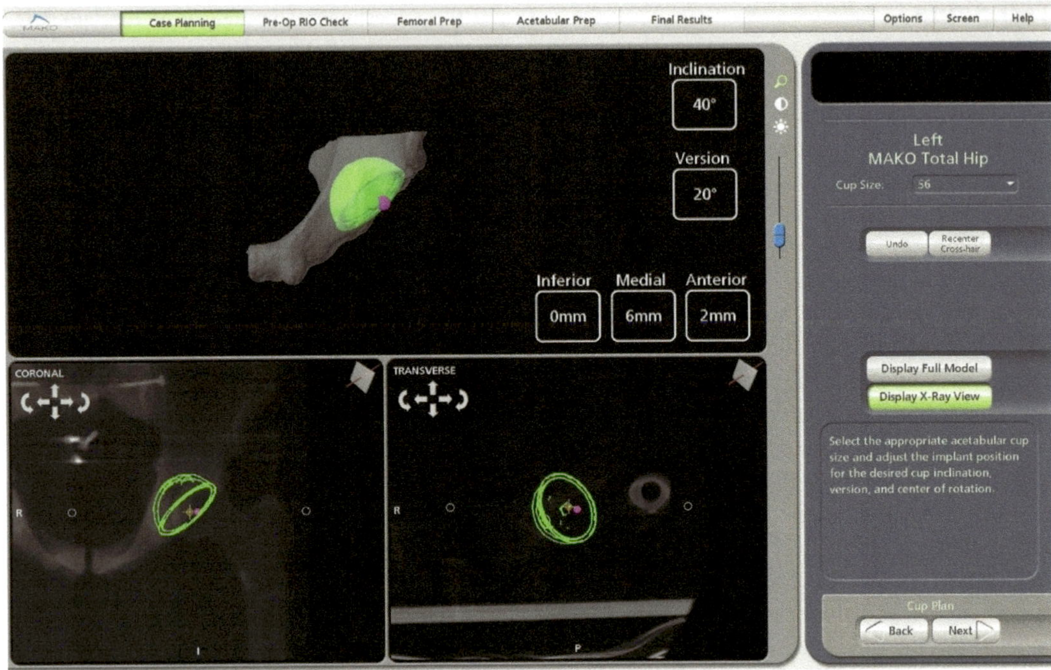

Fig. 20.2 The "planned cup" position often results in a change in the location of the center of rotation with adjustments on the femoral side

A computer prediction of what the final reconstruction should look like can be seen on the computer screen (Fig. 20.3b).

The principle of haptically guided hip arthroplasty requires that there is accurate information flow to and from the robot and the computer that drives its function. Precise knowledge of where the patient is in space as well as the working aspect of the robot, the end effector, is critical for the system to function. Before actual surgical incision occurs, robot registration is performed. To accomplish this, the end effector of the robotic arm is equipped with an array that has a series of reflective markers (Fig. 20.4a, b). In addition to the end effector, the robot position itself is captured by tracking an array attached to the front of the robotic housing (the base array). A light source placed typically at the head of the operating table and the arrays are tracked to establish the location of robotic system in space. Once the robot has been registered, surgical exposure may commence.

Haptically guided total hip arthroplasty may be accomplished using a variety of surgical approaches although it was initially described using the posterolateral approach. The only modification of surgical exposure is the need to place tracking arrays into the pelvis. Most surgeons place tracking pins into the iliac crest although it is possible to place pelvic array pins within the wound. Pelvic tracking pins can be placed at any time of the surgery prior to acetabular preparation.

Following surgical exposure, femoral registration is performed. An array is placed into the proximal femur as well as a smaller checkpoint screw to verify accuracy of registration. Multiple points along the proximal femur, as dictated by the computer software, are obtained using the registration probe (Fig. 20.5). These multiple points verify the anatomy as defined by the preoperatively obtained CT scan. An acceptable error for registration should be less than 0.5 mm. Once the femur has been registered, an exact level of femoral neck osteotomy is determined based upon the preoperative plan.

Based upon the previous concept of combined anteversion, femoral preparation is performed

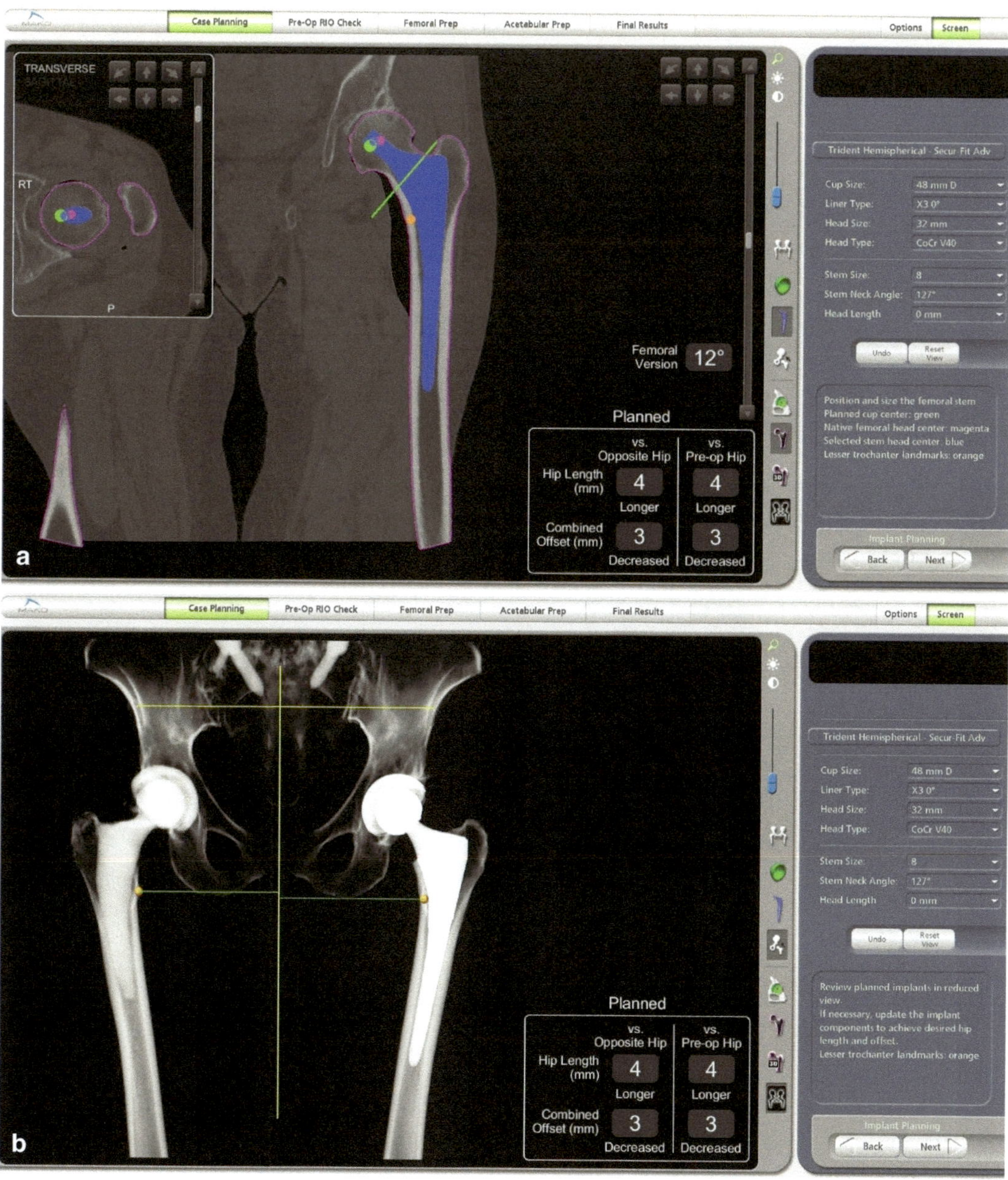

Fig. 20.3 (a) Femoral version must be taken into account in determining the degree of desired acetabular version. (b) A computer prediction of what the final reconstruction should look like can be seen on the computer screen

first. "Ream and broach" or "broach only" techniques may be used. Once the final broach is inserted, a measurement of center of rotation as well as version can be made (Fig. 20.6). Based upon these findings, adjustments in socket orientation such as either increasing or decreasing anteversion may be made. In addition, changes to femoral implant choice which may affect leg length and offset can be considered at this time as well.

Socket preparation begins with pelvic registration. Pelvic tracking pins either in the iliac crest or "in-wound" should be in place. A pelvic check point which can be used at any time to ascertain the integrity of registration and array placement is then inserted. Similar to femoral

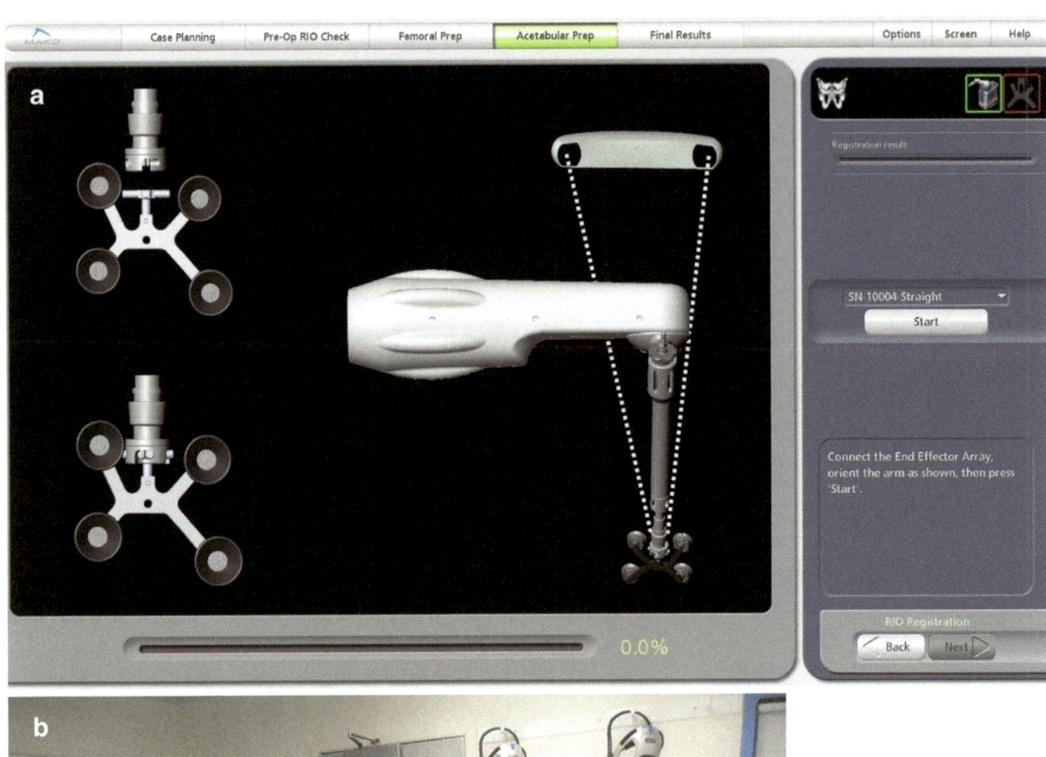

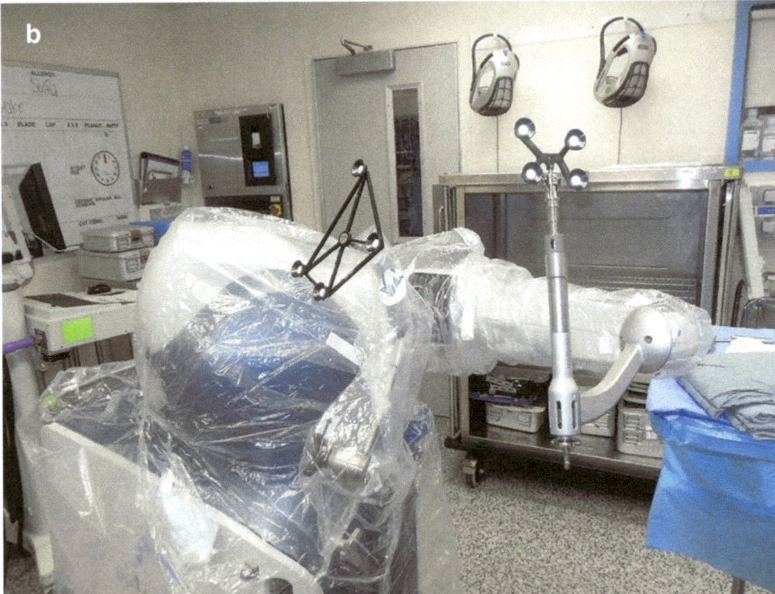

Fig. 20.4 (**a, b**) Before a surgical incision occurs, robot registration is performed by the end effector of the robotic arm, which is equipped with an array that has a series of reflective markers

registration, pelvic registration is accomplished by using the probe to verify multiple bony landmarks in proximity to the acetabular vault (Fig. 20.7). These points again should conform to the anatomic model obtained from the preoperative CT scan. Once registration is complete,

haptically guided acetabular preparation is ready to begin.

Acetabular reaming is performed within a haptic cone: meaning that while the tip of the reamer is constrained, the reamer is permitted to move within a conical area in order to remove

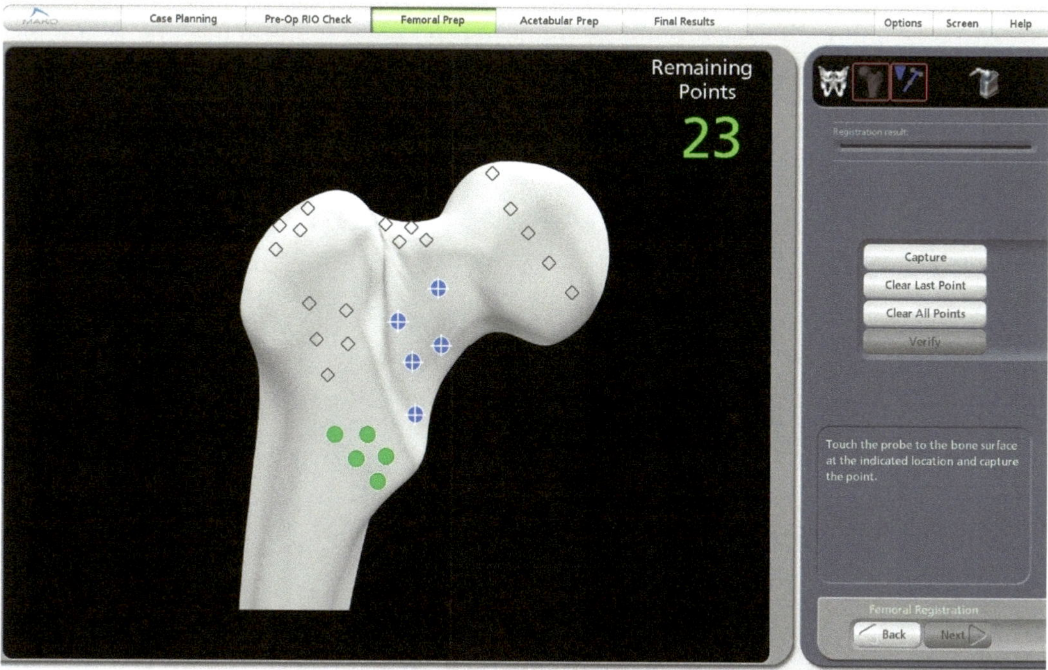

Fig. 20.5 Femoral registration occurs at multiple points along the proximal femur, as dictated by the computer software

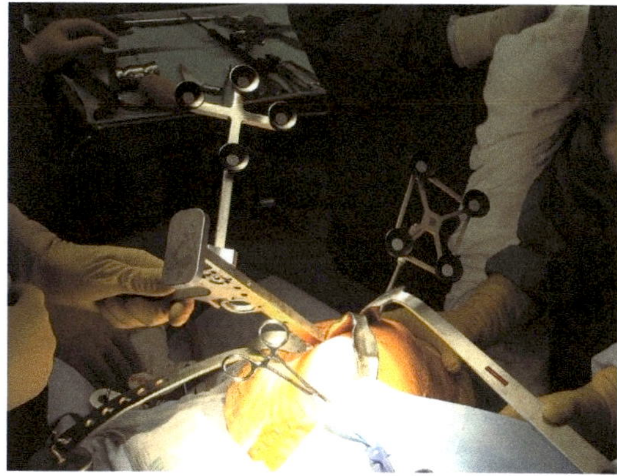

Fig. 20.6 Once the final broach is inserted, a measurement of center of rotation as well as version can be made

predetermined amount of bone. This feature allows the surgeon to remain in control of the reaming function (Fig. 20.8a, b). Some surgeons prefer to use a single reamer of the size compatible with the acetabular component to be inserted. My preference is to use sequential reaming (multiple reamers) to avoid the reaming basket getting overfilled with removed bone and monitor all planes of bone removal. Remember,

if your registration is erroneous, then inadvertent depth and orientation of bone removal is possible.

Following acetabular bone removal, acetabular component insertion proceeds. The acetabular component is attached to the end effector and after final verification of registration error, cup impaction proceeds. Unlike acetabular reaming, cup insertion occurs with line haptics, meaning the system will not allow deviation from the plane and the component orientation is "held" in the predetermined orientation (Fig. 20.9). Once the acetabular component is in place, confirmation of position is established by acquiring 5 points around the periphery of the cup using a probe (Fig. 20.10) and final orientation is established. This typically will conform to the preoperative plan but minor deviations may occur especially upon impaction in instances of extremely dense sclerotic bone. At this point, after placement of the acetabular line, the hip is reduced. With arrays on the femur as well as the pelvis, the reduction results are seen. Change in length as well as offset based upon the new center of rotation is observed. Based upon these

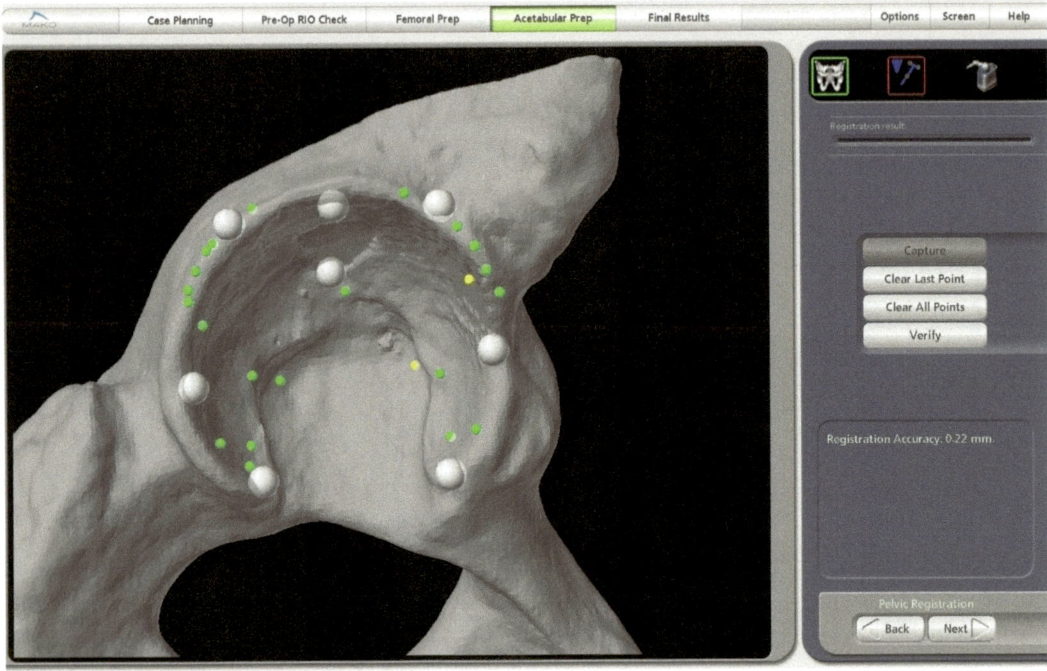

Fig. 20.7 Pelvic registration is accomplished by using the probe to verify multiple boney landmarks in proximity to the acetabular vault

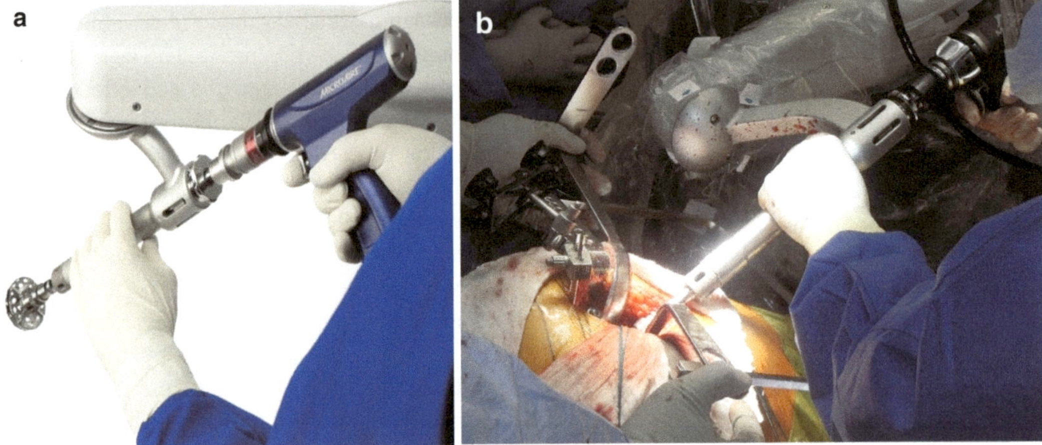

Fig. 20.8 (**a, b**) Acetabular reaming is performed within a haptic cone. (**a** courtesy of Stryker, Kalamazoo, MI, USA)

observations, the surgeon will either replace the trial implant with the actual implant or an implant with differing length or offset as needed to reach the desired goals.

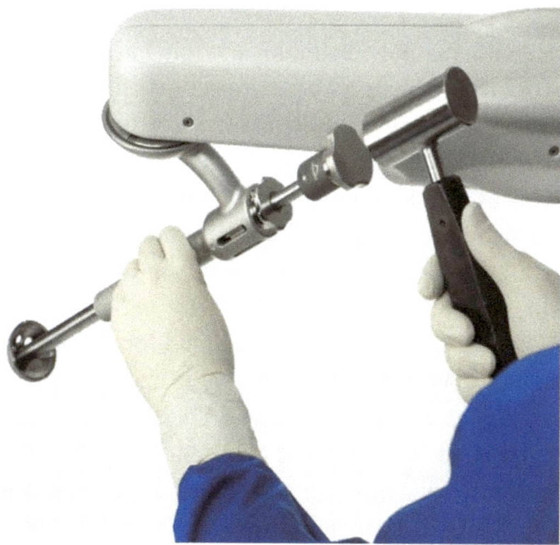

Fig. 20.9 Cup insertion occurs with line haptics, meaning the system will not allow deviation from the plane and the component orientation is "held" in the predetermined orientation. (Courtesy of Stryker, Kalamazoo, MI, USA)

Validation

Preclinical

This type of enabling technology is the culmination of the efforts on the parts of engineers, computer software experts, implant designers and surgeons. Prior to its clinical use, preclinical validation to ensure not only precision and accuracy but safety was essential. Given that the premise of this technology was the superiority to traditional "manually" inserted hip components, the goal of the initial work [18] was to compare and contrast manual versus robotically assisted hip arthroplasty in a series of cadaveric specimens. Six pelvis-to-foot cadaveric specimens (12 paired acetabula) underwent both standard AP radiographs as well as CT scanning according to established protocol as part of the preoperative planning for haptically guided total hip arthroplasty. Variable of socket placement as well as leg length and offset were also included. Each specimen was randomized to receive one manually inserted THR and the opposite would receive a robotically

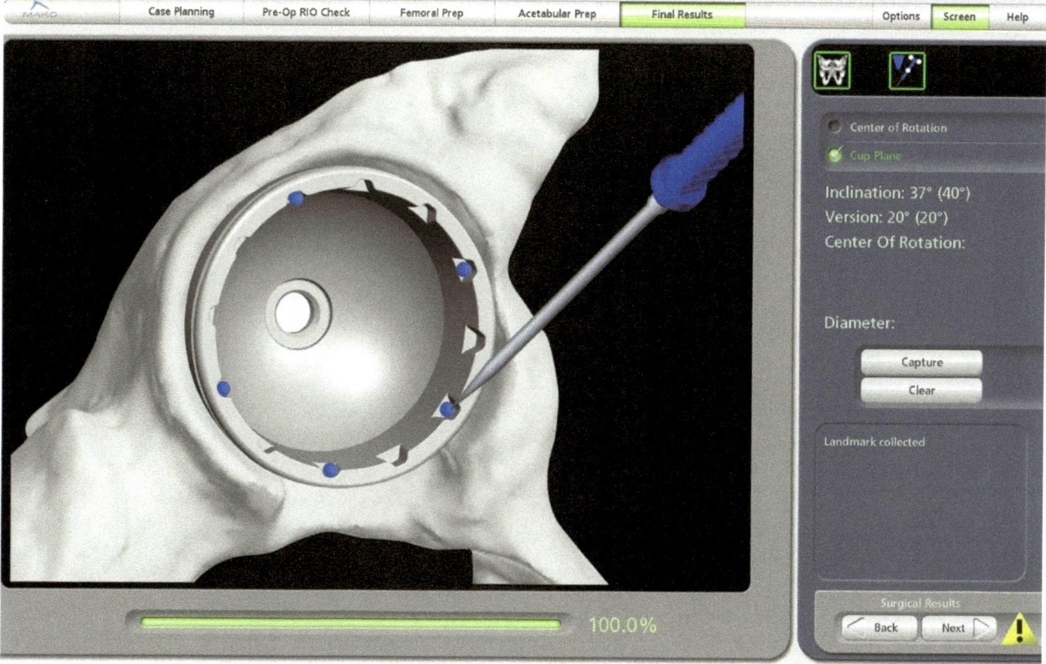

Fig. 20.10 Once the acetabular component is in place, confirmation of position is established by acquiring 5 points around the periphery of the cup using a probe

guided THR. All procedures were performed using a posterolateral approach by a single surgeon experienced with both techniques. The primary outcome of interest was acetabular component position with the target goal of 40° of abduction and 20° of anteversion. The manual procedures were aided by the use of a commercially available hand-held alignment guide. The robotic procedures were performed using the protocol as outlined above. Following implantation, all specimens underwent postoperative CT scanning. The differences between planned and actual were calculated by using a CT-based 3-D registration method (Fig. 20.11). The CT scans were aligned using the same pelvic coordinating plane and the differences between the preoperative plan and the postoperative cup orientation could be determined. Accuracy of cup position was determined by calculating the root mean square (RMS) errors.

The results of this initial validation work demonstrated that errors in component position were 5 times greater for cup inclination and 3.4 times greater for acetabular version using manual insertion techniques than robotic assistance (Fig. 20.12). These results confirmed the improved precision and accuracy of this haptically guided system over manual insertion techniques and supported the enthusiasm for clinical adoption.

Clinical

As with any new technology, while basic science work to establish proof of concept is critical, ultimately translation of novel ideas to clinical practice will be required for widespread adoption. One of the first clinical validation studies performed as a multi-institutional study from four US centers including members of the original surgeon design team [19]. Thirty patients from each site (120 hips) were recruited for this investigation. All patients underwent primary total hip arthroplasty using the RIO® (Robotic Arm Interactive Orthopaedic System, Mako). All patients had surgery performed in the lateral decubitus position using a cementless hemispherical acetabular component. Preoperative CT scanning was performed per protocol. Intended preoperative abduction was 40°. Planned cup anteversion was based upon achieving a combined cup-stem anteversion of 25–40° depending upon clinical parameters such as gender and

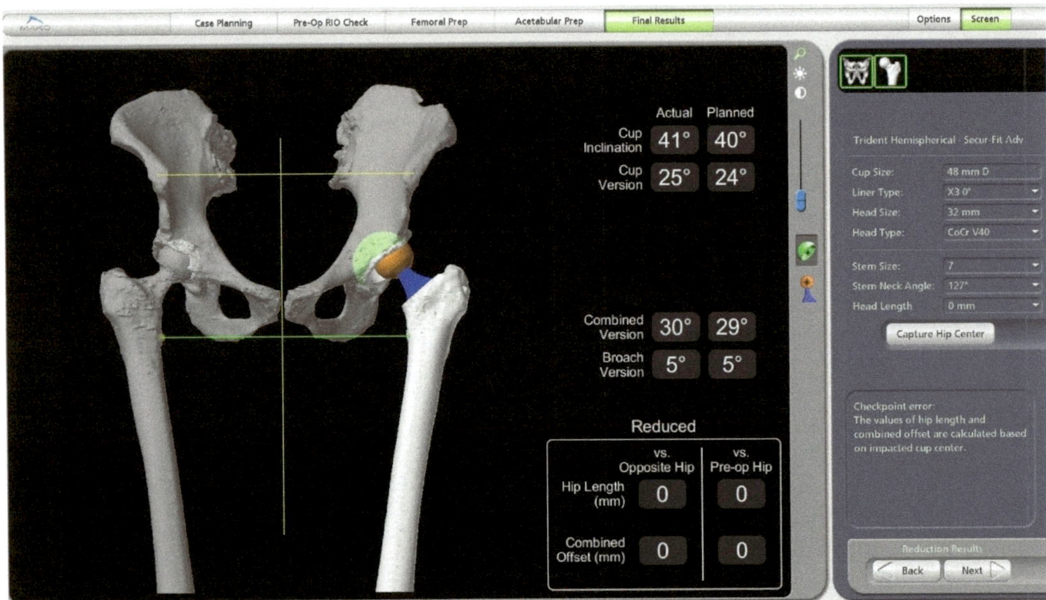

Fig. 20.11 Following implantation, all specimens underwent postoperative CT scanning, with the differences between planned and actual procedure calculated using a CT-based 3-D registration method

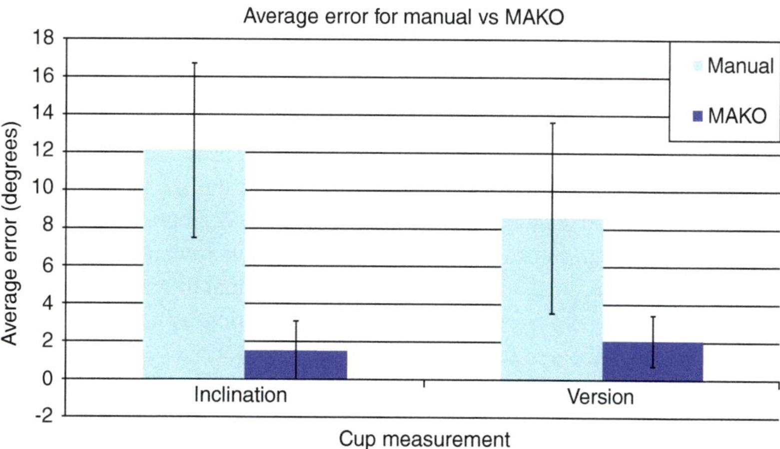

Fig. 20.12 The results of this initial validation work demonstrated that errors in component position were 5 times greater for cup inclination and 3.4 times greater for acetabular version using manual insertion techniques than robotic assistance

Table 20.1 The Average Inclination and Anteversion Values of the Acetabular components in the Study, Showing the Preoperative Plan, Measures Recorded Interoperatively, and Those Measured from Plan Radiographs Using the Martell Method

	Preoperative Plan	Intraoperative Robotic Arm Measurements	Martell Radiographic Measurement
Inclination	40.0 ± 1.2°	39.9 ± 2.0°	40.4 ± 4.1°
Version	18.7 ± 3.1°	18.6 ± 3.9°	21.5 ± 6.1°
Count (n)	119	119	110

From Elson et al. [19], with permission

activity. Postoperative assessment of component position was determined by obtaining anteroposterior (AP) pelvis and cross table lateral radiographs and using the Martell Hip Analysis Suite™ for both abduction and version. The 95% predictive intervals using the preoperative plan and the intra-operative robotic arm measurements were 3.5° for inclination and 3.6° for version. The consistency for inclination and version from preoperative plan to intra-operative measurements and finally to postoperative measurements is seen in Table 20.1. The results of this study clearly demonstrated that vast improvement in acetabular component placement precision contrasted with traditional techniques of insertion relying upon either manual instruments or anatomic landmarks.

Clinical Studies

Since this report, there have several other clinical studies looking at the precision of this technique. Kanawade et al. [20] reported the results of 38 patients undergoing total hip replacements (THRs) using this robotic technique. Using postoperative CT as a measure of implant position, these authors demonstrated that implants were within 5° of intended target 88% for inclination and 84% for version. Domb et al. [21] reported on their early experience using the robot compared to a group of conventionally inserted THRs. These authors found that all (100%) of the robotic-assisted sockets were within the desired "safe zone" contrasted to 80% of the conventionally inserted implants.

The utility of this technology has also been demonstrated in cohorts that have been traditionally associated as outliers for component position. Historically, obesity has been shown to compromise accurate implant positioning, with a higher proportion of outliers, when using conventional methods. Gupta [22] and investigators were able to establish that there was no impact of BMI on the precision and accuracy of socket placement using robotically assisted THR. Some have questioned whether robotic-assisted technology is necessary in light of recent advances in using alternatives such as fluoroscopic guidance. Kamara [23] et al. studied a high volume center's experience achieving component placement using manual, fluoroscopically aided and robotic-assisted techniques for total hip arthroplasty. These authors concluded that in their experience, robotically assisted methods resulted in significant and immediate improvement in component precision compared to the other techniques. These findings were mirrored by Illgen and coauthors [24] who compared socket positions among three cohorts: early career results manually, 10 years later in practice with manual tools and finally his first 100 robotic-assisted THRs. In the robotic-assisted group, 77% of implants were in the "safe-zone" while his early manual results demonstrated only 30% within the desired target and 10 years later only improved to 45%.

While there is clear consensus that robotically assisted hip arthroplasty has improved precision in implant orientation, what is less clear is the impact of this technology upon improvement in clinical outcomes. Bukowski et al. [25] compared to cohorts: a series of 100 robotic aided THRs with a consecutive series of manually performed THAs. Outcome measures of interest included the SF-12, WOMAC, University of California, Los Angeles (UCLA) activity scores and the modified Harris Hip Score. At a mean follow-up of approximately 1 year, the robotic group demonstrated significantly better Harris Hip scores and UCLA activity scores than the manual group. However, there was no difference observed in either the WOMAC or SF-12 outcomes.

In a critical analysis of robotic-assisted hip arthroplasty, Newman et al. [26] performed a systematic review of the literature assessing clinical outcomes. While component position and alignment was statistically improved using the robotic technology, it was difficult to demonstrate short term improvement in patient reported outcomes. Some of the previously mentioned studies [18, 21] have demonstrated that the use of a robotically assisted system for THR results in a reduction in leg length discrepancy; however, improvements in clinical scores is currently not available with this system. Nonetheless, since the effects of improved implant positioning may only

be best appreciated in the long term outcomes assessing wear and function, ongoing monitoring of patient performance is mandatory.

In summary, robotic-assisted total hip arthroplasty using the Mako Robot has without question improved the precision and accuracy of acetabular component position and has been instrumental in improving metrics such as limb length and offset. The 3-D planning and execution using this platform is an exciting new step forward in improving hip arthroplasty. Coupling this technology with improved understanding of functional alignment of the hip as it relates to spinopelvic disorders should be the next logical step in improving outcomes after hip replacement.

References

1. Charnley J. A biomechanical analysis of the use of cement to anchor the femoral head prosthesis. J Bone Joint Surg Br. 1965;47:354–63.
2. Charnley J. An artificial bearing in the hip joint: implications in biological lubrication. Fed Proc. 1966;25(3):1079–81.
3. Schulte KR, Callaghan JJ, Kelley SS, Johnston RC. The outcome of Charnley total hip arthroplasty with cement after a minimum twenty-year follow-up. The results of one surgeon. J Bone Joint Surg Am. 1993;75(7):961–75.
4. Warth LC, Callaghan JJ, Liu SS, Klaassen AL, Goetz DD, Johnston RC. Thirty-five-year results after Charnley total hip arthroplasty in patients less than fifty years old. A concise follow-up of previous reports. J Bone Joint Surg Am. 2014;96(21):1814–9.
5. McLaughlin JR, Lee KR. Total hip arthroplasty with an uncemented tapered femoral component in patients younger than 50 years of age: a minimum 20-year follow-up study. J Arthroplast. 2016;31(6):1275–8.
6. Bozic KJ, Kurtz SM, Lau E, Ong K, Vail TP, Berry DJ. The epidemiology of revision total hip arthroplasty in the United States. J Bone Joint Surg Am. 2009;91(1):128–33. https://doi.org/10.2106/JBJS.H.00155.
7. Padgett DE, Warashina H. The unstable total hip replacement. Clin Orthop Relat Res. 2004;420:72–9. Review
8. Lewinnek GE, Lewis JL, Tarr R, Compere CL, Zimmerman JR. Dislocations after total hip-replacement arthroplasties. J Bone Joint Surg Am. 1978;60(2):217–20.
9. Esposito CI, Gladnick BP, Lee YY, Lyman S, Wright TM, Mayman DJ, Padgett DE. Cup position alone does not predict risk of dislocation after hip arthroplasty. J Arthroplast. 2015;30(1):109–13.

10. Kligman M, Michael H, Roffman M. The effect of abduction differences between cup and contralateral acetabular angle on polyethylene component wear. Orthopedics. 2002;25(1):65–7.

11. Kligman M, Furman BD, Padgett DE, Wright TM. Impingement contributes to backside wear and screw-metallic shell fretting in modular acetabular cups. J Arthroplast. 2007;22(2):258–64.

12. Shon WY, Baldini T, Peterson MG, Wright TM, Salvati EA. Impingement in total hip arthroplasty a study of retrieved acetabular components. J Arthroplasty. 2005;20(4):427–35.

13. Callanan MC, Jarrett B, Bragdon CR, Zurakowski D, Rubash HE, Freiberg AA, Malchau H. The John Charnley Award: risk factors for cup malpositioning: quality improvement through a joint registry at a tertiary hospital. Clin Orthop Relat Res. 2011;469(2):319–29. https://doi.org/10.1007/s11999-010-1487-1.

14. Padgett DE, Hendrix SL, Mologne TS, Peterson DA, Holley KA. Effectiveness of an acetabular positioning device in primary total hip arthroplasty. HSS J. 2005;1(1):64–7.

15. Sendtner E, Schuster T, Wörner M, Kalteis T, Grifka J, Renkawitz T. Accuracy of acetabular cup placement in computer-assisted, minimally-invasive THR in a lateral decubitus position. Int Orthop. 2011;35(6):809–15.

16. Paul HA, Bargar WL, Mittlestadt B, Musits B, Taylor RH, Kazanzides P, Zuhars J, Williamson B, Hanson W. Development of a surgical robot for cementless total hip arthroplasty. Clin Orthop Relat Res. 1992;285:57–66.

17. Dorr LD, Malik A, Dastane M, Wan Z. Combined Anteversion technique for total hip arthroplasty. Clin Orthop Relat Res. 2009;467(1):119–27.

18. Nawabi DH, Conditt MA, Ranawat AS, Dunbar NJ, Jones J, Banks S, Padgett DE. Haptically guided robotic technology in total hip arthroplasty: a cadaveric investigation. Proc Inst Mech Eng H. 2013;227(3):302–9.

19. Elson L, Dounchis J, Illgen R, Marchand RC, Padgett DE, Bragdon CR, Malchau H. Precision of acetabular cup placement in robotic integrated total hip arthroplasty. Hip Int. 2015;25(6):531–6.

20. Kanawade V, Dorr LD, Banks SA, Zhang Z, Wan Z. Precision of robotic guided instrumentation for acetabular component positioning. J Arthroplast. 2015;30(3):392–7.

21. Domb BG, El Bitar YF, Sadik AY, Stake CE, Botser IB. Comparison of robotic-assisted and conventional acetabular cup placement in THA: a matched-pair controlled study. Clin Orthop Relat Res. 2014;472(1):329–36.

22. Gupta A, Redmond JM, Hammarstedt JE, Petrakos AE, Vemula SP, Domb BG. Does robotic-assisted computer navigation affect acetabular cup positioning in total hip arthroplasty in the obese patient? A comparison study. J Arthroplast. 2015;30(12):2204–7.

23. Kamara E, Robinson J, Bas MA, Rodriguez JA, Hepinstall MS. Adoption of robotic vs fluoroscopic guidance in total hip arthroplasty: is acetabular positioning improved in the learning curve? J Arthroplast. 2017;32(1):125–30.

24. Nd IRL, Bukowski BR, Abiola R, Anderson P, Chughtai M, Khlopas A, Mont MA. Robotic-assisted total hip arthroplasty: outcomes at minimum two-year follow-up. Surg Technol Int. 2017;25(30):365–72.

25. Bukowski BR, Anderson P, Khlopas A, Chughtai M, Mont MA, Illgen RL. Improved functional outcomes with robotic compared with manual total hip arthroplasty. Surg Technol Int. 2016;XXIX:303–8.

26. Newman J, Carroll K, Cross MB. Robotic-assisted total hip arthroplasty: a critical appraisal. Dovepress. 2014;2014(1):37–42. https://doi.org/10.2147/RSRR.S54420.

William L. Bargar and Nathan A. Netravali

Total hip arthroplasty (THA) is widely performed to relieve pain and restore function in patients with end-stage osteoarthritis of the hip joint. It is typically a successful surgery with positive clinical outcomes and over 95% survivorship at 10-year follow-up and 80% survivorship at 25-year follow-up [1, 2]. THA continues to grow within the USA with 284,000 primary THAs being performed in 2009, and this number is expected to grow to over 511,000 by 2020 [3]. The success of a hip replacement depends on a number of factors including strong osteointegration to prevent femoral loosening [4, 5] and correct implant alignment which correlate with prolonged implant survivorship and reduced dislocation [6, 7]. Technological developments, including computer-assisted navigation and robotics, can increase the accuracy of implant placement and reduce outliers with the overall goal of improving long-term results. These technologies have shown significant improvements in implant positioning when compared to conventional techniques [8].

The first active robotic system used in THA was ROBODOC (THINK Surgical Inc., Fremont, CA) and was based on a traditional computer-aided design (CAD)-computer-aided manufacturing (CAM) system. The TSolution One system (Think Surgical Inc., Fremont, CA) is based on the legacy technology developed as ROBODOC and provides active preparation of the femoral canal as well as guidance and positioning assistance during acetabular cup reaming and implanting. The preoperative planning and surgical technique for TSolution One are described below in some detail based on the senior author's (WLB) experience.

Technique

The technique begins with preoperative planning based on a CT scan (Fig. 21.1). From this scan, a detailed 3-D reconstruction of the patient's pathologic hip anatomy is created using the preoperative planning software, TPLAN. The user then creates a 3-D template of the surgical plan in TPLAN for both the femoral and acetabular portions of the procedure. The user can select implants from an open library of 510(k) cleared implants, meaning that the user is not limited to a single implant design or manufacturer. The surgeon can control every aspect of implant positioning including rotation, version, fit and fill on the femoral side, and anteversion and inclination on the acetabular side (Fig. 21.2). Once the desired plan has been achieved, it is uploaded to TCAT.

W. L. Bargar (✉)
Department of Orthopaedic Surgery, University of California at Davis School of Medicine, Sutter General Hospital, Sacramento, CA, USA
e-mail: wbargar@jointsurgeons.com

N. A. Netravali
Think Surgical, Inc., Fremont, CA, USA

© Springer Nature Switzerland AG 2019
J. H. Lonner (ed.), *Robotics in Knee and Hip Arthroplasty*,
https://doi.org/10.1007/978-3-030-16593-2_21

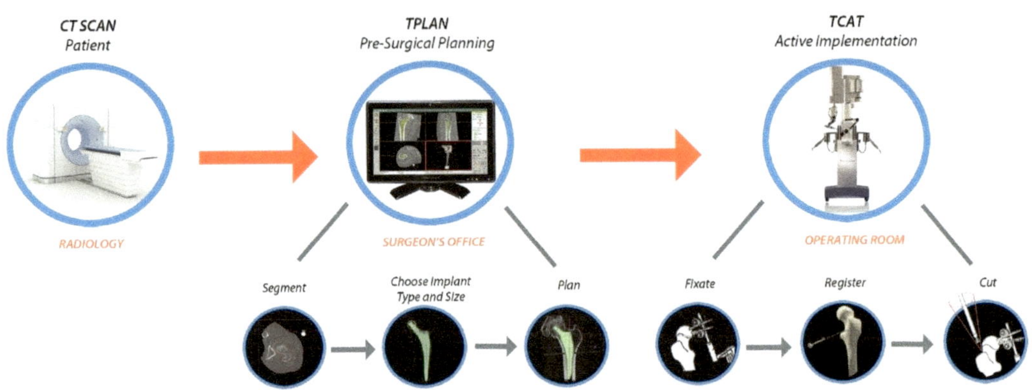

Fig. 21.1 Workflow with TSolution One. (Courtesy of Think Surgical Inc., Fremont, CA, USA)

Fig. 21.2 Implant positioning with TPLAN. The surgeon controls every aspect of implant positioning including rotation, version, fit and fill on the femoral side, and anteversion and inclination on the acetabular side

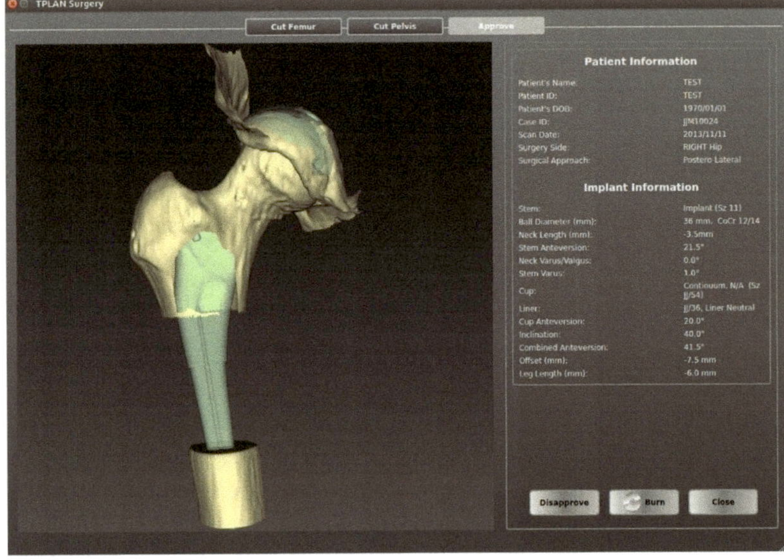

The TCAT robot is an active system based on CAD-CAM principles such that the robot follows a predetermined path. More specifically, it actively mills out the femoral cavity as planned within sub-millimeter accuracy. This is in contrast to a haptic system, where the user manually guides the robotic arm within a predefined boundary. The acetabular portion of the procedure currently uses a standard reamer system and power tools, but TCAT guides the surgeon to the planned cup orientation such that its position is maintained during reaming and impaction.

In the OR, the plan is uploaded into TCAT via a transfer media. The software requires the user to confirm the plan and patient as part of the surgical "time out." The system currently supports a posterolateral approach with a standard OR table, but the direct anterior approach is in development. Once the hip joint is exposed and dislocated, retractors are placed to protect the soft tissues and allow the robot its working space.

One procedural difference from the typical THA is that the femoral head is initially retained to fixate the femur relative to the robot (Fig. 21.3). A Schanz pin is placed in the femoral head and then rigidly attached to the base of the robot (Fig. 21.3). A point-to-surface registration method is used to digitize the surface of the exposed bone

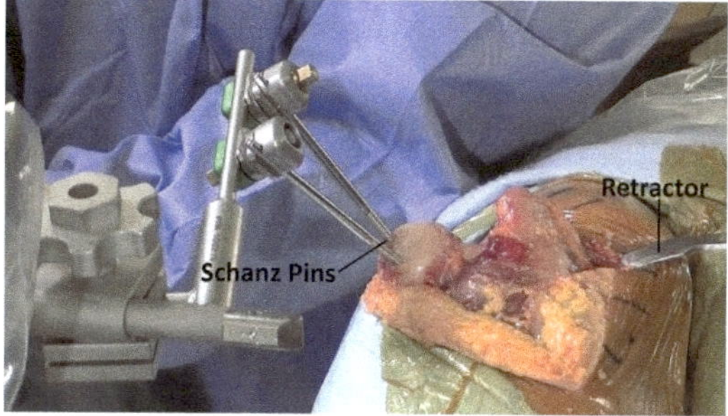

Fig. 21.3 Intraoperative fixation. Once the hip joint is exposed and disarticulated, retractors are placed to protect the soft tissues and allow the robot its working space. Schanz pins are placed in the femoral head and then rigidly attached to the base of the robot

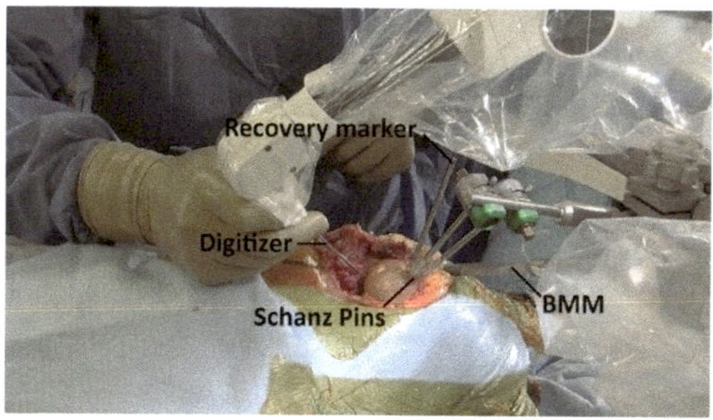

Fig. 21.4 Intraoperative registration process. A point-to-surface registration method is used to digitize the surface of the exposed bone using a probe attached to the robot called the digitizer. As safety feature, a bone motion monitor (BMM) is also attached to the femur along with two recovery makers

using a probe attached to the robot called the digitizer (Fig. 21.4). The TCAT monitor guides the surgeon through point collection by showing regions on the 3-D bone model based on the CT images. Once registration is complete, the milling begins with the cutter spinning at 80,000 rpm, and saline is used as irrigation to remove bone debris (Fig. 21.5). The actual milling process takes from 5 to 15 minutes depending on the model and size of the implant.

As a safety feature, a bone motion monitor (BMM) is also attached to the femur along with two recovery markers (Fig. 21.5). The BMM immediately pauses the robot during any active bone milling if it senses femoral motion from the original position. The surgeon then digitizes the recovery markers to re-register the bone's position and resume the milling process.

For the acetabular portion of the procedure, the robot is again rigidly fixed to the patient's pelvis along with the recovery markers. Once the surgeon has registered the acetabular position using the digitizer, the robotic arm moves into the preoperatively planned orientation (Fig. 21.6). A universal quick release allows the surgeon to attach a standard reamer to the robot arm and ream while the robot holds the reamer in place. Once the acetabular preparation is complete, the cup impactor is attached to the robotic arm, once again in the preoperatively planned orientation, and the implant is impacted into the patient (Fig. 21.7). Thereafter, the digitizer can be used to collect points on the surface of the cup and confirm the exact cup placement in comparison to the preoperative plan.

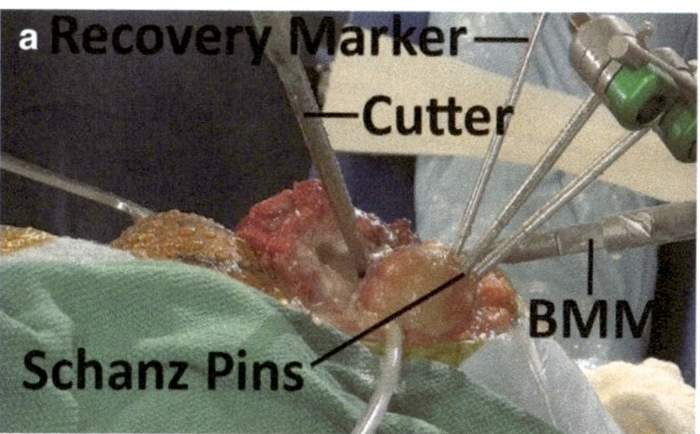

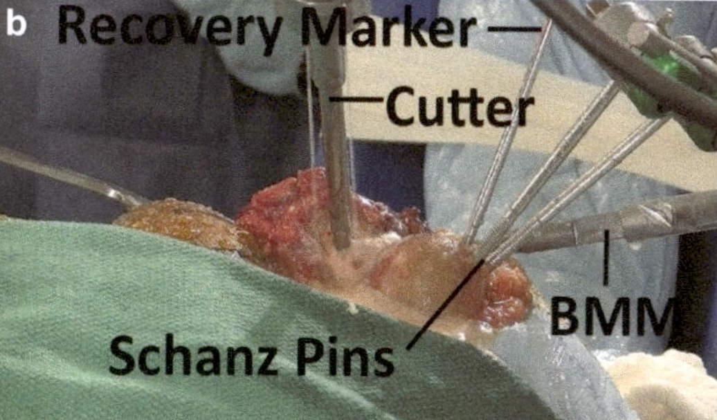

Fig. 21.5 Intraoperative cutting process. Once registration is complete, the milling begins with the cutter spinning at 80,000 rpm (**a**), and saline is used as irrigation to remove bone debris (**b**)

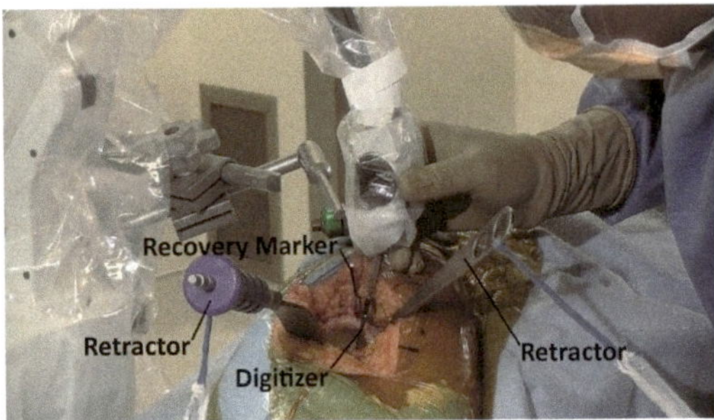

Fig. 21.6 Intraoperative acetabular registration. For the acetabular portion of the procedure, the robot is again fixed to the patient's pelvis along with the recovery markers, and the surgeon registers the acetabular position using the digitizer

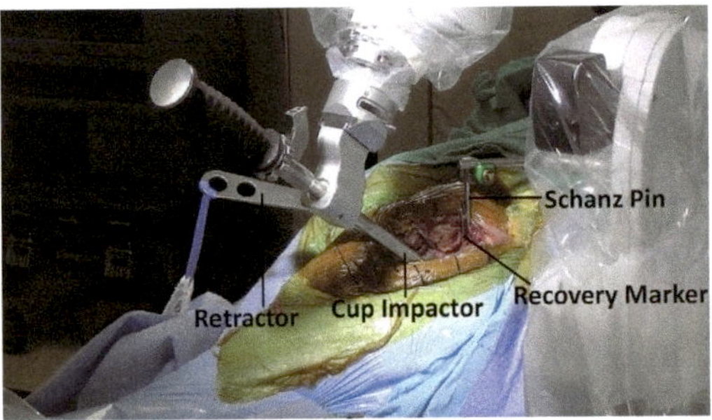

Fig. 21.7 Intraoperative cup placement. Once the acetabular preparation is complete, the cup impactor is attached to the robotic arm, once again in the preoperatively planned orientation, and the implant is impacted into the patient

Outcomes

Although the TSolution One system is new to the market, it shares fundamental principles of operation with the legacy system, ROBODOC, which has been used in thousands of clinical cases for both THA and TKA. The data presented below represents a summary of the THA clinical studies (Table 21.1). The ROBODOC system only had the active preparation of the femoral canal and did not provide any guidance for the acetabular cup.

The first clinical cases in the USA with ROBODOC were described by Bargar et al. [9] along with the first 900 THA procedures performed in Germany. In the USA, these cases were part of a prospective, randomized control study with 65 robotic cases and 62 conventional control

Table 21.1 Summary of clinical studies using ROBODOC for THA. All values presented are for ROBODOC/conventional where available

Study	Procedure	No. cases
Bargar et al. US [9]	THA	65/62
Bargar et al. Germany [9]	THA	900/–
Honl et al. [10]	THA	61/80
Nishihara et al. [14]	THA	75/–
Nishihara et al. [12]	THA	78/78
Hananouchi et al. [13]	THA	31/27
Schulz et al. [16]	THA	143/–
Nakamura et al. [11]	THA	75/71

cases. The study demonstrated no differences between the groups when looking at functional outcomes at 3 months, 1 year, and 2 years, postoperatively. Radiographically, the robot group had improved fit and component positioning. The robot group also had significantly increased surgical time and blood loss but no femoral fractures, while there were three fractures in the control group. In Germany, they reported on 870 primary THA's and 30 revision THA cases. The Harris hip scores rose from 43.7 preoperatively to 91.5 postoperatively in the primary cases at 24 months. Complication rates were similar to conventional techniques, except there were no intraoperative femoral fractures in these robot cases.

There have been several prospective randomized clinical studies comparing the ROBODOC system with a conventional technique. Honl et al. [10] included 74 robotic cases and 80 conventional cases and found statistically significant improvements in limb-length equality and varus-valgus orientation of the stem in the robotic cases. Excluding the revision cases, they found that Harris hip scores, limb length differentials, and prosthetic alignment were improved in the robotic group at both 6 and 12 months. Nakamura et al. [11] compared at 75 robotic cases and 71 conventional cases. They found that the robotic group had improved JOA scores at 2 and 3 years, postoperatively, but by 5 years, the differences were gone. The robotic group had a smaller range for leg length inequality (0–12 mm) compared to the conventional group (0–29 mm). They also found that at both 2 and 5 years, postoperatively, there was more significant stress shielding of the proximal femur suggesting greater bone loss in the conventional group. Nishihara et al. [12] compared two groups that each had 78 subjects and found significantly better Merle D'Aubigné hip scores at 2 years postoperatively in the robotic group. There were five intraoperative fractures in the conventional group compared with none in the robotic group. The conventional group also had greater estimated blood loss, higher than expected vertical seating, an increased use of undersized stems, and less accurate femoral anteversion. However, the robotic cases did take 19 minutes longer than the conventional cases. Hananouchi et al. [13] looked at how precise robotic milling could lead to effective load transfer from implant to bone. They compared periprosthetic bone remodeling in 31 robotic hips and 27 and used dual energy X-ray absorptiometry (DEXA) to measure bone density. They found significantly less bone loss in the proximal periprosthetic areas in the robotic group compared to the conventional group; however, there were no differences in the Merle d'Aubigné hip scores.

In 2004, Nishihara et al. [14] evaluated the accuracy of femoral canal preparation with the original pin-based version of ROBODOC. Instead of the point-to-surface registration used in other studies, this version required fiducial markers to be placed in the bone prior to the CT scan. They found, in 75 cases of THA, that the differences between the preoperative plan and the postoperative CT were less than 5% in terms of canal fill, less than 1 mm in gap, and less than 1° in mediolateral and anteroposterior alignment with no reported fractures or complications.

Lim et al. [15] looked specifically at short-term femoral stem implants to determine alignment accuracy and clinical outcomes. In a group of 24 robotic cases and 25 conventional cases, the robotic cases had significantly improved stem alignment and leg length inequality with no statistically significant differences in Harris Hip, WOMAC scores, or complications at 24 months.

Complications with the use of ROBODOC have been reported in some studies. Schulz et al. [16] reported on 97 of 143 consecutive cases performed from 1997 to 2002 and stated that 9 technical complications that occurred. They classified five instances of the BMM pausing cutting and

requiring the user to re-register as a complication, when this safety system worked as designed to prevent unwanted bone cuts and harm to the patient. The remaining complications included two femoral shaft fissures requiring wire cerclage, one case of damage to the acetabular rim from the milling device, and one defect of the greater trochanter that was milled. These four complications were in contrast to other studies with ROBODOC [9, 11, 12, 14] which did not report similar complications, and the rate found in this study was comparable to a conventional technique. Despite these reported complications, functional outcomes and radiographic outcomes were comparable to conventional techniques.

In the study by Honl et al. [10] mentioned above, they found that dislocation was more frequent in the group treated with robotic implantation since it occurred in 11 of the 61 patients compared with 3 of 80 in the control group. Also, recurrent dislocation and pronounced limping were indications for revision surgery in 8 of the 61 patients treated with robotic implantation compared with none of the 78 treated with manual insertion. Rupture of the gluteus medius tendon was observed during all of the revision operations.

The complications reported in both of these papers can be attributed to human error rather than robot error. The surgeon has certain responsibilities when using the system, among them are selecting an appropriate implant for each case, constructing an appropriate plan, giving the robot its workspace by retracting and protecting the soft tissues, as well as continuously monitoring the cutting with the control pendant in hand with the ability to stop the system at any point. By executing these responsibilities, the reported complications in these studies are considered preventable.

Conclusion

Since 1992, when the first robotic surgery was performed in the USA using the ROBODOC system upon which the current TSolution One is based, thousands of robotic hip replacements have been performed worldwide. The clinical results have demonstrated that robotics clearly offers clear benefits in terms of accuracy and reproducibility. These benefits will likely translate into improved long-term outcomes for patients [17].

Although much debate still exists regarding the "ideal position" for hip implants for each individual patient, it is clear that active robotic technology can help surgeons hit their targets. This technology may be the tool that will help determine ideal implant position since its use can help eliminate surgeon variability and allow various alignment techniques to be compared. In any case, surgical robots have demonstrated clear improvements in precision that will likely translate into improved long-term outcomes.

References

1. Kurtz S, Ong K, Lau E, Mowat F, et al. Projections of primary and revision hip and knee arthroplasty in the United States from 2005 to 2030. J Bone Joint Surg. 2007;89(4):780–5.
2. National Joint Registry for England and Wales. 7th annual report. National Joint Registry: Hemel Hempstead, 2010.
3. Kurtz SM, Ong KL, Lau E, et al. Impact of the economic downturn on total joint replacement demand in the United States. J Bone Joint Surg. 2014;96(8):624–30.
4. Paul HA, Bargar WL, Mittlestadt B, Musits B, Taylor RH, Kazanzides P, Zuhars J, Williamson B, Hanson W. Development of a surgical robot for cementless total hip arthroplasty. Clin Orthop Relat Res. 1992;285:57–66.
5. Bobyn JD, Engh CA. Human histology of bone-porous metal implant interface. Orthopedics. 1984;7(9):1410–21.
6. Barrack RL. Dislocation after total hip arthroplasty: implant design and orientation. J Am Acad Orthop Surg. 2003;11(2):89–99.
7. Miki H, Sugano N, Yonenobu K, Tsuda K, Hattori M, Suzuki N. Detecting cause of dislocation after total hip arthroplasty by patient-specific four-dimensional motion analysis. Clin Biomech. 2013;28:182–6.
8. Sugano N. Computer-assisted orthopaedic surgery and robotic surgery in total hip arthroplasty. Clin Orthop Surg. 2013;5:1–9.
9. Bargar WL, Bauer A, Börner M. Primary and revision total hip replacement using the Robodoc® system. Clin Orthop Relat Res. 1998;354:82–91.
10. Honl M, Dierk O, Gauck C, Carrero V, Lampe F, Dries S, Quante M, Schwieger K, Hille E, Morlock M. Comparison of robotic-assisted and manual implantation of primary total hip replacement: a prospective study. J Bone Joint Surg. 2003;85:1470–8.
11. Nakamura N, Sugano N, Nishii T, Kakimoto A, Miki H. A comparison between robotic-assisted and manual implantation of cementless total hip arthroplasty. Clin Orthop Relat Res. 2010;468:1072–81.
12. Nishihara S, Sugano N, Nishii T, Miki H, Nakamura N, Yoshikawa H. Comparison between hand rasping and robotic milling for stem implantation in Cementless Total hip arthroplasty. J Arthroplast. 2006;21(7):957–66.
13. Hananouchi T, Sugano N, Nishii T, Nakamura N, Miki H, Kakimoto A, Yamamura M, Yoshikawa H. Effect of robotic milling on periprosthetic bone remodeling. J Orthop Res. 2007;25(8):1062–9.
14. Nishihara S, Sugano N, Nishii T, Tanaka H, Nakamura N, Yoshikawa H, Ochi T. Clinical accuracy evaluation of femoral canal preparation using the ROBODOC system. J Orthop Sci. 2004;9:452–61.
15. Lim S-J, Ko K-R, Park C-W, Moon Y-W, Park Y-S. Robot-assisted primary cementless total hip arthroplasty with a short femoral stem: a prospective randomized short-term outcome study. Comput Aided Surg. 2015;20(1):41–6.
16. Schultz A, Seide K, Queitsch C. Results of total hip replacement using the Robodoc surgical assistant system: clinical outcome and evaluation of complications for 97 procedures. Int J Med Robot. 2007;3(4):301–6.
17. Bargar WL, Parise CA, Hankins A, Marlen NA, Campanelli V, Netravali NA. Fourteen year follow-up of randomized clinical trials of active robotic-assisted total hip arthroplasty. J Arthroplast. 2018;33:810e–814.

Part IV

Emerging Uses

Robotics in Spine Surgery: Uses in Development

Anthony E. Bozzio, Xiaobang Hu,
and Isador H. Lieberman

Since the emergence of surgical robotic technology in the 1980s, an obvious application of its uses has been in spinal surgery, where complex anatomy and the need for accurate implant position exist. The additional goals of less invasive surgery, decreased operating time and radiation exposure, as well as the aim to improve patient outcomes have fueled the development of both guidance and navigation systems in spinal surgery.

Guidance Versus Navigation

There are several commercially available systems used for spinal surgery that are either robotic guidance systems or navigation systems, and there are several key differences between the two.

Navigation systems in use today, such as SteathStation® combined with the O-arm® (Medtronic, USA), are based on intraoperative CT scans of the patient with stereotactic markers attached to fixed points, such a spinous process or posterior superior iliac spine. After the intraopera- tive scan is complete, the CT scanner is taken away from the operative field, the stereotactic markers are left attached to the patient, and tools with additional stereotactic markers are registered to the patient using the SteathStation® which then gives real-time feedback displaying position and distances relative to the CT scan images. The surgeon then positions pedicle awls or drills in space and adjusts trajectories. A stylus can also be registered to the system to find anatomic landmarks prior to performing decompressions, or using a burr at the level of a pseudoarthrosis. Navigation systems rely on intraoperative imaging and real-time image feedback in a virtual environment with surgeon adjustment to findings. In terms of accuracy, these systems have been found to be accurate and safe, although there can be differences of up to 5.92 mm in projected versus final screw tip position as detected in a study of 158 screws placed with navigation [1].

In comparison to navigation, robotic guidance systems rely on a preoperative plan that is created by the surgeon to position a guide in space for placement of instrumentation. Similar to navigation software, a separate workstation running an interface software facilitates the preoperative planning, intraoperative image acquisition and registration, kinematic calculations, and real-time motion control of the guidance system. Rather than adjustment by the surgeon with a pedicle awl in response to images, the guidance system aligns predetermined trajectories for the

A. E. Bozzio
Texas Back Institute, Plano, TX, USA

X. Hu · I. H. Lieberman (⊠)
Scoliosis and Spine Tumor Center, Texas Back Institute, Texas Health Presbyterian Hospital, Plano, TX, USA
e-mail: xhu@texasback.com;
ilieberman@texasback.com

© Springer Nature Switzerland AG 2019
J. H. Lonner (ed.), *Robotics in Knee and Hip Arthroplasty*,
https://doi.org/10.1007/978-3-030-16593-2_22

implants based on advance planning. The robotic systems do allow for intraoperative planning by obtaining an intraoperative CT scan. Likewise, should the need arise, robotic systems allow for intraoperative changes of the preoperative plan to facilitate intraoperative unanticipated variables.

Robotic Systems

There are several robotic systems being developed for spinal surgery. The first system that was approved by FDA and currently in use is the Renaissance® and its second-generation Mazor X™ (Mazor Robotics Ltd, Caesarea, Israel) systems (Fig. 22.1). These are robotic guidance systems that work by pairing a preoperative CT scan to intraoperative fluoroscopy. The techniques of robotic spine surgery have been described previously [2, 3]. The basic steps include a preoperative CT scan for preoperative planning on a 3D computer model. The plan is created by the surgeon prior to surgery and includes screw trajectories, lengths, and widths (Fig. 22.2). This plan is then uploaded to the workstation. Next, the stabilization platform is mounted to the patient, either to spinous processes or posterior superior iliac spine (Fig. 22.3). The robotic system is then attached to the platform, thus linking it to the patient. Imaging registration and referencing are then performed with fluoroscopy and a reference frame that serves to position each individual vertebra in 3-dimentional space with respect to the mounting platform (Fig. 22.4). The referencing works by identifying vertebrae as individual segments. Trajectories are then placed by sending the robotic guidance arm to each position as determined by the preoperative plan (Fig. 22.5). It is possible to alter these trajectories based on intraoperative decision-making.

Recently, FDA approved the ROSA robotic system (Zimmer Biomet, Warsaw, IN) and the Excelsus system (Globus Medical, Audubon, PA) for use in spine surgery. Both systems include a robotic arm with six degrees of freedom attached to a mobile floor-fixed base. A navigation camera is mounted to a second mobile base. They use intraoperative fluoroscopy or CT scan for planning. The robotic arm moves in concordance with the patient based on the navigation camera and tracking pins placed on the patient's bony anatomy in reference to tracking spheres affixed to the robot [4].

Clinical Applications

Robotic guidance systems can in theory be applied to almost any area of spinal surgery, but are most useful in situations that demand accurate trajectories. Some examples of clinical uses, either open or percutaneous, include the following:

1. Pedicle screws
2. Translaminar screws
3. Facet screws
4. S2 alar and S2 alar iliac screws
5. Drill paths for sacroiliac joint fusion
6. Biopsies
7. Drilling pseudoarthroses
8. Tumor surgery
9. Osteotomy planning

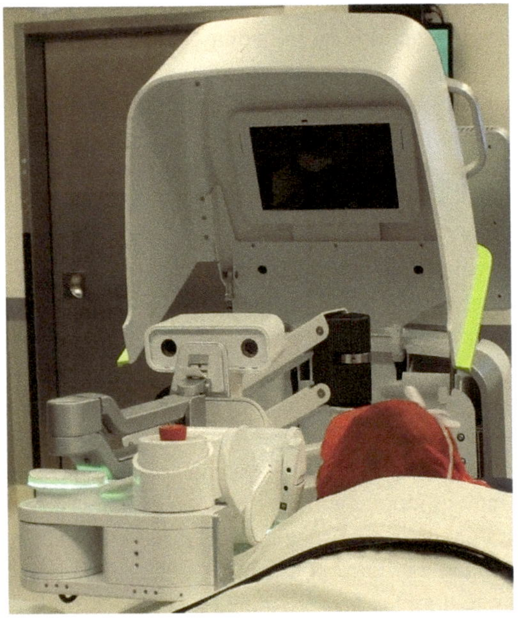

Fig. 22.1 The Mazor X robot system

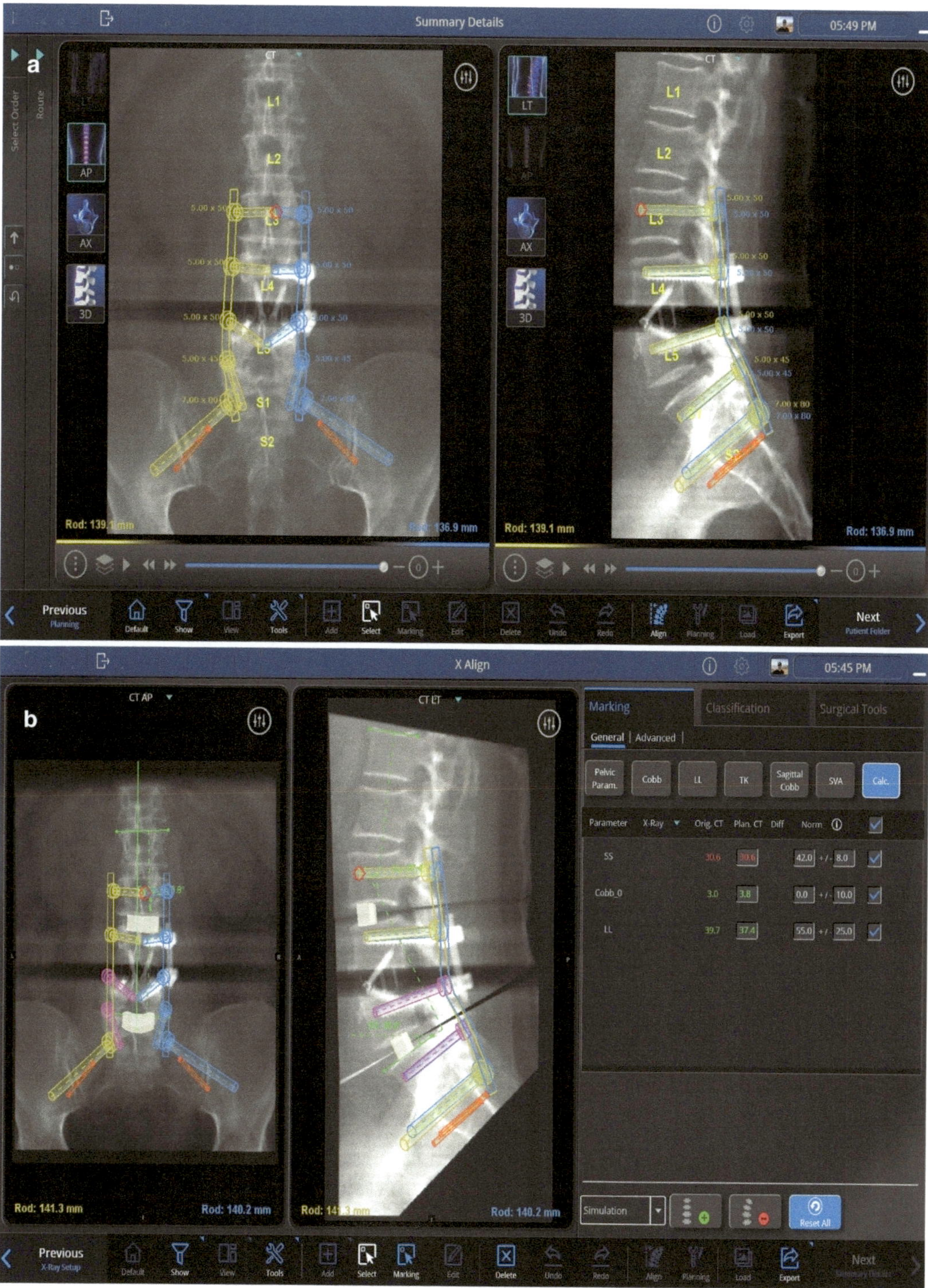

Fig. 22.2 (**a, b**) The preoperative planning using the Mazor X system

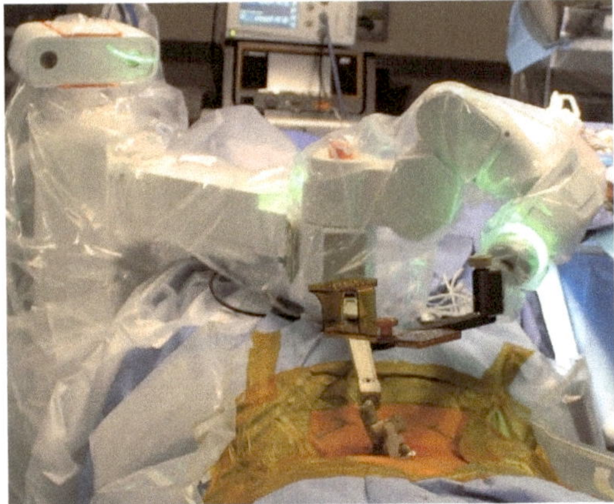

Fig. 22.3 Mounting the stabilization platform on patient

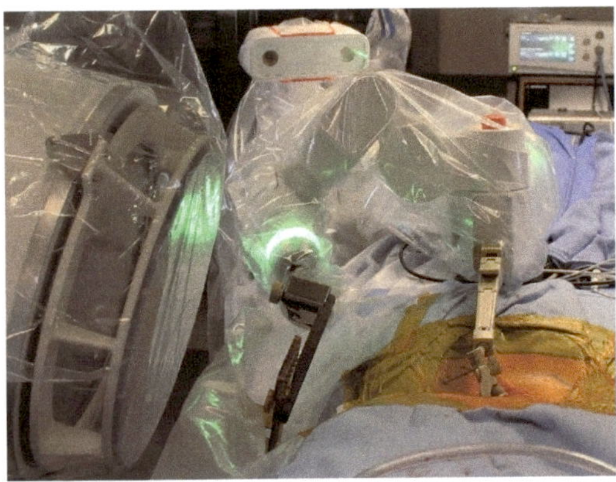

Fig. 22.4 Automatic image registration for the robotic system

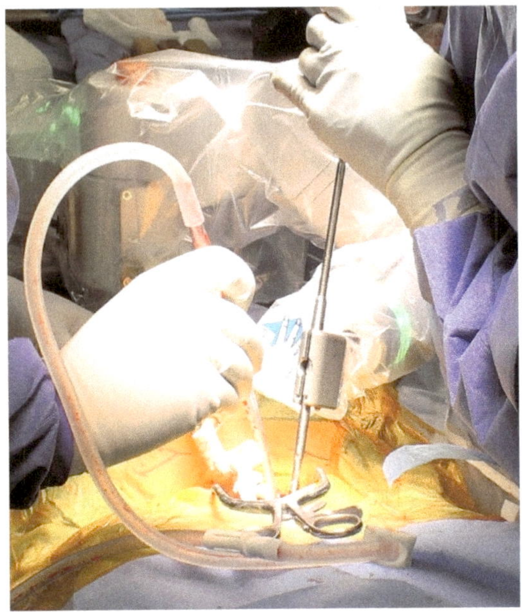

Fig. 22.5 Placing the pedicle screw with robotic guidance

State of the Art (Available Literature)

The most common of all uses of guidance is pedicle screw placement as pedicle screws are the foundation of spinal fixation, providing both multidimensional control and necessary rigidity to facilitate fusion. These advantages have led to the widespread use of pedicle screws in different spinal diseases, such as degenerative, traumatic, and developmental spinal conditions [5].

Accuracy and Safety

Pedicle screw placement is especially challenging in patients with severe deformities and/or prior surgeries. The rate of malpositioned pedicle screws has been reported to range from 4.2% to 15.7% [6, 7]. In a 2010 article by Devito et al., 80 patients with adolescent scoliosis curves averaging 66.5 degrees (range 46–95) underwent posterior spinal fusion with robotic-assisted pedicle screw placement. They found that of the 1163 screws placed, 95.9% were in their precise locations, while 99.9% were clinically acceptable. There were no device complications or screw revisions [8]. In a CT to CT comparison study by van Dijk et al., 178 robotically placed screws were compared in a CT overlay to the preoperative template. They found that 97.9% were within 2 mm of the templated plan comparing start point and angle of insertion and no screws were revised [9].

In a 2013 study by Hu et al., the accuracy of robotic-assisted screw placement in a consecutive series of 102 patients was studied. Robotic-guided screw placement was successful in 95 patients. Of the 960 screws that were implanted using the robot, 949 (98.9%) were successfully and accurately implanted, and 11 (1.1%) were malpositioned, despite the fact that the majority of patients had significant spinal deformities and/or previous spine surgeries. One of the inciting issues thought to cause this was "tool skiving". This occurs when the drill guide is placed onto a sloping part of the bone and the sharp teeth do not engage fully; rather, they slide or skive off target prior to drilling the pedicle. Intraoperative anteroposterior and oblique fluoroscopic imaging used for registration was the limiting issue in four of the seven aborted cases as adequate registration could not be obtained [10]. Recently, Cannestra et al. retrospectively analyzed the outcome of 705 adult degenerative spine patients who were operated either with robotic-guided MIS approach or with fluoroscopic-guided MIS or open approaches. They found that robotic-guided MIS procedures are associated with significantly decreased rate of surgical complications and revision surgeries [11].

Learning Curve and Pitfalls

In terms of learning curve for this relatively new and advancing technology, Hu and Lieberman looked at this in a 2014 paper which found that after 30 cases, the need to abandon robotic guidance and use manual techniques diminished sharply. They also noted that the overall rate of malpositioned screws was relatively similar over time. They used 162 consecutive cases in which the robotic system was used and divided them into five comparison groups representing different time points. In the first group, they found a 17% switch to manual screw placement, but in subsequent groups, the rates were between 4% and 7% [12].

As mentioned previously, tool skiving can cause malpositioned screws. This can occur when there is too much tension on the robotic guidance sleeve from soft tissues or when placing on a sloped part of the bone and allowing the tools to slide off target. Additional issues can arise if vigorous retraction that moves the patient or robot occurs. It is essential to ensure that when doing open cases, the dissection is complete prior to the registration process, and in percutaneous cases to ensure the soft tissues are not pulling the aiming arm off target.

Emerging Technologies

With the two complimentary technologies of navigation and robotic guidance currently in use, a desirable technology would be one that utilizes both the preoperative planning and guidance benefits of the robotic systems while also allowing the freedom of motion and surgeon adjustment that navigation systems provide. Pairing components of systems that work well together is the next step in advancing this type of surgery.

The O-arm® has been used intraoperatively to obtain CT scans for robotic planning purposes already. This type of surgery that allows real-time operative imaging and planning will be a future direction as these two technologies merge together. Combining this with more rigid and longer reaching robotic guidance arms, as well as the potential for patient specific implants has the potential to improve accuracy, ease of use, and efficiency of the navigation/guidance systems.

The current robotic applications in spine surgery are passive in the sense that they provide guidance as determined by the surgeon beforehand. As the technology advances, there will be more semi-active and active robotics integrated which could be useful for osteotomies, decompressions, and other applications where the robot can perform predetermined and templated portions of the surgery.

Summary

The use of robotic systems in spine surgery can facilitate the accurate placement of spinal instrumentation, potentially reduce surgical complications, and improve the patient's outcome. The systems can also be useful for other procedures such as kyphoplasty, biopsies, osteotomy planning, or tumor resection due to the advanced planning of trajectories. These systems have shown some advantages in minimally invasive spine surgery by allowing precise placement of pedicle screws while limiting radiation exposure in the operation room. At the meantime, further well-designed studies are needed to advance the full role of robotics in spine surgery.

Surgeons must appreciate that the robot is not designed to replace the surgeon, rather to enhance the surgeon's ability to treat patients [13]. It is merely a tool and not actually performing the surgery. It is the surgeon who must understand how to both plan and perform the surgery and use the robotic guidance to enhance accuracy.

References

1. Kleck CJ, Cullilmore I, LaFleur M, Lindley E, Rentschler ME, Burger EL, et al. A new 3-dimensional method for measuring precision in surgical navigation and methods to optimize navigation accuracy. Eur Spine J. 2016;25(6):1764–74.
2. Lieberman IH, Togawa D, Kayanja MM, Reinhardt MK, Friedlander A, Knoller N, et al. Bone-mounted miniature robotic guidance for pedicle screw and translaminar facet screw placement: part I--Technical development and a test case result. Neurosurgery. 2006;59(3):641–50; discussion -50.
3. Togawa D, Kayanja MM, Reinhardt MK, Shoham M, Balter A, Friedlander A, et al. Bone-mounted miniature robotic guidance for pedicle screw and translaminar facet screw placement: part 2--Evaluation of system accuracy. Neurosurgery. 2007;60(2 Suppl 1):ONS129–39; discussion ONS39.
4. Lonjon N, Chan-Seng E, Costalat V, Bonnafoux B, Vassal M, Boetto J. Robot-assisted spine surgery: feasibility study through a prospective case-matched analysis. Eur Spine J. 2016;25(3):947–55.
5. Gaines RW Jr. The use of pedicle-screw internal fixation for the operative treatment of spinal disorders. J Bone Joint Surg Am. 2000;82-A(10):1458–76.
6. Hicks JM, Singla A, Shen FH, Arlet V. Complications of pedicle screw fixation in scoliosis surgery: a systematic review. Spine (Phila Pa 1976). 2010;35(11):E465–70.
7. Ledonio CG, Polly DW Jr, Vitale MG, Wang Q, Richards BS. Pediatric pedicle screws: comparative effectiveness and safety: a systematic literature review from the Scoliosis Research Society and the Pediatric Orthopaedic Society of North America task force. J Bone Joint Surg Am. 2011;93(13):1227–34.
8. Devito DP, Gaskill T, Erickson M. Robotic-based guidance for pedicle screw instrumentation of the scoliotic spine. In: Spine Arthroplasty Society (SAS) 10th annual global symposium on motion preservation technology; 2010.
9. van Dijk JD, van den Ende RP, Stramigioli S, Kochling M, Hoss N. Clinical pedicle screw accuracy and deviation from planning in robot-guided spine surgery: robot-guided pedicle screw accuracy. Spine (Phila Pa 1976). 2015;40(17):E986–91.
10. Hu X, Ohnmeiss DD, Lieberman IH. Robotic-assisted pedicle screw placement: lessons learned from the first 102 patients. Eur Spine J. 2013;22(3):661–6.
11. Cannestra A, Sweeney T, Poelstra K, Schroerlucke S. Surgical outcomes of robotic-guidance vs. freehand instrumentation: a retrospective review of 705 adult degenerative spine patients operated in minimally invasive and open approaches. Society for Minimally Invasive Spine Surgery (SMISS) Annual Forum, 2016.
12. Hu X, Lieberman IH. What is the learning curve for robotic-assisted pedicle screw placement in spine surgery? Clin Orthop Relat Res. 2014;472(6):1839–44.
13. Taylor R. A perspective on medical robotics. Proc IEEE. 2006;94:1–13.

Emerging Robotic Technologies and Innovations for Hospital Process Improvement

Jess H. Lonner, Julian Zangrilli, and Sundeep Saini

...automation can be the ally of our prosperity if we will just look ahead, if we will understand what is to come, and if we will set our course wisely after proper planning for the future. (President Lyndon Johnson, August 19, 1964 [1])

The era of collaborative robots is upon us, impacting industries from manufacturing to warehousing and other industries. While surgical robots are making a substantial impact on patient care, presently robots programmed for autonomous hospital logistical support or for augmenting physical therapy, nursing, perioperative services, pharmacy, and other areas of healthcare are lagging far behind. However, a number of emerging robotic innovations may increasingly play a role in various hospital-based operational processes [2]. Indeed, healthcare is on the verge of transformative innovations as a result of automation and robotics [3].

In healthcare, perhaps more than other industries, the greatest potential value of robots is not necessarily in whether or how they can autonomously perform a myriad of functions, but rather in how they can complement or augment human capabilities and tasks [4]. Initially slow to enter the healthcare space, the global medical and surgical robotics market is expected to grow annually at 21% [5]. If realized, emerging and future nonsurgical applications of autonomous and collaborative robots may revolutionize comprehensive healthcare delivery in the hospital setting by reducing errors, enhancing efficiencies and productivity, increasing employee and patient satisfaction, improving safety, and allowing personnel to focus on the most important elements of patient-centric care by "rehumanizing time" [4].

It is estimated that roughly 36% of healthcare activities and processes have the potential to become automated, even robotized in many cases. This will depend on the technical feasibility of automating the activity/process; the costs to automate; the scarcity, skills, and costs of workers who otherwise perform the activity; the potential benefits of automation such as efficacy, efficiency, and safety; and acceptance considerations by regulatory bodies, administrators, care providers, and patients [3]. While some worry

J. H. Lonner (✉)
Department of Orthopaedic Surgery,
Rothman Orthopaedic Institute, Sidney Kimmel
Medical College, Thomas Jefferson University,
Philadelphia, PA, USA
e-mail: jess.lonner@rothmanortho.com

J. Zangrilli · S. Saini
Department of Orthopaedic Surgery, Rowan
University School of Osteopathic Medicine,
Stratford, NJ, USA

© Springer Nature Switzerland AG 2019
J. H. Lonner (ed.), *Robotics in Knee and Hip Arthroplasty*,
https://doi.org/10.1007/978-3-030-16593-2_23

about job displacement with broad adoption and incorporation of robots for hospital logistics and process support, reports have shown that they have the potential to do just the opposite. The 2016 Economic Report of the President noted that the increased prevalence of robotics and automation positively affects both worker welfare and overall productivity [6]. Others have found wage increases in industries where robots were utilized to collaborate with, rather than substitute for, the work force [4, 7, 8].

Logistical support robots are being utilized with increasing prevalence across a spectrum of in-hospital clinical settings in order to improve operational efficiencies and relieve the burden on medical and support personnel by preparing and delivering supplies and medications; by augmenting the role of nurses, clerks, and physical therapists; and by collaborating in perioperative processes such as instrument sterilization and scrub technician support. To be clear, however, the full potential of incorporation of robots into hospital processes is still far from being realized [5, 9–13].

Simplistically, there are three primary categories of robots that can be incorporated to support healthcare workers and care providers. These include robots to perform or augment direct patient care, indirect patient care, and home healthcare [14]. Examples of direct patient care robots are surgical robots, nursing care robots, exoskeletons, and prosthetics. Exoskeletons are at the forefront of robotic rehabilitative medicine helping patients obtain mobility and independence after functional limb loss, due to stroke or other causes, but which may prove to have a role in joint replacement rehabilitation [14]. Indirect patient care robots are meant to accomplish the repetitive, sometimes menial, but necessary tasks required to support care of patients, logistics, or other processes in a hospital setting. For instance, pharmacy robots prepare and track medication administration to patients which help reduce errors, maintain sterility, protect pharmacists from accidental needle sticks, and prevent exposure to toxic substances during preparation. Delivery robots can transport medications, linens, medical supplies, meals, empty beds, or waste, effectively allowing providers to focus their time to patient

needs [14]. And disinfection robots cruise halls and patient rooms to maintain a sterile environment within the hospital. Finally, home healthcare robots encompass telepresence equipment enabling physicians to monitor, examine, and treat patients in remote locations. For example, physical therapists can monitor home rehab sessions performed by patients using robotic equipment to ensure safe and proper progression of therapy. This application of telepresence also gives patients or other care providers access to specialists who may work far away [14].

This chapter will highlight some of the current and potential future direct and indirect robot applications that may synergistically support care and other crucial processes within the hospital. Some of these concepts are currently in use; others are concepts in various stages of development and commercialization.

Nursing

Economists at the Bureau of Labor and Statistics rank "registered nurse" as the occupation that will experience the greatest job growth between 2016 and 2026 [15]. The concerning paradox, however, is that there is an ongoing shortage of nurses which some predict to increase by more than 1 million jobs by 2020 [16], suggesting a real need for process improvement to augment nurses' work capacity and reduce workload burden over the forthcoming decade. Nurses assume a pivotal role in healthcare delivery and are often the first to assess patient needs. However, their direct patient care responsibilities are often sidetracked by the need to perform clerical, support, logistics, and transportation tasks. Some of these, such as scheduling, room allocation, and staffing assignments, may be effectively managed with robotic intervention [17]. In one study, a robot from the Computer Science and Artificial Intelligence Lab at the Massachusetts Institute of Technology was programmed to automatically generate assignments for nursing coverage. The robot generated coverage assignments that demonstrated 90% agreement with those made by its human counterparts. By automating such decision-making processes, the nursing and clerical staff can be unburdened and freed up to perform other more necessary direct patient-related tasks. Automating certain nursing and clerical tasks, such as medication delivery and charting, may also ultimately prove to make workflow more efficient and reduce errors, much like pilot errors have been reduced by automating key components of flight [9, 17–19].

Nurses are commonly subjected to physical stresses and strain that can lead to musculoskeletal injuries at some point in their careers as a result of manually lifting or moving patients [20]. Efforts are being made to ease the physical workload and improve ergonomics necessary for comprehensive patient care with the application of robotic nursing assistance. One such mobile robotic device, the Robotic Nurse Assistant (HStar Technologies, Burlington, MA), is designed to provide nurses with physical assistance for patient repositioning and transportation, thereby reducing the risk of work-related injuries and potentially increasing job satisfaction [21]. Other examples of occupational hazards that can jeopardize the health of nurses include respiratory disease spread by droplet transmission or blood-borne disease due to needle stick injuries. Engineers have attempted to limit occupational hazards by using robots in crisis situations caused by infectious disease or toxic materials. Inspired by the Ebola outbreak in 2014, Duke Engineers began working on a Tele-Robotic Intelligent Nursing Assistant, meant to serve as a surrogate nurse – helping to deliver materials, supplies, or medicines or to adjust a patient's position – in areas that are deemed too dangerous for healthcare personnel [22]. The status of these sorts of robots in terms of commercialization or clinical use is unclear at this time, although their potential is immense.

Transportation

Transportation and logistical support of supplies within the hospital require a complex interaction of planning, organization, scheduling, coordination, and physical flow of materials. Despite the critical nature of hospital logistics, in this regard hospitals are often woefully inefficient and disorganized. Integration of autonomous information technologies for ordering of supplies, planning of resources, and coordination with robotic transportation systems may have a profound effect on logistical process improvement [23].

With regard to transportation of materials and supplies in the hospital setting, expenditures are unnecessarily inflated from manpower hours and inefficiencies. In fact, hospital logistics account for nearly 30% of all hospital expenses [23, 24]. For nurses, time spent dealing with logistics issues may account for 12% of their time spent during the day [25]. By automating transportation of medications, supplies, food, instruments, linens, beds, waste, and clothing, operational costs per delivery may be reduced by as much as 80% [25], and staff members can devote more time focused on high-quality direct patient care activities. One such system, the TUG robot (Aethon, Pittsburgh, PA), is an example of a robotic transportation system that has been recently implemented in multiple hospitals across the United States [25]. In one case study, the University of Maryland Medical Center set a goal of controlling medication inventory losses by implementing a network of three mobile TUG robots to deliver, track, and retrieve medications in a hospital trauma department [26]. After 1 year of use, medication delivery times decreased by 40%, and delivery reliability improved by 23%. Based on these positive findings, the hospital system subsequently added six additional robotic TUG systems, and with improved monitoring and delivery efficiencies, the incorporation of these robots have proved to optimize staff utilization and availability for patient care, as well as contain costs [26]. Despite the up-front capital cost concerns, cost savings have been realized by a number of hospitals and health systems that have incorporated mobile robotic transport systems. For instance, in 2010, a hospital in Mountain View, CA, leased 19 delivery robots at an annual cost of roughly $350,000, which amounted to an annual savings of $650,000 compared to paying the hospital employees to do those same tasks [27].

Pharmacy

One of the earliest examples of automation in healthcare was the tablet counter used in pharmacies, the first of which was invented by John Kirby in England in 1970 [28]. Rapid evolution of these devices in the ensuing decades resulted in more widespread adoption of this technology in both clinical and industrial pharmacies [29]. The first truly robotic pharmacy devices came to market in 1997. In addition to tablet counting, these robots are now also able to pick, label, dispense, and package a variety of medications [29]. The use of modern prescription-filling robots has been shown to increase safety, accuracy, and efficiency of medication preparation and allocation compared to traditional systems [30, 31]. The early success of automation in the pharmacy realm proved the potential benefits of robotics in healthcare and served as a foundation for automation in other medical settings. Computer-controlled dispensing units termed automated dispensing systems (ADS) have been shown to provide secure drug distribution, helping to reduce overall medication errors in unstable critical care patients. For instance, in 2010, a university hospital implemented one such ADS (Omnicell, Mountain View, CA) in a medical ICU directly comparing it to the former distribution system over a 4-month period. Data showed that this system significantly reduced the incidence of medical errors related to selecting, preparing, and delivering drugs in an ICU, and the technology was also well received by the ICU staff, over 96% of which recommended its ongoing use [32].

Surgical Scrub Technicians/Nurses

Collaboration between surgeons, anesthesiologists, scrub nurses/technicians, and circulating nurses in the operating room is critical for the safe performance of surgery, as well as influencing workflow and team well-being. We have seen how robots can augment and improve the capabilities of surgeons. Education, preparation, repetition, engagement, and reinforcement can also improve the performance of the surgical team. Despite the fact that most surgical procedures other than highly complex and less common surgeries follow the same basic steps, with little variability between the same types of cases, there are naturally some demonstrable differences in experience, skill, and engagement of scrub nurses and technicians that can impact the surgical experience, pace, effort, and workflow and which may be an opportunity for robotic intervention.

Small errors in the interaction between scrub nurses/technicians and surgeons – from ambiguity of instructions, to failure to provide necessary instruments, to inattentiveness and intraoperative or setup delays – can have a negative impact on the flow or outcome of the surgery [33]. Recent research assessing verbal and nonverbal exchanges in the operating room (OR) have shown that communication failures between scrub team members are frequent and commands are often delayed, incomplete, or not received at all and frequently left unresolved. Thirty-six percent of failures resulted in visible effects on system processes including inefficiency, team tension, resource waste, work-around, delay, patient inconvenience, and procedural error [34]. One study found that 31% of all communications in the OR represent failures [35], a third of which had a negative impact on the patient. Another study found that 36% of communication errors were related to equipment use [36], sometimes caused by team inexperience, lack of resources (limited staffing), lack of staff engagement, and distractions [37]. Additionally, there is measurable variability in scrub nurse engagement, which impacts the need for verbal requests and effort by the surgeon, as well as OR time. In one observational study, scrub nurses spent an average of 74% of OR time watching surgery and 35% of OR time performing surgery-related activities. Greater skilled or engaged nurses spent less time watching surgery, performed more anticipatory movements per procedure, and required fewer verbal cues and prompts from the surgeon. Additionally, depending on case complexity, duration of surgeries may vary by as much as 5–30 minutes in some specialties depending on experience and engagement of the scrub nurse/technician [38]. One intriguing field of investigation is whether these errors, inefficiencies, and overall work effort could potentially be improved by introducing robots into the operating room to serve as automated scrub technicians.

Treat et al. described the first documented surgical procedure in which a semiautonomous robotic "instrument server" (Penelope Surgical Instrument Server, Robotic Surgical Tech, New York, NY) delivered and retrieved surgical instruments during a lipoma excision in 2005, in response to voice commands [39]. The authors documented 100% successful instrument deliveries among 16 requests, although 25 verbal requests were necessary, meaning that 36% of the time, 2 or 3 requests were needed to receive the instruments. Additionally, the mean instrument delivery time was 12.4 seconds, far slower than human scrub nurse or technician times [39]. This preliminary work was intriguing, although it is unclear where the technology stands in terms of further development, refinement, and commercialization. Since then, additional robotic scrub technician systems have been developed to assist in surgical procedures, and preliminary preclinical studies are encouraging.

The Quirubot Robotic Scrub Nurse (nBIO lab, Miguel Hernandez University, Alicante, Spain) has a speech recognition system sophisticated enough to recognize requests for 27 instruments and 82 different instructions [40]. The Quirubot's objective is to locate the instrument on a tray among an array of other instruments using computer vision and pattern recognition. The robot then delivers the instrument within reach of its human surgeon counterpart. In one study, the Quirubot was tested against human scrub nurses in a simulated operating room. Both were subjected to the same 1200 commands, with the robot successfully selecting and passing the correct surgical instrument 94.2% of the time compared to the human scrub nurses' success rate of 89.1%. The robot could also be trained to optimize anticipatory movements during surgery as it became accustomed to the procedural order. That feature could potentially augment the abilities of a less experienced scrub nurse/technician if paired with the robot during surgery. This particular technology demonstrated increased overall surgical instrument delivery time, sometimes taking up to three times longer when compared to human scrub nurses during experimentation. Therefore, the authors speculated that the utility of the robotic scrub nurse might be greatest when an experienced scrub nurse was not available for an urgent procedure where the anticipatory movements of the machine could offset its decreased delivery speed [40].

An alternative robotic scrub nurse, Gestonurse (Purdue University, West Lafayette, IN), is programmed to respond to basic hand gestures from the surgeon to indicate the desired surgical instruments to be passed. A series of experiments found that the robot reliably picked instruments from a Mayo stand when instruments were separated by at least 25 mm, with slight variability in accuracy based on instrument size. Ninety-five percent of the gestures were recognized correctly, with a mean of 4.06 seconds between requesting the instrument and receiving it, which on average was 0.83 seconds slower than human scrub nurses tested [33]. In another study, comparing the variance in position of a passed instrument relative to the surgeon requestor's hand, the authors found 89% less variance in position of the tool when the instrument was passed by the robotic scrub nurse compared to a human scrub nurse, suggesting the potential for improved economies of movement, energy expenditure, and risk of injury when using the robotic scrub nurse assistance [41]. Clearly the potential for improvements in workflow and ergonomics, as well as for augmenting the skill and performance of less experienced or engaged scrub nurses/technicians with robotic intervention, is intriguing, but further work is still to be done on optimizing accuracy and decreasing instrument transaction times before commercialization is likely to occur.

Surgical Sterilization and Processing

Improper handling, processing, and sterilization of reusable surgical instruments have been attributed to approximately 44–52% of avoidable surgical complications such as infection and perioperative morbidity, as well as surgical delays [42, 43]. Much of the sterilization process requires a team of workers to perform hundreds of repetitive quality control measures throughout the day. This leaves significant room for human error given the monotonous nature of the work [44]. The problem is compounded when considering the high rate of turnover among the typically poorly trained, overworked, underpaid personnel charged with the responsibility of sterile processing of instruments [45]. A pilot program orchestrated by the Centers for Medicare and Medicaid Services found that 28% of 1500 outpatient surgery centers inspected across the country had multiple infection control deficiencies directly related to equipment tracking and sterilization [44]. Surgical instrument processing errors can occur in approximately 3% of surgical cases [46]. Although employing formalized Lean methodologies may reduce some of these errors, such as incorrect assembly, sterilization, and damage during transportation, others, such as processing of incorrect instruments and retained debris, have been shown to persist [46]. Errors may result from poor training, inattention, poor visibility within elements of the instruments, time constraints/pressures, and complicated instructions regarding complex instrument care [47].

Furthermore, even with appropriate protocols for manual instrument cleaning – several repeated cycles of manual brushing and scrubbing, soaking in a commercial enzymatic solution according to manufacturer's specifications, placement in a sterilization reprocessor for at least two cycles – some instruments may still contain remnants of blood, bone, tissue, and rust. Manual washing and brushing does not consistently clean the difficult to reach interior lumens of cannulated instruments in particular. The extent of debris, brush size, brushing time, and human error all reduce the likelihood of consistent cleaning and increase the risk of leftover bioburden remaining in the instrument. One study found that despite strict adherence to protocols, fewer than 5% of 350 suction tips analyzed were free of residual debris [48]. These potentially non-sterile remnants might contaminate the surgical field and increase risk of postoperative infection.

In an attempt to reduce the incidence of retained debris, improve processing efficiencies, and decrease the rate of contamination, some have sought to implement robotic technology in instrument processing. Automated cleaning technology may more effectively clean debris from surgical tools, and particularly the lumens of challenging instruments such as laparoscopic, arthroscopic, and robotic cannulae, and suction tips than current manual instrument washing techniques [49, 50]. One robotics company (Robotic Systems and Technologies, Bronx, NY) has applied lean manufacturing principles to automation techniques aiming to improve efficiency and quality in hospitals. Their robot is designed to automate key functions in the hospital's sterile supply department and is able to count, sort, and inspect already sterile instruments, ensuring that each tray sent to the operating room contains correct, functioning instruments. The robot is also capable of updating the hospital's inventory system to provide total accountability for instruments, optimize trays, and reduce workload for personnel [51]. Furthermore, by automating the loading and unloading of surgical tools into washers and disinfectors, perioperative efficiencies and ergonomics in a central processing department might be improved, thereby enhancing safety, lowering the risk of physical strain or crush injuries, and accelerating the pace of work so employees could focus on other initiatives such as organization and scheduling [52]. In addition to instrument sterilization, robotic technology has also been applied to cleaning and sterilizing the operating rooms themselves. Studies have shown that some surfaces in the operating room may be contaminated even after standard disinfection, with approximately 50% of surfaces containing organisms such as *Pseudomonas*, *Acinetobacter*, and *Klebsiella* [53, 54]. A robotic disinfection system that uses pulsed-xenon ultraviolet (UV) light to reduce the contamination that remains in operating rooms after they are manually cleaned (Xenex, San Antonio, TX) was found to reduce the rate of surgical site infections by 46% in clean procedures when used once a day. This was estimated to have potentially saved the hospital

$478,055 in costs [55]. Inadequacies in surgical sterilization and processing lead to increased patient morbidity and mortality. By automating some of these steps of the perioperative process with robotic technologies, hospitals and surgery centers may further improve management and sterilization of instruments.

Physical Therapy and Rehab Services

Physical therapy (PT) and rehabilitation practices are undoubtedly a critical component to optimizing a patient's recovery from knee and hip arthroplasty procedures. In some instances, the rehabilitation component of care is equally important for recovery as the medical or surgical intervention itself. However, it is uncertain whether there will be adequate numbers of physical therapists to provide these services adequately to patients in the near future. In 2017, the American Physical Therapy Association (APTA) projected the supply and demand of physical therapists from 2010 to 2025, estimating a potential shortage of physical therapists by 2025 that could be as high as 26,000, due to an increase in the numbers of insured individuals, growing numbers of patients undergoing knee and hip arthroplasty (and other procedures requiring PT), and growing population with medical ailments requiring PT, without a matched increase in trained physical therapists in the United States [56]. The initial few days after surgery are particularly impactful for training patients to ambulate, maintain reasonable balance, and minimize the risk of falling. Most often, in the acute postoperative period while hospitalized, two physical therapists (or a PT with one aid) will assist a patient while ambulating to ensure a reasonable level of safety after TKA, THA, and hip fracture surgery. Nonetheless, despite appropriate protocols and precautions after knee and hip arthroplasty, the risk of falling during the hospitalization is roughly 0.4–2.7% [57, 58], and those numbers are even greater in patients transferred to inpatient rehabilitation centers or skilled nursing facilities [59]. When analyzing patient falls, 74% of patients are using an ambulatory assistive device at the time of the fall [60], and 27% fall while ambulating with staff supervision/assistance [61]. The risk of falling after surgical repair of hip fractures in geriatric patients is even more concerning, occurring in as many as 31% of patients during the hospitalization [62]. These statistics suggest the need for some sort of supplemental method to augment physical therapists, aids, and nursing personnel when mobilizing patients, particularly on the first 2 or 3 days after knee and hip arthroplasty, when most falls occur [63, 64].

If we consider the need to reconcile the increased number of knee and hip arthroplasty surgeries performed annually with the impending shortage of physical therapists and the risk of falling in the postoperative period, the rationale behind some sort of robotic assistance for postoperative rehabilitation gains clarity. Robotic assistance may serve a role in reducing the burden on physical therapists, improving the safety and efficacy of the rehabilitation process for countless patients, and perhaps reducing the risk of falling [65].

Seemingly optimal for performing and quantifying repetitive, reproducible, and guided limb movements with continuous sensorimotor feedback, and monitoring and quantifying performance metrics, automated rehabilitation robots should be studied as a vehicle for augmenting conventional physical therapy, preventing falls [65], enhancing gait retraining, facilitating return of knee range of motion and strength, and enhancing the efficacy and efficiency of rehabilitation programs [66]. The penetration of robotics in rehabilitation is already being realized. In fact, in 2015, 42% of the global revenue share of the healthcare assistive robot industry was in the rehabilitation space, with a predicted annual growth rate of more than 19% over the next 7 years [67]. While clearly the emphasis on robot-assisted rehabilitation has been for patients with neuromuscular diseases or injury, such as cerebral palsy, stroke, traumatic brain injury, and spinal cord injury [68, 69], there may be an additional untapped role for patients after knee and hip joint arthroplasty and hip fracture surgery [70–77].

While the precise application of robotics in orthopedic rehabilitation is not yet clear, it is likely that it has the potential to change the paradigm of rehabilitation in the next 5 years [78]. In 1992, the hybrid assistive limb (HAL, Cyberdyne Corporation, Tsukuba, Japan), a lower extremity exoskeletal suit, was developed to aid users with physical support and gait assistance. Bioelectric signals generated by contracting muscles around the limb are detected by electrodes attached to the surface of the skin, which then prompt an assistive force to be initiated by the HAL power unit [79, 80]. Several early studies comparing robot-assisted rehabilitation using the HAL exoskeleton versus conventional methods after TKA found improved walking speed, stride length and quadriceps strength, as well as less knee pain, within the first few weeks after surgery when robot assistance was used for postoperative physical therapy [81, 82]. While exoskeletons are an option to consider as an adjunct to manual PT for TKA and THA, these are unlikely to become commonplace for this application. Other forms of collaborative robots, not yet common for lower extremity arthroplasty patients, may eventually play a role in safe ambulation training and help reduce the fall risk in hospitalized patients after surgery of the knee and hip [76, 77].

Conclusion

Collaborative robots have the potential to revolutionize healthcare delivery far beyond the current paradigm in which we think of robots simply as surgical aids. While the surgical robotics sector has enjoyed the greatest attention, relatively untapped nonsurgical healthcare-related robotic applications may prove to have immeasurable value as well. Nonetheless, while intellectually we can envision the next robotic frontier in healthcare to be the application of robots for process improvement, logistical support, operations management, and perioperative services, there will undoubtedly be challenges that will inhibit rapid adoption. These will include biases against and skepticism toward automation and robotics,

fear of job displacement, and appropriate desire for proof regarding metrics of need, safety and reliability, robot capability and function, and cost and clinical effectiveness [83]. Clearly a cost-benefit analysis is necessary before embracing emerging and future robotic technologies, and barriers to adoption will need to be addressed. Robots may or may not ultimately prove to be effective means of augmenting some of the logistical and operational processes within the hospital that we've addressed in this chapter.

Indeed, currently service and logistical robots are not commonly used in hospitals. However, their active development and commercialization continue and will likely become more prevalent in a greater number of hospitals for a spectrum of services within the next 5–10 years. Regardless of one's averseness or proclivity toward the broadening possibilities for robots within the hospital setting, there is no reason to think that the greater societal impact of robots that is occurring at the present time will not soon occur to some extent in healthcare, outside of the operating room. Given the success of robots in a number of industries, it is our expectation that as more hospitals integrate robotic technology, hospital-based services will become more streamlined, efficient, safe, and cost-effective, staff and patient satisfaction will be improved, and quality of care optimized. Time will tell.

References

1. Peters G, Woolley JT. The American presidency project, https://www.presidency.ucsb.edu/documents/remarks-upon-signing-bill-creating-the-national-commission-technology-automation-and.
2. One Hundred Year Study on Arti cial Intelligence (AI100), Stanford University, https://ai100.stanford.edu/sites/default/files/ai100report10032016fnl_singles.pdf. Accessed Sept 2018.
3. Chui M, Manyika J, Miremadi M. Where machines could replace humans – and where they can't (yet). McKinsey Quarterly July 2016. https://www.mckinsey.com/business-functions/digital-mckinsey/our-insights/where-machines-could-replace-humans-and-where-they-cant-yet. Accessed Sept 2018.
4. Daugherty PR, Wilson HJ. Human + machine. Reimagining work in the age of AI. Boston: Harvard Business Review Press; 2018.

5. https://www.marketresearchengine.com/medical-robots-market Accessed 3 Sept 2018.
6. The 2016 Economic report of the president. National Archives and Records Administration, National Archives and Records Administration, obamawhitehouse.archives.gov/blog/2016/02/22/2016-economic-report-president.
7. Graetz G, Michaels G. Robots at work London School of Economics and Political Science, 2015, Robots at Work, cep.lse.ac.uk/pubs/download/dp1335.pdf.
8. Melanson A. Three ways robots boost wages. Aethon, 11 Mar 2016, www.aethon.com/three-ways-robotics-boost-wages/.
9. Gombolay M, Yang XJ, Hayes B, Seo N, Liu Z, Wadhwania S, Yu T, Shah N, Golen T, Shah J. Robotic assistance in coordination of patient care http://people.csail.mit.edu/gombolay/Publications/Gombolay_RSS_2016.pdf.
10. Bloss R. Mobile hospital robots cure numerous logistic needs. Indust Robot Int J. 2011;38(6):567–71.
11. DiGiose N. Hospitals hiring robots, February 2013. URL http://www.electronicproducts.com/Computer Peripherals/Systems/Hospitalshiringrobots.aspx.
12. Hu J, Edsinger A, Lim YJ, Donaldson N, Solano M, Solochek A, Marchessault R. An advanced medical robotic system augment- ing healthcare capabilities-robotic nursing assistant. In: Robotics and Automation (ICRA), 2011 IEEE international conference on: IEEE; 2011. p. 6264–9.
13. Murai R, Sakai T, Kawano H, Matsukawa Y, Honda Y, Campbell KC, et al. A novel visible light communication system for enhanced control of autonomous delivery robots in a hospital. In: System integration (SII), 2012 IEEE/SICE international symposium on: IEEE; 2012. p. 510–6.
14. Research report: healthcare robotics 2015–2020. Robotics Business Review, 26 Jan 2015, www.roboticsbusinessreview.com/download/research-report-healthcare-robotics-2015-2020/.
15. US Department of Labor, Bureau of Labor Statistics, Occupational Outlook Handbook, December 10, 2018, http://www.bls.gov/ooh/About/Projections-Overview.htm.
16. Kuehn BM. No end in sight to nursing shortage: bottleneck at nursing schools a key factor. JAMA. U.S. National Library of Medicine, 10 Oct. 2007, www.ncbi.nlm.nih.gov/pubmed/17925507.
17. CSAIL, Adam Conner-Simons I. Robot helps nurses schedule tasks on labor floor. MIT News, 13 July 2016, news.mit.edu/2016/robot-helps-nurses-schedule-tasks-on-labor-floor-0713.
18. Dismukes RK, Berman BA, Loukopoulous LD. The limits of expertise: rethinking pilot error and the causes of airline accidents: Ashgate Publishing; 2007.
19. Dixon SR, Wickens CD. Automation reliability in unmanned aerial vehicle control: a reliance-compliance model of automation dependence in high workload. Hum Factors. 2006;48(3):474–86.
20. Meier E. Ergonomic standards and implications for nursing. Nurs Econ. 2001;19(1):31–2.
21. Hu J. et al. An advanced medical robotic system augmenting healthcare capabilities - robotic nursing assistant. 2011 IEEE international conference on robotics and automation, 2011, https://doi.org/10.1109/icra.2011.5980213.
22. Liu E. Duke engineers, nurses develop robotic nursing assistant. The Chronicle, 22 Nov 2016., www.dukechronicle.com/article/2016/11/duke-engineers-nurses-develop-robotic-nursing-assistant.
23. Ozkil AG, et al. Service robots for hospitals: a case study of transportation tasks in a hospital. 2009 IEEE international conference on automation and logistics, 2009, https://doi.org/10.1109/ical.2009.5262912.
24. Poulin E. Benchmarking the hospital logistics process a potential cure for the ailing health care sector. CMA Manag. 2003;77(1):20–3.
25. "Aethon - TUG™: the automated robotic delivery system," http://www.aethon.com/products/logistics.php.
26. "University of Maryland Medical Center DECREASES CYCLE TIME, INCREASES NURSE SATISFACTION with TUG Robots and MedEx System 'Chain of Custody' Solutions." www.aethon.com/Wp-Content/Uploads/2014/08/UMMC-Case-Study-2011b.Pdf, Aethon.
27. King R, "Soon, that nearby worker might be a robot," Bloomberg Businessweek, June 2, 2010, http://www.businessweek.com/stories/2010-06-02/soon-that-nearby-worker-might-be-a-robotbusinessweek-business-news-stock-market-and-financial-advice.
28. Kirby J. Patent: counting machines. England 8 September 19070. Patent #: GB1358378.
29. Thomsen C. Automation and Robotics - Practical Technology. September 2004. http://thethomsengroup.com/TTGI%20Pages/Articles%20Studies%20&%20Presentations/2005%20Business%20Briefings.pdf. Accessed 5 Apr 2017.
30. Walsh KE, Chui MA, Kieser MA, Williams SM, Sutter SL, Sutter JG. Exploring the impact of an automated prescription-filling device on community pharmacy technician workflow. J Am Pharm Assoc (2003). 2011;51(5):613–8. https://doi.org/10.1331/JAPhA.2011.09166.
31. Lin AC, Huang Y-C, Punches G, Chen Y. Effect of a robotic prescription-filling system on pharmacy staff activities and prescription-filling time. Am J Health Syst Pharm. 2007;64(17):1832–9. https://doi.org/10.2146/ajhp060561.
32. Chapuis C, et al. Automated drug dispensing system reduces medication errors in an intensive care setting. Crit Care Med. 2010;38(12):2275–81. https://doi.org/10.1097/ccm.0b013e3181f8569b.
33. Jacob M, Li YT, Akingba G, Wachs JP. Gestonurse: a robotic surgical nurse for handling surgical instruments in the operating room. J Robot Surg. 2012;6:53–63.
34. Lingard L, Espin S, Whyte S, et al. Communication failures in the operating room: an observational classification of recurrent types and effects. Qual Saf Health Care. 2004;13:330–4.

35. Firth-Cozens J. Why communication fails in the operating room. Qual Saf Health Care. 2004;13(5):327.

36. Halverson AL, Casey JT, Andersson J, Anderson K, Park C, Rademaker AW, Moorman D. Communication failure in the operating room. Surgery. 2010;149(3):305–10.

37. Carthey J, de Laval MR, Wright DJ, et al. Behavioural markers of surgical excellence. Saf Sci. 2003;41:409–25.

38. Zheng B, Taylor MD, Swanstrom L. An observational study of surgery-related activities between nurses and surgeons during laparoscopic surgery. Am J Surg. 2009;197:497–502.

39. Treat MR, et al. Initial clinical experience with a partly autonomous robotic surgical instrument server. Surg Endosc. 2006;20(8):1310–4. https://doi.org/10.1007/s00464-005-0511-0.

40. Perez-Vidal C, Carpintero E, Garcia-Aracil N, Navarro-Sabater JM, Azorin JM, Candela A, Fernandez E. Steps in the development of a robotic scrub nurse. Robot Auton Syst. 2012;60(6):901–11. https://doi.org/10.1016/j.robot.2012.01.005.

41. Wachs JP, Jacob MG, Li YT, Akingba AG. Does a robotic scrub nurse improve economy of movements? Proc SPIE. 2012;8316:8316E.

42. Levinson DR. Adverse events in Hospitals: National Incidence among Medicare Beneficiaries. Washington, DC: US Department of Health & Human Services, Office of the Inspector General; 2010. Accessed Jan 26, 2013. https://oig.hhs.gov/oei/reports/oei-06-09-00090.pdf.

43. Lefevre F, et al. Iatrogenic complications in high-risk, elderly patients. Arch Intern Med. 1992;152(10):2074–80.

44. Eaton J. Filthy surgical instruments: the hidden threat in America's operating rooms. In: MedTechMentor's value equations. 2012. http://www.ideasforsurgery.com/2012/02/23/filthy-surgical-instruments-the-hidden-threat-in-americas-operating-rooms/.

45. Chobin N. The real costs of surgical instrument training in sterile processing revisited. AORN J. 2010;92:185–93.

46. Blackmore CC, Bishop R, Luker S, Williams BL. Applying lean methods to improve quality and safety in surgical sterile instrument processing. Jt Comm J Qual Patient Saf. 2013;39(3):99–105.

47. AAMI. Reprocessing. 2011 Summit. Priority issues from the AAMI/FDA medical device Reprocessing Summit. https://www.aami.org/meetings/summits/reprocessing/Materials/2011_Reprocessing_Summit_publication.pdf.

48. Azizi J, Anderson SG, Murphy S, Pryce S. Uphill grime: process improvement in surgical instrument cleaning. AORN J. 2012;96:152–62.

49. The TEMPEST - the colossally effective new washer for industry-leading surgical and laparoscopic instrument cleaning. In: Tempest surgical instrument washer - laparoscopic instrument washer. 2011. http://www.fisherbiomedical.com/tempest/surgical-instrument-washer.htm.

50. Automated cleaning technology for cannulated & robotic surgical instruments. In: Southwest Solutions Group. 2017. http://www.southwestsolutions.com/infection-control-systems/automated-cleaning-technology-cannulated-robotic-surgical-instruments.

51. Madhavan R. Robotic tools in hospitals. IEEE Robot Automat. 2011;11:99.

52. Fully automated loading/unloading solution: an ergonomic revelation. 2013. http://ic.getinge.com/Documents/hc/knowledge-education/case-studies/Getinge%20case%20study%20Varberg%20EN.pdf.

53. Munoz-Price LS, Birnbach DJ, Lubarsky DA, Arheart KL, Fajardo-Aquino Y, Rosalsky M, et al. Decreasing operating room environmental pathogen contamination through improved cleaning practice. Infect Control Hosp Epidemiol. 2012;33:897–904.

54. Carling PC, Briggs JL, Perkins J, Highlander D. Improved cleaning of patient rooms using a new targeting method. Clin Infect Dis. 2006;42:385–8.

55. Catalanotti A, Abbe D, Simmons S, Stibich M. Influence of pulsed-xenon ultraviolet light-based environmental disinfection on surgical site infections. Am J Infect Control. 2016;44:e99. https://doi.org/10.1016/j.ajic.2015.12.018.

56. Ellerbe R. A model to project the supply and demand of physical therapists 2010–2025. www.apta.org, 17 Apr 2017, www.apta.org/WorkforceData/ModelDescriptionFigures/.

57. Memtsoudis SG, Dy CJ, Ma Y, Chiu YL, Della Valle AG, Mazumdar M. In-hospital patient falls after total joint arthroplasty: incidence, demographics, and risk factors in the United States. J Arthroplasty. 2012;27:823–8.

58. Wasserstein D, Farlinger C, Brull R, Mahomed N, Gandhi R. Advanced age, obesity and continuous femoral nerve blockade are independent risk factors for inpatient falls after primary total knee arthroplasty. J Arthroplast. 2013;28:1121–4.

59. Vlahov D, Myers AH, al-Ibrahim MS. Epidemiology of falls among patients in a rehabilitation hospital. Arch Phys Med Rehabil. 1990;71:8.

60. Mandl LA, Lyman S, Quinlan P, Bailey T, Katz J, Magid SK. Falls among patients who had elective orthopaedic surgery: a decade of experience from a Musculoskeletal Specialty Hospital. J Orthop Sports Phys Ther. 2013;43:91–6.

61. Pelt CE, Anderson AW, Anderson MB, Dine CV, Peters CL. Postoperative falls after total knee arthroplasty in patients with a femoral nerve catheter: can we reduce the incidence? J Arthroplast. 2014;29:1154–7.

62. Berggren M, Englund U, Olofsson B, Nordström P, Gustafson Y, Stenvall M. Effects of geriatric interdisciplinary home rehabilitation on complications and readmissions after hip fracture: a randomized controlled trial. Clin Rehabil. 2018:1–10.

63. Johnson RL, Duncan CM, Ahn KS, Schroeder DR, Horlocker TT, Kopp SL. Fall-prevention strategies and patient characteristics that impact fall rates after total knee arthroplasty. Anesth Analg. 2014;119:1113–8.

64. Jørgensen CC, Kehlet H. Fall-related admissions after fast-track total hip and knee arthroplasty -- cause of concern or consequence of success? Clin Interv Aging. 2013;8:1569–77.

65. Geok Chua KS, Keong Kuah CW. Innovating with rehabilitation technology in the real world: promises, potentials, and perspectives. Am J Phys Med Rehabil. 2017;96(Suppl):S150–6.

66. Iosa M, Morone G, Cherubini A, et al. The three laws of neurorobotics: a review on what neurorehabilitation robots should do for patients and clinicians. J Med Biol Eng. 2016;36:1–11.

67. https://www.gminsights.com/industry-analysis/healthcare-assistive-robot-market.

68. Marchal-Crespo L, Reinkensmeyer DJ. Review of control strategies for robotic movement training after neurologic injury. J. Neuroeng Rehabil. 2009;6:20. http://www.pubmedcentral.nih.gov/articlerender.fcgi?artid=2710333&tool=pmcentrez&rendertype=abstract (Online).

69. Milot M-H, Spencer SJ, Chan V, Allington JP, Klein J, Chou C, Bobrow JE, Cramer SC, Reinkensmeyer DJ. A crossover pilot study evaluating the functional outcomes of two different types of robotic movement training in chronic stroke survivors using the arm exoskeleton BONES. J Neuroeng Rehabil. 2013;10:112.

70. Ali SA, Miskon MF, Shukor AZ, Bahar MB, Mohammed MQ. Review on application of haptic in robotic rehabilitation technology. Int J Appl Eng Res. 2017;12(12):3203–13. ISSN 0973-4562, © Research India Publications. http://www.ripublication.com.

71. Solis J. Development of a human-friendly walking assisting robot vehicle designed to provide physical support to the elderly. Science Direct IFAC-PapersOnLine. 2016;49-21:656–61.

72. Shirota C, van Asseldonk E, Matjačić Z, Vallery H, Barralon P, Maggioni S, Buurke JH, Veneman JF. Robot-supported assessment of balance in standing and walking. J Neuroeng Rehabil. 2017;14:80. https://doi.org/10.1186/s12984-017-0273-7.

73. Schuck A, Labruyere R, Vallery H, Riener R, Alexander Duschau-Wicke A. Feasibility and effects of patient-cooperative robot-aided gait training applied in a 4-week pilot trial. J Neuroeng Rehabil. 2012;9:31.

74. Krebs HI, Hogan N. Robotic therapy: the tipping point. Am J Phys Med Rehabil. 2012;91(11 0 3):S290–7. https://doi.org/10.1097/PHM.

75. Henderson KG, Wallis JA, Snowdon DA. Active physiotherapy interventions following total knee arthroplasty in the hospital and inpatient rehabilitation settings: a systematic review and meta-analysis. Physiotherapy. 2018;104:25–35.

76. Esquenazi A, Packel A. Robotic-assisted gait training and restoration. Am J Phys Med Rehabil. 2012;91(11 Suppl 3):S217–27. ; quiz S228-31. https://doi.org/10.1097/PHM.0b013e31826bce18.

77. van Hedel HJA, Severini G, Scarton A, O'Brien A, Reed T, Gaebler-Spira D, Egan T, Meyer-Heim A, Graser J, Chua K, Zutter D, Schweinfurther R, Möller JC, Paredes LP, Esquenazi A, Berweck S, Schroeder S, Warken B, Chan A, Devers A, Petioky J, Paik NJ, Kim WS, Bonato P, Boninger M, ARTIC network. Advanced Robotic Therapy Integrated Centers (ARTIC): an international collaboration facilitating the application of rehabilitation technologies. J Neuroeng Rehabil. 2018;15:30. https://doi.org/10.1186/s12984-018-0366-y.

78. Barry DT. Innovations influencing physical medicine and rehabilitation: adaptation, artificial intelligence, and physical medicine and rehabilitation. PM R. 2018;10:S131–43. www.pmrjournal.org.

79. Lee S, Sankai Y. Virtual impedance adjustment in uncon- strained motion for an exoskeletal robot assisting the lower limb. Adv Robot. 2005;19:773–95.

80. Kawamoto H, Taal S, Niniss H, Hayashi T, Kamibayashi K, Eguchi K, et al., editors. Voluntary motion support control of robot suit HAL triggered by bioelectrical signal for hemiplegia. Conf Proc IEEE Eng Med Biol Soc. 2010; 2010:462–6.

81. Yoshikawa K, Mutsuzaki H, Sano A, Koseki K, Fukaya T, Mizukami M, Yamazaki M. Training with hybrid assistive limb for walking function after total knee arthroplasty. J Orthop Surg Res. 2018;13:163.

82. Tanaka Y, Oka H, Nakayama S, Ueno T, Matsudaira K, Miura T, Tanaka K, Tanaka S. Improvement of walking ability during postoperative rehabilitation with the hybrid assistive limb after total knee arthroplasty: a randomized controlled study. SAGE Open Med. 2017;5:1–6.

83. Riek LD. Healthcare robotics. Commun ACM. 2017;60(11):68–78. https://doi.org/10.1145/3127874.

Index

© Springer Nature Switzerland AG 2019
J. H. Lonner (ed.), *Robotics in Knee and Hip Arthroplasty*,
https://doi.org/10.1007/978-3-030-16593-2